Clinical Atlas of PET

Clinical Atlas of PET
With Imaging Correlation

Michael S. Kipper, MD

Radiology Medical Group
Scripps-Mercy Hospital
San Diego, California

Assistant Clinical Professor
Department of Radiology
University of California at San Diego
San Diego, California

Marie Tartar, MD

Medical Director, PET and Breast Imaging
North County Radiology
Tri City Medical Center
Oceanside, California

Assistant Clinical Professor
Department of Radiology
University of California at San Diego
San Diego, California

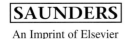

An Imprint of Elsevier

SAUNDERS
An Imprint of Elsevier

The Curtis Center
Independence Square West
Philadelphia, Pennsylvania 19106

CLINICAL ATLAS OF PET   ISBN 0-7216-3926-7
© 2004, Elsevier Inc. All rights reserved.

Notice

Radiology is an ever-changing field. Standard safety precautions must be followed, but as new research and clinical experience broaden our knowledge, changes in treatment and drug therapy may become necessary or appropriate. Readers are advised to check the most current product information provided by the manufacturer of each drug to be administered to verify the recommended dose, the method and duration of administration, and contraindications. It is the responsibility of the treating physician, relying on experience and knowledge of the patient, to determine dosages and the best treatment for each individual patient. Neither the publisher nor the editor assumes any liability for any injury and/or damage to persons or property arising from this publication.

The Publisher

Library of Congress Cataloging-in-Publication Data

Kipper, Michael S.
    Clinical atlas of PET: with imaging correlation / Michael S. Kipper, Marie Tartar.—1st ed.
    p. ; cm.
    ISBN 0-7216-3926-7
    1. Tomography, Emission—Atlases. 2. Diagnostic imaging—Atlases. I. Tartar, Marie. II.
Title.
    [DNLM: 1. Tomography, Emission-Computed—Atlases. 2. Fludeoxyglucose F
18—diagnostic use—Atlases. 3. Heart Diseases—radionuclide imaging—Atlases. 4.
Neoplasms—radionuclide imaging—Atlases. 5. Nervous System Diseases—radionuclide
imaging—Atlases. 6. Radiopharmaceuticals—diagnostic use—Atlases. WN 17 K57c 2004]
    RC78.7.T62K55 2004
    616.07'575—dc21   2003050588

Publishing Director: Rich Lampert
Acquisitions Editor: Allan Ross
Developmental Editor: Christy Bracken
Production Manager: Norman Stellander
Designer: Gene Harris

Printed in the United States of America

Last digit is the print number: 9   8   7   6   5   4   3   2   1

Preface

The second half of the twentieth century saw remarkable developments in medical imaging with the advent of CT and MRI. These anatomic-based modalities represented quantum leaps in our ability to noninvasively localize and monitor disease. The new millennium has begun with the recognition of positron emission tomography (PET) as a powerful technique for functional imaging. PET has recently evolved from a research tool at academic centers to a valuable clinical modality available worldwide.

It is almost inconceivable to us that oncologic imaging was practiced so recently without PET. The overwhelming majority of diagnostic PET studies are currently performed to diagnose and evaluate cancer; however, clinical applicability has been demonstrated in the evaluation of neurologic and cardiac disorders. Preliminary work is also ongoing in evaluation of infection as well as other diseases.

Our purpose in writing this atlas is to provide imagers and interested clinicians with an indepth understanding of the complementary roles of PET and anatomic-based imaging modalities. We have chosen case presentations from a large cross-section of oncologic, neurologic, and cardiac referrals. Pathologic, surgical, and long-term follow-up are documented for each case. Teaching points are directed at the busy imager in a typical "real world" practice. References cited are limited by design rather than exhaustive. Excellent books on PET are now available that provide critically important technical information as well as lengthy literature references.

Our goal is to provide the beginning and experienced PET reader with a comprehensive guide to interpretation and correlation with CT, MRI, and other modalities. Of crucial importance is an understanding of normal variants and potential pitfalls, in part due to the relative nonspecificity of fluorodeoxyglucose (FDG). This glucose analogue, the mainstay of oncologic imaging with PET, allows evaluation of many cancers based on the increased metabolism of malignant cells. In addition, many benign conditions (e.g., infection, inflammation, fracture, granulomatous disease, activated bone marrow, etc.) result in enhanced FDG accumulation. The wide range of examples chosen should shorten the learning curve for new readers and broaden the knowledge base of the more experienced reader.

The field of PET is growing exponentially. FDG is only one of many radiopharmaceuticals now in production or under active investigation. Current PET scanners are rapidly evolving as well, with new crystal materials, PET/CT combination systems, and other technical innovations already in use. The future use of PET for genetic and drug research, therapy planning, and disease monitoring is exciting. We hope that the material provided in this atlas will facilitate the reader's ability to interpret PET studies and generate the same enthusiasm with which we approach PET.

Michael S. Kipper, MD
Marie Tartar, MD

Acknowledgments

It is with great pleasure and gratitude that I thank the following people. First and foremost, to my wife Chris. Her patience and willingness to sacrifice so many nights and weekends are a tribute to her understanding and compassion. Next, to my radiology colleagues, whose help and enthusiasm dramatically enhanced my PET reading skills. To our technologists and support staff who were critical to the success of our program. To our medical colleagues who showed such confidence in PET and whose input was vital to patient evaluation. Finally, and most importantly, to our patients. They are the reason I am a physician. They remain, after thirty years, a constant source of inspiration and motivation. If the end result of this atlas, a true labor of love, is improved care for them, it is worth all our efforts.

Michael S. Kipper, MD

The idea for this atlas came after hours, in a trailer behind Tri City Hospital, where our first PET practice was born. Waiting for a case to finish, I looked over the shoulder of my colleague, Mike Kipper, MD, as he labored diligently at the workstation on which we review studies.

"What are you doing?"

"Oh, I'm just making up some teaching examples for Alliance (our mobile PET vendor), a thank you for all their help."

As I looked closer, I could see he was filming selected images, carefully annotating them with clinical and outcome data, demonstrating how useful PET had proven in these cases.

"Great marketing material, all right—looks like a lot of work," I said, thinking it was too bad more people wouldn't benefit from this effort.

Some time later, after finding a dearth of teaching file books at meetings, I ventured: "As long as you are doing all that work, you should turn that material into an atlas."

Silence.

Eventually, I persisted: "I could help you with the imaging correlation."

Only a truly naïve person could think it isn't that great a leap from collecting teaching file cases to writing a book, but this is probably just as well. If one knew at the outset the true scope of a project of this type, no one would knowingly embark on such a course.

That was in the early days of prime-time PET. Our hospital had been the first to establish clinical PET services in the San Diego area. When I joined North County Radiology shortly afterward, I had to get up to speed quickly on PET. Fortunately for me, I had the benefit of Mike's earlier start and experience to shorten my personal learning curve. As I sought additional reference material, I found only a limited selection of my favorite textbook type, the atlas or teaching file, so dear to time-pressed and visually oriented imagers.

Mike and I quickly fell into a routine of reviewing cases together, and we found there was a valuable synergy in combining our approaches to PET. Mike is a nuclear medicine physician, with an internal medicine background, while I am a radiologist, specializing in head to toe cross-sectional imaging, nuclear medicine, and breast imaging. For my part, I was amazed by my introduction to PET—to me, the image quality and ease of anatomic localization made PET seem more analogous to cross-sectional imaging than to traditional nuclear medicine. At the same time, the benefits of its functional basis and ability to demonstrate "sub-radiographic" disease were immediately apparent. My initial reaction: "Amazing! So black and white!"

Which is true—sometimes. It turns out there truly is a learning curve to PET interpretation, and in fact the best interpretations employ many shades of gray. They also require incorporation of detailed clinical history and rigorous imaging correlation. In researching the outcomes of these selected cases, we have learned where we were right and wrong, and where we overcalled and undercalled. Along the way, we've learned pitfalls and blind spots. Fine-tuning this knowledge is an ongoing process, essential for optimizing care for our patients.

There are many to whom thanks are due. For me, this work would not have been possible without my husband, Steven S. Eilenberg, MD, my constant companion since residency at Mallinckrodt. In addition to teaching me the rudiments of digital camera operation and Photoshop image management, he graciously accepted the time intrusion into both our lives and his necessarily expanded culinary duties. For supporting and nourishing me in all possible ways, my deepest thanks.

Thanks also go to my former North County Radiology colleagues, who provided essential support through the services of one tireless research nurse, Jeanine Coffman, RN. Jeanine's persistence, tenacity, and thoroughness in chasing down clinical data, pathology reports, and other forms of follow-up made this work possible.

Many staff members of the Tri City Hospital community contributed as well, from film librarians who requested off-site correlation studies to technologists who filmed essential illustrative imaging studies. Special thanks are extended to Linda Musarra, who piloted our fledgling PET program as our first PET coordinator, and Zuchel Contrarez, who ably succeeded her, aided by our former nuclear medicine scheduler, Misty Fenton. Transcription support in manuscript preparation was provided by Suzan Bentley. The PET technologists from Alliance Imaging were always willing to bring up yet another case to be reviewed and filmed. Thanks go as well to our referring clinicians and their hard-working staffs, who provided the access necessary for what is in essence a large-scale quality-assurance project.

Finally, thanks go to our editorial team. Most particularly, Christy Bracken demonstrated meticulous attention to detail in the editing process, and this work is strengthened by her participation.

Marie Tartar, MD

Contents

Color plates follow page 274

CHAPTER
4
Lymphoma .143

CHAPTER
5
Melanoma .173

CHAPTER
6
Colorectal Cancer 193

The Basics of PET

Positron emission tomography (PET) is an imaging technique utilizing radionuclides, with broad clinical application in oncology as well as neurologic and cardiac disorders. This brief overview will highlight the technical aspects of PET imaging and the performance of a PET scan. Selected references are provided for the reader who is interested in greater detail.

TECHNICAL ASPECTS

Most radioisotopes used for nuclear medicine imaging procedures decay by releasing energy as gamma rays with energies less than 400 keV. These photons are detected by gamma cameras using either the planar or single photon emission computed tomography (SPECT) mode. Other radioisotopes decay by positron emission. These positively charged electrons are emitted from the nucleus and travel a very short distance (1 to 2 mm) before colliding with local electrons. The subsequent annihilation reaction results in the emission of two gamma rays of very high energy (511 keV). The high-energy photons are emitted at 180 degrees to each other and detected simultaneously (coincidence) by opposite detectors on the PET scanner (Figure 1). The PET image is a representation of large numbers of these coincidence events. Reconstruction algorithms, which include correction factors for attenuation and scatter, generate cross-sectional images through the body, reliably reflecting the concentration of the positron-emitting radionuclide.[1-3] The accuracy of the method is in large part secondary to the high energy of the emitted photons. This results in reduced scatter and attenuation within the body and measurement of only those photons that strike opposing crystals simultaneously.

RADIONUCLIDES

The four most commonly used radioisotopes for PET imaging are fluorine-18, carbon-11, nitrogen-13, and oxygen-15. The latter three have very short physical half-lives (20.3 minutes, 9.97 minutes, and 2 minutes, respectively), which necessitates their use in close proximity to the site of production (i.e., biomedical cyclotron). Fluorine-18 has a 109.8-minute half-life

and can be transported to scanners remote from the cyclotron. The shorter the half-life of the radioisotope, the less time available for the chemical incorporation of the radionuclides into suitable compounds for clinical use. Fluorine-18 can be substituted for hydrogen atoms and is most commonly used as 2-(^{18}F)-fluoro-2-deoxy-D-glucose (FDG). Utilized to measure glucose metabolism, this compound is the mainstay for current oncologic imaging. FDG uptake in cancer is based on enhanced glycolysis associated with malignant cells.[4] This phenomenon is related to at least two factors: an increase in glucose membrane transporters and an upregulation of enzymes controlling glycolytic pathways. Overexpression of glucose transporters results in an increase in intracellular transport of glucose (FDG). Once intracellular, FDG is a substrate for hexokinase, the first enzyme of glycolysis. This results in phosphorylation to FDG-6-phosphate. The next enzyme along the glycolytic pathway, glucose-6-phosphate isomerase, does not react with FDG-6-phosphate. Therefore, FDG-6-phosphate remains trapped intracellularly and its concentration is an accurate reflection of the glycolytic activity of exogenous glucose (Figure 2). It is important to realize that tumor uptake of FDG may be complex and multifactorial. These factors include histologic grade, proliferative activity, doubling time, the number of viable cells, tissue oxygenation, blood flow, local inflammatory reactions, etc.[4] Whereas other positron-emitting radionuclides are used in research protocols (especially carbon-11), clinical PET is nearly always performed with FDG. An exception is myocardial perfusion imaging, which is best performed with either nitrogen-13 ammonia or rubidium-82 (generator produced).

PET SCANNER

Currently, dedicated PET systems consist of multiple complete rings of small crystals with two-dimensional imaging (septa in place) and three-dimensional imaging (septa retracted). Crystal materials include sodium iodide, bismuth germinate (BGO), lutetium oxyorthosilicate (LSO), and gadolinium oxyorthosilicate (GSO). A detailed explanation of the technical differences between cameras and crystals can be found in references 3 and 5. Most modern PET scanners provide resolution in the 8- to 10-mm

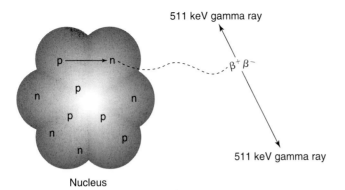

FIGURE 1. The annihilation principle. The nucleus consists of protons (p) and neutrons (n). As decay of proton-rich nucleus occurs, a proton is converted to a neutron, with the resultant emission of a positron (+). This + travels a short distance (1 to 2 mm) and then collides with an electron (−). This produces two 511-keV gamma rays that are emitted 180 degrees apart. If both of these photons escape the patient, they can be detected simultaneously by the camera's detectors (coincidence imaging).

range for clinical studies. Among the many variables for image acquisition and processing are the issues of attenuation correction and quantification. Attenuation correction is necessary for quantitative tracer uptake determination. For qualitative assessment, arguments have been advanced for both non-attenuation and attenuation-corrected imaging.[6,7] As outlined by Wahl,[6] the arguments in favor of attenuation correction include the following:

1. Radioactivity concentrations in the body and tumors are accurately measured, helping to differentiate benign from malignant lesions.
2. There is no distortion of lesion size, shape, or location.
3. Lesion intensity is similar between deep and superficial sites.
4. Image interpretation may be easier for inexperienced readers.
5. Transmission maps can be reconstructed as images that can be useful for image fusion and tumor localization.

6. Clinical studies with attenuation correction show the superiority of PET to CT.

Arguments against attenuation correction include the following[6]:

1. The attenuation scan adds time and radiation exposure to the patient.
2. Transmission scans are noisy and may degrade image quality.
3. Patient motion between attenuation measurements and emission data (misregistration) can lead to serious artifacts.
4. Methods to perform attenuation correction after tracer injection can lead to quantitative artifacts.
5. Segmentation methodology can produce artifacts.
6. Attenuation correction methods vary.
7. Time spent acquiring attenuation data may be better spent.

A number of the arguments against using attenuation correction are obviated by the recent development of the combination PET-CT scanner. Using CT for attenuation correction reduces study time, reduces patient radiation, and significantly improves registration. Throughput increases, and more precise location of pathologic FDG uptake in relation to anatomical structures is possible. Many believe that the use of combined PET-CT will become standard practice in the near future. Visual qualitative assessment of PET images is generally satisfactory for routine clinical work. However, semi-quantitative analysis is often performed using tumor to non-tumor uptake ratios or the standardized uptake value (SUV). The SUV essentially compares the concentration of FDG in the suspected tumor site with the average concentration of FDG in the body. SUV is dependent on many variables, including glucose level, body weight (lean body mass), region of interest size, time of measurement after FDG injection, and even scanner resolution.[4] In general, the higher the SUV, the more likely the lesion represents malignancy. Many authors use a cutoff value of 2.5 for thoracic lesions, such as solitary pulmonary nodules. However, it is well recognized that small lesions and low metabolic rate tumors may have SUVs less than 2.5. Additionally, many benign lesions (e.g., granulomas, inflammatory foci) have SUVs greater than 2.5. Although data are preliminary, there may be benefit in serial determination of SUVs to monitor tumor response to therapy.

PERFORMANCE OF A PET SCAN

The technical aspects vis-à-vis camera parameters are manufacturer specific. Some PET scanners allow both two-dimensional and three-dimensional acquisition. Choice of one over the other is most often a personal preference. The use of attenuation correction is also an issue; recall that to perform SUV measurements, attenuation correction is necessary. One of the most important aspects of scan performance is patient preparation. For oncologic patients, it is recommended the patient fast for a minimum of 4 to 6 hours before FDG injection. This will reduce serum insulin levels, minimizing FDG accumulation in skeletal muscle and cardiac muscle. Water is permitted (along with necessary medications) to promote hydration. Blood glucose level is measured before administration of FDG. Hyperglycemia can interfere with tumor targeting owing to competitive inhibition of FDG by D-glucose. Diabetic patients present a special challenge. Although there is no uniform consensus, many recommend fasting for diet-controlled patients,

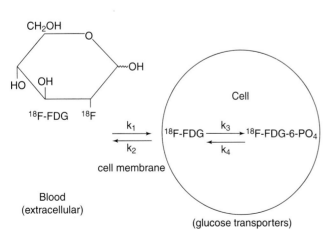

FIGURE 2. FDG metabolism. Extracellular FDG is transported across the cell membrane by one or more glucose transporters. Once intracellular, it is phosphorylated by hexokinase to FDG-6-phosphate. FDG-6-phosphate accumulates within the cell, owing to a low concentration of glucose-6-phosphatase, a necessary enzyme for dephosphorylation (low levels in most cancers). k_1 to k_4 = rate constants.

fasting with no added insulin or one-half normal dose in insulin-dependent diabetics, and fasting for diabetics on oral agents. Caution is recommended in administering insulin to these patients if their measured glucose level is high (i.e., >150 to 200 mg/dL). This may promote muscular uptake of FDG. In patients referred for a myocardial viability study, the goal is to enhance cardiac uptake. Multiple protocols are in use, all attempting to maximize heart uptake of FDG. These range all the way from fasting to carbohydrate loading before the scan. Unfortunately, lack of consensus has led to confusion rather than clarity.

The University of California at Los Angeles (UCLA), which has performed pioneering work in cardiac PET, recommends the following[8]:

For nondiabetic patients:
1. Overnight fast
2. Light breakfast (high protein)
3. Measurement of blood glucose level 1 hour before FDG administration
4. If glucose level is less than 110 mg/dL, give 50 g Trutol, and remeasure glucose level 1 hour later.
5. If initial glucose level is greater than 110 mg/dL, do not give Trutol.
6. If glucose level is greater than 150 mg/dL, give 3 to 5 U of insulin and then remeasure glucose level.

For diabetic patients:
1. Stay on regular diet and medications
2. Measure glucose
3. If glucose level is greater than 150 mg/dL, give 3 to 5 U insulin and monitor patient and recheck.

Other centers ask their patients to consume a high carbohydrate meal approximately 30 minutes before administration of FDG. In spite of careful attention to site-specific protocols and measured glucose values in the desired range, myocardial uptake may still vary considerably. If initial imaging demonstrates minimal or no uptake, consideration may be given to repeat scanning after 2 to 3 hours, administration of a small amount of intravenous insulin (e.g., 2 to 3 U) with reimaging or repeat study. Cardiac imaging is typically performed 30 minutes after FDG injection. For our protocol, please refer to Chapter 12.

For oncologic patients, a 60- to 90-minute uptake phase is recommended after FDG administration. The longer time frame may improve tumor to background ratio. During the uptake phase, the patient should remain quiet without activities that would stimulate muscular uptake of FDG (including chewing or excessive talking). In fact, most centers prefer that their patients minimize physical exertion for the day before the study (again, to decrease uptake in skeletal muscles). For neurologic studies, brain stimulation should be minimized (quiet, low-lit uptake area). Anxious or tense patients may be given low dose muscle relaxants or sedatives. Transportation home accompanied by an adult is mandatory.

SCAN INTERPRETATION

Normal FDG uptake, variations of normal, benign causes of FDG accumulation, and potential pitfalls are discussed in depth in Chapter 2. Briefly, normal tracer distribution includes the brain (gray matter), myocardium (in part dependent on substrate availability), urinary tract (especially the bladder), oculomotor muscles, mouth, nasopharynx, liver, spleen, bone marrow, gastrointestinal tract (may be quite variable), thyroid, and genitalia.[9,10] In an attempt to decrease urinary bladder activity, many modifications have been proposed. Some recommend hydration with frequent voiding, emptying the bladder just before the imaging, and beginning at the pelvic level and proceeding cephalad. Others recommend intravenous furosemide (10 to 20 mg) 20 minutes after FDG administration. Still others suggest catheterization (with some advocating instillation of sterile saline to "dilute" the radioactive urine). Lastly, if pelvic images are suboptimal, the pelvis can be re-imaged after voiding. Even with current reconstruction algorithms, including sagittal views, it seems prudent to consider hydration (intravenous during uptake phase) and furosemide when evaluating gynecologic patients or when the bladder area is critical. A minority of physicians resort to catheterization. Bowel activity is more difficult to deal with, because it can be quite unpredictable. Because this activity is likely caused by bowel wall accumulation along with bacterial concentration, cathartics or enemas offer little benefit. Fortunately, most benign activity tends to be tubular and of only moderate intensity. With this in mind, focal, intense increased FDG uptake should be viewed with suspicion and prompt further investigation.

Additional factors that are crucial to proper scan interpretation include knowledge of patient history (proximity of study to prior surgery, chemotherapy, or radiation therapy), intercurrent sites of active inflammation or infection, prior malignancies (some may recur years later such as breast, melanoma, thyroid, colon, etc.), results of serum tumor markers, knowledge of the typical biologic behavior of the patients' tumor, and, most importantly, comparison with other pertinent imaging studies. This cannot be overemphasized. Although PET is extremely sensitive, FDG accumulation may be relatively nonspecific and lack of anatomic landmarks is problematic. Comparison to anatomic-based modalities such as CT or MRI enhances interpretive ability immeasurably. Most of the case presentations in this atlas document the complementary nature of these imaging modalities.

RADIATION DOSIMETRY

In-depth estimates of radiation absorbed dose for FDG have been presented.[11,12] The urinary bladder wall is the critical organ (0.27 rads/mCi), followed closely by the heart wall (0.25 rads/mCi). Absorbed doses for the red marrow, ovaries, and testes are low, and FDG-PET is clearly within the range of other routinely performed nuclear medicine studies.

REFERENCES

1. Maisey M, Jeffery P: Clinical applications of positron emission tomography. Br J Clin Pract 1991;45:1-8.
2. Cherry SR: Fundamentals of positron emission tomography and applications in preclinical drug development. J Clin Pharm 2001;41:482-491.
3. Thompson CJ: Instrumentation. In Wahl RL, Buchanan JW (eds): Principles and Practice of Positron Emission Tomography. Philadelphia, Lippincott Williams & Wilkins, 2002, pp 48-64.
4. Rigo P, Paulus P, Kaschten BJ, et al: Oncological applications of positron emission tomography with fluorine-18 fluorodeoxyglucose. Eur J Nucl Med 1996;23:1641-1674.

5. Patton JA: Physics of PET. In Delbeke D, Martin WH, Patton JA, et al (eds): Practical FDG Imaging: A Teaching File. New York, Springer-Verlag, 2002, pp 18-36.

6. Wahl RL: To AC or not to AC: That is the question. J Nucl Med 1999;40:2025-2028.

7. Bleckmann C, Dose J, Bohuslavizki KH, et al: Effect of attenuation correction on lesion detectability in FDG PET of breast cancer. J Nucl Med 1999;40:2021-2024.

8. Schelbert HR: PET in myocardial imaging. Presented at Academy of Molecular Imaging 2002 Annual Conference, San Diego, CA, October 27, 2002.

9. Gordon BA, Flanagan FL, Dehdashti F: Whole-body positron emission tomography: Normal variations, pitfalls, and technical considerations. Am J Roentgenol 1997;169:1675-1680.

10. Cook GJR, Fogelman I, Maisey MN: Normal physiological and benign pathological variants of 18-fluoro-2-deoxyglucose positron-emission tomography scanning: Potential for error in interpretation. Semin Nucl Med 1996;26:308-314.

11. Mejia AA, Nakamura T, Masatoshi I, et al: Estimation of absorbed doses in humans due to intravenous administration of fluorine-18 fluorodeoxyglucose in PET studies. J Nucl Med 1991;32:699-706.

12. Hays MT, Watson EE, Thomas SR, et al: MIRD dose estimate report no. 19: Radiation absorbed dose estimates from 18F-FDG. J Nucl Med 2002;43:210-214.

Approach to PET Image Interpretation, Normal Variants, and Benign Processes

KEYS TO SUCCESS

I. Accurate, Detailed Clinical History
  A. Sources
    1. Information from referring physician (consultations, chart notes, history and physical examination, progress notes, pathology reports)
    2. Patient questionnaires (including diagnoses; dates of related surgery, chemotherapy, and irradiation; recent trauma, current symptoms (e.g., localized pain, lumps noted); sites of catheters, stomas, prostheses; prior cancers)
    3. Interview with patient and family members
II. Imaging Correlation (reports and films [x-rays, ultrasound, CT, MRI])
  A. Distribution of normal, physiologic activity of FDG
    1. Normal (almost always)
      a. Brain (intense)
      b. Myocardium (variable)
      c. Liver (low level—frequently diffusely mottled)
      d. Kidneys (collecting systems—intense; parenchyma —low level)
      e. Bladder (intense)
    2. Normal (frequently seen)
      a. Stomach
      b. Intestine
    3. Variable (almost always normal)
      a. Muscle
      b. Laryngeal
      c. Salivary gland
      d. Tonsils
      e. Thyroid
      f. Breast (parenchymal and nipple)

USUAL DISTRIBUTION OF FDG

A typical body or truncal study includes the neck, chest, abdomen, and pelvis (Figure 1). The most intense normal activity is in the brain, with intense activity of excreted FDG outlining the collecting systems of the kidneys, variably the ureters, and the urinary bladder. Normal renal parenchymal activity is comparatively of low-level intensity (Figures 2 to 4).

Myocardial uptake is variable and ranges from negligible to intense. It can vary considerably even in the same patient, scanned on different occasions (Figure 5). An attempt is made to minimize myocardial activity by having the patient fast for 4 to 6 hours before PET imaging, because fasting reduces insulin levels (myocardial uptake is increased in the presence of insulin). However, even with fasting, myocardial activity is highly variable. In theory, intense myocardial activity could make the evaluation of a nearby lesion, such as esophageal carcinoma, more difficult. In practice, this rarely occurs. On the contrary, it could be argued that some myocardial activity serves a practical localization function, as an anatomic landmark.

Mildly intense, uniformly mottled activity is seen throughout the liver and may limit the sensitivity of PET for small, pathologic lesions. Normal bowel activity can be seen in the stomach, small bowel, and colon, and, on occasion, in the esophagus. Bowel activity varies in intensity, even in the same patient on different occasions (see Figure 5), but it is typically low level and uniform. Most often it is readily recognizable either by its characteristic location and/or serpiginous, tubular pattern of activity. Differentiating normal intra-abdominal bowel activity from pathologic uptake can occasionally be difficult. Focally intense activity, particularly if different from the remainder of bowel activity in that patient, should be regarded with suspicion (Figures 6 and 7). Inflammatory processes of the bowel can result in increased intensity of bowel activity. There is overlap with the relatively intense diffuse bowel activity seen in asymptomatic patients being evaluated for other reasons.

Occasionally, it can be difficult to differentiate normal ureteral activity from pathologic retroperitoneal nodal activity, such as from metastatic disease or lymphoma. Just as on intravenous urography or enhanced abdominal CT, where ureteral opacification depends on timing and peristalsis, the ureters may or may not be identifiable on PET. Usually, they are readily recognized by their characteristic location and can be traced on sequential sections to the intrarenal collecting systems and/or to the bladder for confirmation (see Figure 2). Occasionally, when the ureters are distended and redundant, this distinction may be more difficult. Conversely, when retroperitoneal adenopathy consists of confluent lymph node chains, this activity may appear surprisingly linear and continuous and mimic ureteral activity. Typically, retroperitoneal adenopathy will be more "lumpy-bumpy" than ureteral activity, as well as more medial than the paraspinal course of the ureters (Figure 8). If available, correlation with a current imaging study, such as CT, will help ensure the most accurate interpretation possible.

Another potential problem in interpretation is the infrequent but not rare occurrence of focal ureteral activity, which presents as an isolated focus of intense activity along the course of the ureter, usually distal (Figure 9). Focal ureteral activity, from excreted FDG, displays a predilection for hang up at the iliac vessel crossing level. Location is the key to correctly identifying this uptake, but, on occasion, confident differentiation from a pathologic site of activity may be difficult. Asymmetry of intrarenal collecting system activity can be another clue to pathologic, rather than physiologic, distal ureteral uptake (Figure 10).

Muscular activity, like myocardium, varies with insulin level (Figure 11). In addition to fasting, muscular activity can be minimized by encouraging patients to avoid strenuous exercise on the day before PET scanning. By this same reasoning, it may be desirable to transport patients to the scanner via wheelchair if the scanner is not close by.

Even small muscles, such as the vocal cords, may display FDG activity if exercised after injection (Figure 12). If the area of interest is in the neck, it may be advisable to discourage the patient from talking during the uptake period. In practice, low-level activity in the larynx can provide a useful landmark for anatomic localization in the neck.

The neck is a frequent site for benign muscular activity, especially when patients are imaged with arms overhead. Usually, the characteristic location and longitudinal orientation poses no diagnostic dilemma (see Figure 12). On occasion, relatively focal cervical, thoracic inlet or supraclavicular muscular activity can be difficult to differentiate from pathologic activity in lymph nodes (Figure 13).

Other physiologic sites of low-level, but variable, FDG accumulation are noted regularly in the oropharynx and neck, including in tonsillar tissues, salivary glands, and the thyroid gland. This activity can range up to moderate intensity and may be potentially confusing, particularly when evaluating patients with head and neck cancer (Figure 14).

Physiologic, low-level breast parenchymal activity is also seen regularly, with nipple uptake (variable in intensity and not always symmetrical) seen on occasion (Figure 15).

Bone marrow activity is also generally low level, is frequently subtle and diffusely mottled, and seen most reliably in the vertebral bodies (Figure 16). On occasion, uptake is noted in the extremities and pelvis. Focal activity greater than the overall background level of the bone marrow should be regarded with suspicion as abnormal. Of course, focal regions of increased activity may be noted within or related to bone that are benign in etiology, such as that due to fractures (Figure 29) and arthritis (Figure 30), analogous to bone scans. Activated or recovering bone marrow, such as might be seen in a patient undergoing chemotherapy with colony-stimulating factors or with anemia, is recognized by an overall increase in bone marrow activity, which is usually fairly uniform and diffuse (see Figure 16B and D). At times, it may be difficult to differentiate between relatively patchy activated marrow and bone metastases (see Figure 16C).

Correlation with MRI may be necessary to confirm osseous metastatic disease.

LOCALIZATION OF DISEASE SITES

The importance of imaging correlation to accurate localization and characterization of disease processes cannot be overemphasized. Review of PET scans in a vacuum can be misleading at worst and imprecise at best. At times, without CT or other imaging study for correlation, it can be difficult to clearly assign a location to an active focus (see Figure 17). Peripheral lung nodules can be difficult to differentiate from chest wall or pleural lesions, whereas focal intra-abdominal foci of activity could be within bowel, studding mesenteric surfaces or within lymph nodes. In the chest, review of both non-attenuation and attenuation-corrected data may aid in lesion localization.

Very extensive disease, such as within one hemithorax, can sometimes be difficult to categorize. It could be due to a primary lesion with satellite lesions and/or hilar and mediastinal nodal involvement and at other times may prove to be predominantly pleural. Similarly, extensive pleural disease, particularly in the inferior costophrenic sulci, can extend so far inferiorly in pleural reflections as to suggest disease below the diaphragm (see Figure 18). Correlation with imaging studies, especially CT, safeguards against such errors. Knowledge of the most frequently encountered patterns of metastatic spread of particular tumors aids in predicting where metabolically active tumor foci may be expected to be distributed anatomically.

Not infrequently, the information derived from PET can lead to identification of anatomic correlates that are subtle and that may not have been recognized prospectively on other studies (see Figure 18H).

UTILITY OF REVIEW OF NON-ATTENUATION CORRECTED DATA

In general, studies are reviewed with attenuation correction. Occasionally, it may be helpful to review the non-attenuation corrected image set as well. Some centers routinely view only attenuation-corrected images, whereas others prefer non-attenuation corrected images, or both. We recommend that readers familiarize themselves with both types of images. This will provide a better understanding of the nuances of each and permit more effective correlation with other studies.

As noted earlier, the increased activity of the lung fields on non-attenuation corrected images may occasionally aid in localizing a lesion to within the lung periphery versus pleura or even within the chest wall. In addition, reconstruction artifacts, particularly in large patients, may contribute to a diffusely mottled appearance of the liver, which may hamper its evaluation on attenuation corrected images. In such cases, review of the non-attenuation corrected images may increase the confidence level regarding the status of the liver. On occasion, a subtle lesion may be more readily recognized on the non-attenuation corrected images (Figure 19). For these reasons, it may be advisable to routinely process the non-attenuation corrected data set (if not an automatic feature of the PET unit) so it is available for review. Particularly when no abnormality is identified and clinical suspicion is high (e.g., rising carcinoembryonic antigen level and suspicion of recurrent colon carcinoma), review of the non-attenuation corrected images may be helpful.

Other imaging artifacts to be aware of include reconstruction artifacts related to dose extravasation and patient motion (Figure 20).

IMPORTANCE OF DETAILED CLINICAL DATA IN INTERPRETATION

A detailed clinical history is essential to accurate PET interpretation. The high sensitivity of the study for all metabolically active processes makes it inevitable that other clinically irrelevant findings will be visualized. Accordingly, in interviewing the patient and the family, an attempt is made to anticipate questions that may arise when the study is reviewed subsequently (Figure 21). Ideally, studies are reviewed before the patient's departure, but in practice this can be difficult to achieve. Therefore, we throw out the widest possible net in questioning to ensure we have the full clinical picture. The patient is asked to bring all recent imaging studies with him or her, if imaging was performed at another facility. The referring physician's office is asked at the time of scheduling to send relevant consultations or history and physical examination results, pathology reports, imaging study results (if from another facility), office notes, and other pertinent information. Often, oncologic consults provide a clear picture of the clinical questions to be answered. If not, a questionnaire and interview with the patient and accompanying family members will be necessary to delineate the history and to anticipate other sources of activity, such as recent procedures, prior surgery, and trauma. The goal is to answer more questions than are raised. To this end, it is important in oncologic cases to have an understanding of the diagnosis, the apparent clinical and imaging stage, and the time course and anatomic distribution of therapies, including surgery, chemotherapy, and radiation. It is also necessary to elicit any history of other malignancies, other major medical problems (especially diabetes, chronic obstructive pulmonary disease, coronary artery disease), prior surgeries (especially recent), and the location of lines, tubes, ports, and ostomy sites. It is important to ask about recent trauma and location of any localized aches or pains and helpful to know about particularly symptomatic joints.

BENIGN CAUSES OF INCREASED ACTIVITY ON FDG PET IMAGING

There are many sources of benign activity that may be seen on PET scans. Significant FDG uptake may also be seen with inflammatory processes, from sinuses to lungs to bowel and soft tissue. The degree of activity is nonspecific and correlates with the activity of the process. Generally, inflammatory processes are less active than neoplastic ones. However, there clearly is overlap. Again, careful correlation with clinical history and imaging studies is necessary to avoid being misled.

Iatrogenic processes are a frequent source of mild to moderately intense activity, which often occurs in characteristic locations. Knowledge of the patients' prior surgical and treatment history is invaluable in recognizing these common, benign sources of activity. Low-level activity is frequently noted at sites of prior surgical biopsies and incisions and can persist for months to a year or more (Figure 22). Other iatrogenic sources of activity can be seen at injection sites (Figure 23), at ostomy sites (Figure 24), and around prostheses. Periprosthetic activity at established joint replacements correlates well with symptomatic replaced joints (Figure 25). Dental work can also produce maxillary and mandibular foci of activity, analogous to bone scans (see Figure 22E). Prolonged effects of radiation therapy may be seen in previously treated patients, most commonly in the lung and spine (Figure 26). Another benign, potentially confounding source of new activity in a young patient after chemotherapy is thymic rebound (Figure 27).

Musculoskeletal sources of benign activity are noted regularly (Figure 28). Again, the clinical history usually provides a ready explanation for observed variations in muscular activity. Patients with advanced chronic obstructive pulmonary disease and increased work of respiration may display increased activity of intercostal and diaphragmatic musculature (see Figure 28F and G). Iatrogenic sources of musculoskeletal activity may also be found, such as after cervical corpectomy (see Figure 28H), Achilles tendon release (see Figure 28I), and bone graft harvest (see Figure 28J).

A history of recent trauma, falls, fractures, or injuries should always be sought in reviewing the patient's clinical data. Unexpected activity in a bone raises the specter of osseous metastatic disease, unless an explanatory trauma history has been previously elicited (see Figures 21 and 29). Similarly, it is helpful to know about particularly symptomatic joints in the event joint-centered activity is noted (see Figures 28L and 30).

Benign thyroid processes may be noted on PET imaging, including goiter, Graves' disease, and thyroiditis (Figures 31 and 34). Benign normal thyroid activity can be seen as a variant (see Fig. 2-4). Markedly increased activity and prominent gland size may indicate Graves' or Hashimoto's thyroiditis (see Figure 34I). Focal thyroid activity in a nodule may be seen in benign and malignant lesions and is an indication for further evaluation.

Variations in cardiac activity from coexisting heart disease, such as cardiomyopathy or pulmonary hypertension, may be incidentally noted when reviewing whole-body studies obtained for oncologic purposes (Figure 32). For this reason, it is helpful to elicit information about a patient's cardiopulmonary or other major medical problems when reviewing the patient's history. Normal myocardial activity varies considerably, despite efforts to minimize such uptake. Depending on the intensity of myocardial activity in any one patient, it may be possible in individual cases to identify disease processes that directly involve the myocardium, such as metastases (see Figures 32D and E).

Benign gastrointestinal sources of unexpected activity include hiatal hernia and intrathoracic stomach, esophagitis and gastroesophageal reflux disease, and abdominal wall hernias containing bowel (Figure 33). As on other imaging modalities, renal congenital and other benign variants can be observed, including ectopic positioning, duplication, ureteropelvic junction disorders, and horseshoe kidney (Figure 34). Imaging correlation is essential to characterize unusual patterns of activity.

REFERENCES

1. Cook GJR, Maisey MN, Fogelman I: ^{18}F-Fluorodeoxyglucose and ^{11}C-methionine PET imaging in clinical practice: Normal variants, pitfalls, and artifacts. In Freeman LM (ed): Nuclear Medicine Annual. Philadelphia, Lippincott Williams & Wilkins, 2000, pp 85-110.

2. Cook GJR, Fogelman I, Maisey MN: Normal physiologic and benign pathological variants of 18-fluoro-2-deoxyglucose positron emission tomography scanning: Potential for error in interpretation. Semin Nucl Med 1996;26:308-314.
3. Sun S-S, Tsai S-C, Hsieh J-F, et al: False positive uptake of ^{18}F-fluorodeoxyglucose in the hilar region and mediastinum. Semin Nucl Med 2001;31:84-86.
4. Gordon BA, Flanagan FL, Dehdashti F: Whole-body positron emission tomography: Normal variations, pitfalls, and technical considerations. AJR Am J Roentgenol 1997;169:1675-1680.
5. Bakheet SM, Powe J: Benign causes of 18-FDG uptake on whole-body imaging. Semin Nucl Med 1998;28:352-358.

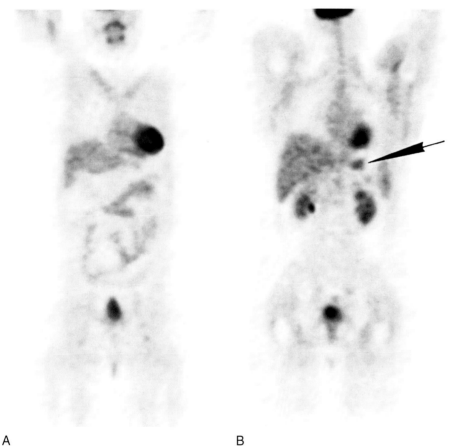

A   B

FIGURE 1. Typical truncal normal PET study. **A,** Anterior view. Intense myocardial activity is seen in this example, and excreted FDG in urine delineates the bladder. The mediastinum is low in activity level. Relatively low-level, diffusely mottled activity is noted in the liver. Normal bowel activity is readily recognized by the typical serpiginous configuration and location and often is fairly uniform in overall intensity. **B,** Posterior view. The included inferior brain is most active, with intense activity also in heart and bladder. Excreted FDG activity also is seen in the intrarenal collecting systems, with lower-level activity in the renal parenchyma. The typical, uniformly mottled pattern of liver activity is well demonstrated. A focal region of gastric activity is seen in the LUQ (*arrow*). The spleen can now be visualized and displays a low-to-medium level of activity, comparable to liver.

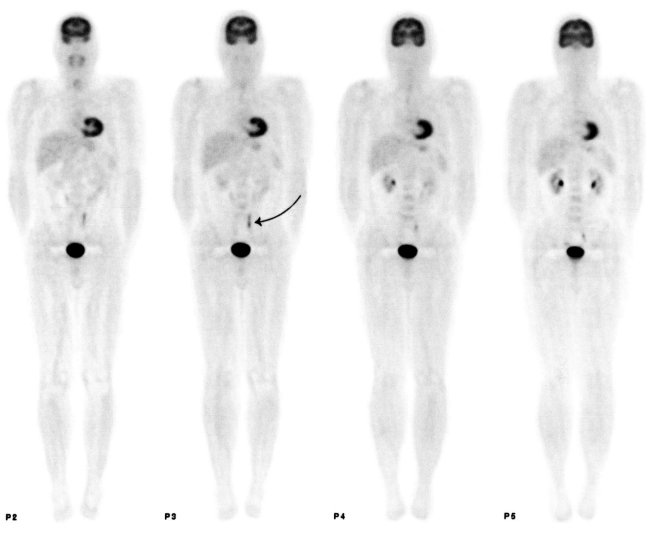

P2   P3   P4   P5

FIGURE 2. Whole-body normal PET study. Contiguous coronal images from a normal study, obtained for melanoma follow-up, show the most intense activity of FDG in brain, heart, and urinary collecting systems, particularly the bladder. Excreted FDG in the renal pelves and ureters is well demonstrated in this example (*arrow*). Low-level activity delineates the liver, spleen, and renal parenchyma. Bowel activity level is modest in this patient, including the stomach .

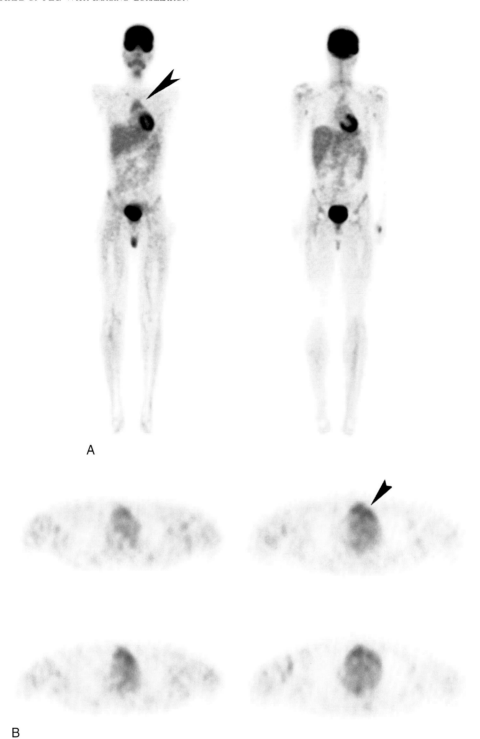

FIGURE 3. Whole-body normal PET study; thymic activity. **A,** Coronal PET images from a normal study of a 31-year-old man referred for melanoma follow-up show normal variant thymic uptake as low-level, triangular, anterior mediastinal activity *(arrowhead)*. Brain and bladder are again most active. Lower-level liver activity is seen, with negligible bowel uptake. Activity at the level of the genitalia is seen in this example. This is variable in presence and intensity from patient to patient. Contiguous transaxial (**B**) images confirm the anterior mediastinal location of the thymic *(arrowhead)* activity. Multiple follow-up studies showed similar findings.

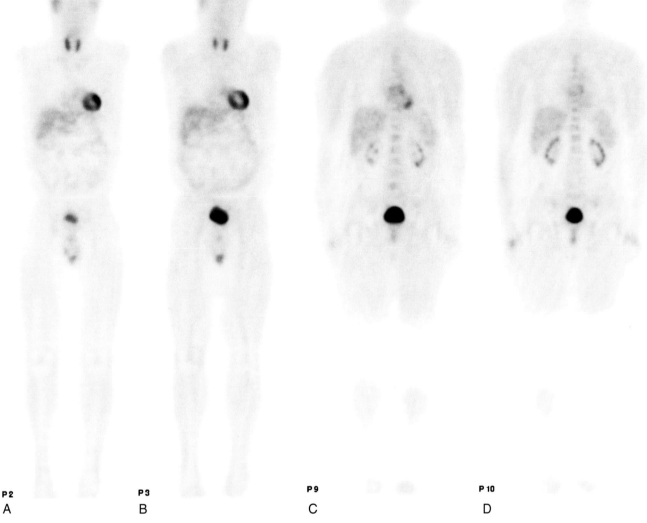

P 2

P 3

P 9

P 10

A   B   C   D

FIGURE 4. Whole-body normal PET study; thyroid activity. **A** and **B**, Anterior coronal images from a 60-year-old man being followed for melanoma show medium intensity, symmetrical, paramedian thyroid gland activity in the low anterior neck. This activity is regularly seen as a normal variant, but it could be seen in inflammatory conditions of the thyroid. Clues to differentiation are symmetry and intensity of uptake. As usual, the most intense FDG uptake is in heart and bladder, with lower level activity noted in liver, bowel, and genitalia. **C** and **D**, More posterior images of this same patient again show the bladder with the greatest activity, with lesser activity in mediastinum, liver, spleen, renal parenchyma, and interosseus muscles of the hands.

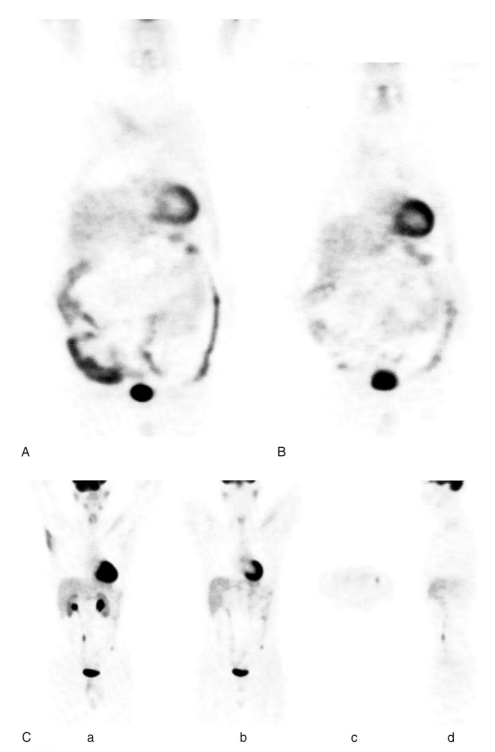

A   B

C   a   b   c   d

FIGURE 5. **A** and **B**, Variability of myocardial and bowel activity in the same patient on different studies. **A**, Treated lung cancer follow-up study shows intense bladder activity, followed in intensity by bowel and myocardium. **B**, PET study in the same patient, approximately 3 months later, shows more intense cardiac activity, with very low level bowel uptake. **C** and **D**, Variability of normal bowel activity in a different patient. **C**, A 58-year-old man is being followed for non-Hodgkin's lymphoma (NHL). Two studies, 9 months apart, show marked variation of bowel activity in the same patient on different occasions. The earlier study shows faint colonic activity, with no evidence of active NHL. Projection image (**a**) and coronal (**b**), transaxial (**c**), and sagittal (**d**) views are shown.

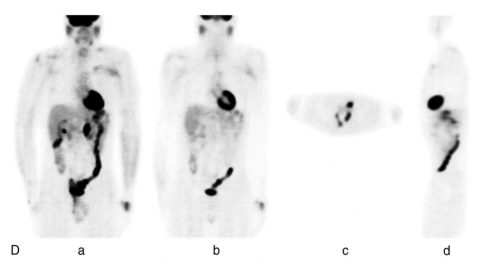

D   a   b   c   d

FIGURE 5. cont'd D, Nine months later, the patient remains asymptomatic and PET imaging again shows no evidence of lymphoma but left colon activity is strikingly intense. This pattern is nonspecific, and its significance must be assessed in light of clinical data. In this asymptomatic patient, a normal variant is presumed. These same findings could reflect a diffuse active inflammatory process (colitis). Projection image (**a**) and coronal (**b**), transaxial (**c**), and sagittal (**d**) views are shown.

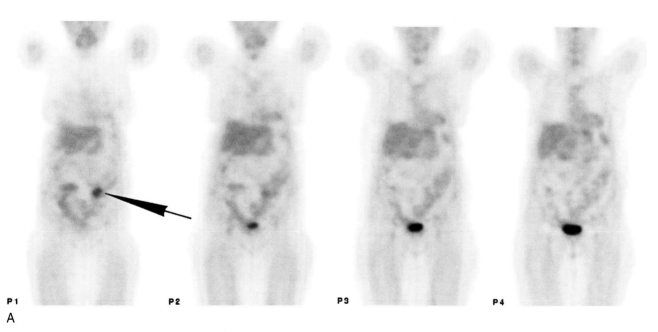

P1   P2   P3   P4

A

FIGURE 6. Focal intra-abdominal activity; differentiating normal bowel activity from pathologic intra-abdominal activity. **A,** Sequential coronal PET images from a 76-year-old woman evaluated after chemotherapy for ovarian cancer. She had presented with an obstructing omental mass and a CA-125 of 3000, which declined to 90 after chemotherapy. PET shows a focus of moderately intense left lower quadrant activity (*arrow*), which differs from the lower overall level of normal bowel activity. *Continued*

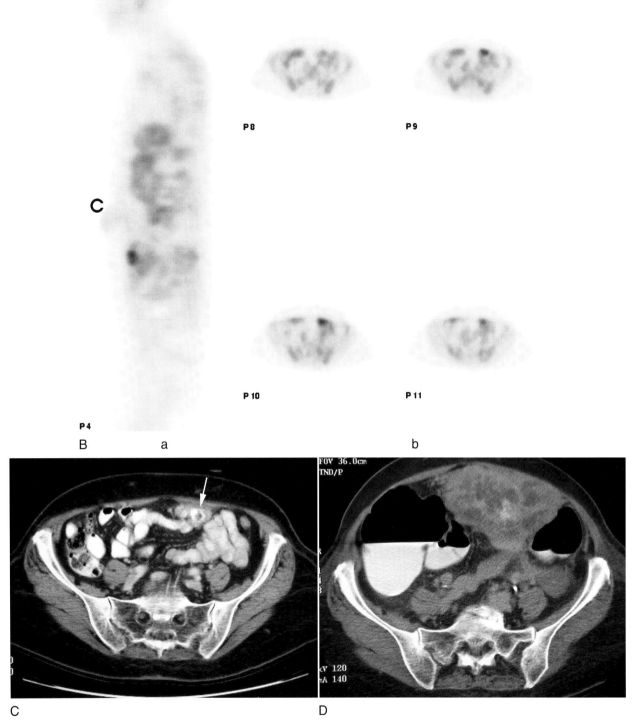

FIGURE 6. cont'd B, A sagittal (a) and four contiguous axial (b) sections from the PET study again show the area in question to be suspiciously focal in activity. The sagittal section also shows an anterior abdominal wall protuberance, a double barrel colostomy (C), providing a landmark for localization. Confident confirmation of the LLQ focus as a pathologic site of persistent disease activity requires correlation with an imaging study. **C,** CT image shows a corresponding focus beneath the left anterior abdominal wall, which differs in appearance from the well-opacified normal bowel. The focus shows a soft tissue collar surrounding a high-density center (*arrow*). Differential diagnosis based on CT appearance includes an abnormal, thick-walled opacified bowel loop versus a centrally calcified bowel or mesenteric mass. To be certain this was the site corresponding to PET finding, all available anatomic localization clues were used, including measuring down from the colostomy level (visual fusion). Software fusion of CT with PET information or combined simultaneous CT and PET imaging eases making such correlations. **D,** If only the most recent CT study on this patient (**C**) was available for correlation, the significance of this focus might have remained somewhat in doubt. The availability of sequential CT studies on this patient makes the story clear. CT at 3 months previously, at the time the patient presented with bowel obstruction, shows a much larger soft tissue mass at this site, with faint central calcification.

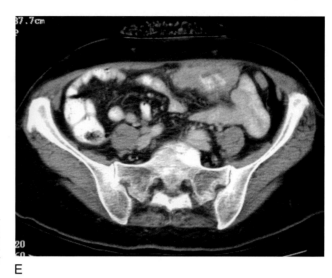

FIGURE 6. cont'd E, A follow-up CT 2 months later (1 month before the PET scan), during chemotherapy, shows a shrinking, progressively calcifying omental mass, which had shrunk further but not resolved at the time of the third CT and the PET scan. The residual mass, corresponding PET scan activity, and persistently elevated CA-125 level all suggest persistent active ovarian cancer at this site.

E

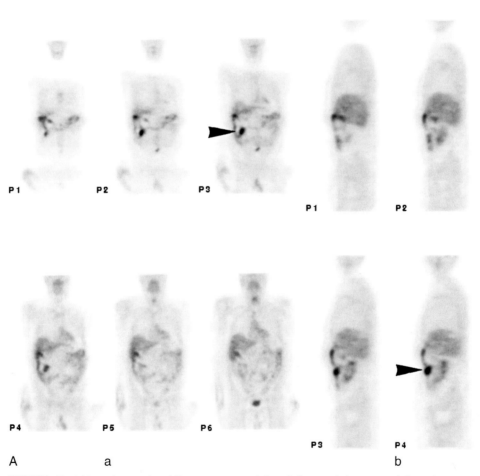

A   a   b

FIGURE 7. Additional examples differentiating normal bowel from pathologic intra-abdominal activity. **A,** Coronal (**a**) and sagittal (**b**) PET images from a 76-year-old man with a history of colon cancer and rising carcinoembryonic antigen level. PET images show a right mid-abdominal hypermetabolic region *(arrowheads),* which is both more focal and more intense in activity than the background bowel activity and should be regarded with suspicion for a site of recurrent tumor. No other etiology was identified in liver or lung for this patient's tumor marker elevation. A second possible intra-abdominal site of increased activity is suggested at the hepatic flexure level, but correlation with the sagittal sections shows this to be more serpiginous and representative of bowel.

Continued

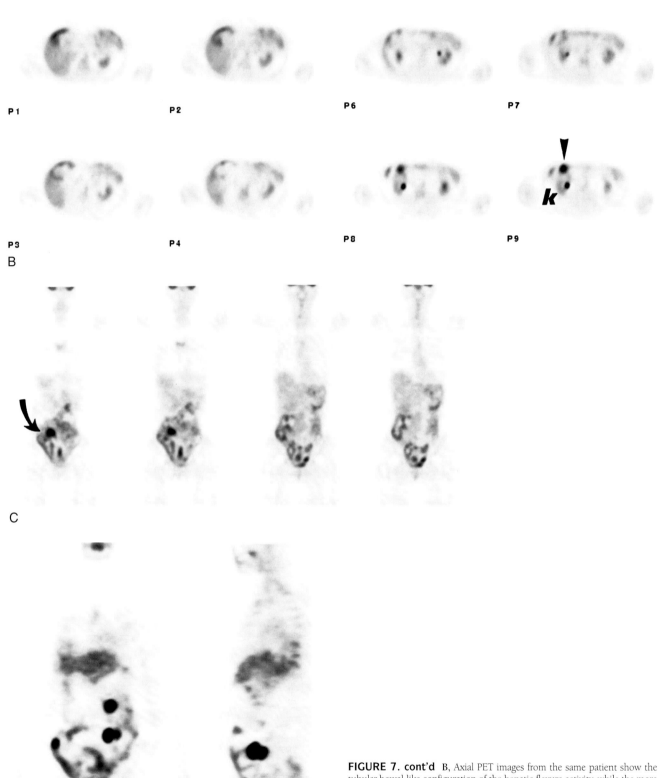

FIGURE 7. cont'd B, Axial PET images from the same patient show the tubular bowel-like configuration of the hepatic flexure activity, while the more suspicious and focal uptake *(arrowhead)* is seen again, anterior to the right kidney (k). **C,** Coronal PET images from another patient, a 61-year-old woman with gastric carcinoma metastatic to peritoneum, demonstrates a RLQ focus of suspicious activity *(arrow),* which stands out from the more tubular background bowel activity by virtue of its focality, size greater than the caliber of adjacent bowel, and intensity. **D,** Coronal (**a**) and sagittal (**b**) PET images of a 69-year-old man with recurrent melanoma within the abdomen: multiple hyperintense foci of activity differ in focality, size, and intensity of activity from lower level normal bowel activity and are consistent with mesenteric metastases.

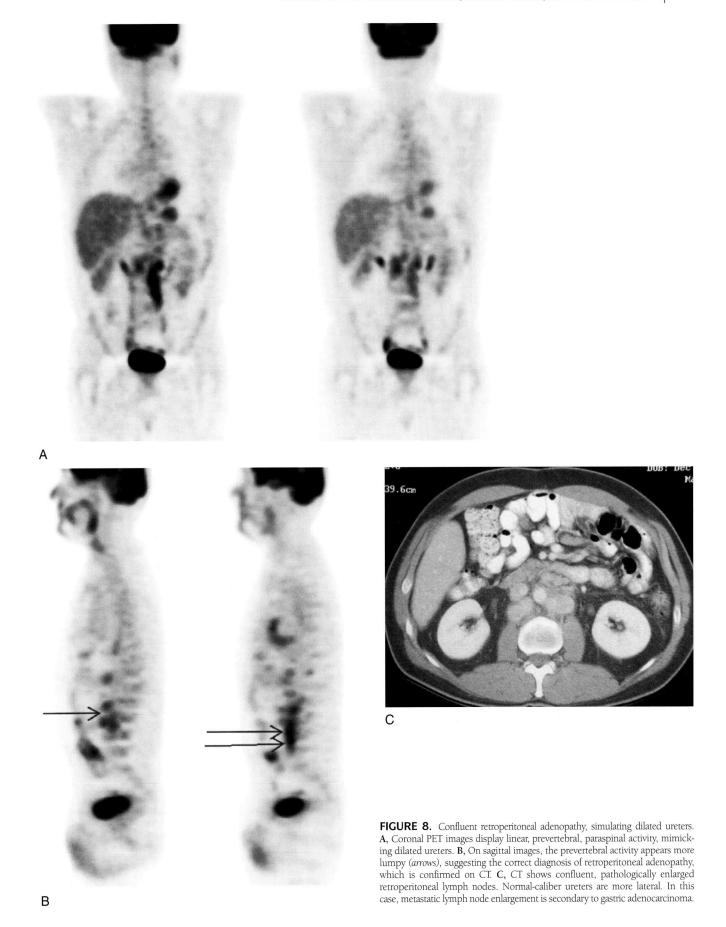

FIGURE 8. Confluent retroperitoneal adenopathy, simulating dilated ureters. **A,** Coronal PET images display linear, prevertebral, paraspinal activity, mimicking dilated ureters. **B,** On sagittal images, the prevertebral activity appears more lumpy *(arrows),* suggesting the correct diagnosis of retroperitoneal adenopathy, which is confirmed on CT. **C,** CT shows confluent, pathologically enlarged retroperitoneal lymph nodes. Normal-caliber ureters are more lateral. In this case, metastatic lymph node enlargement is secondary to gastric adenocarcinoma.

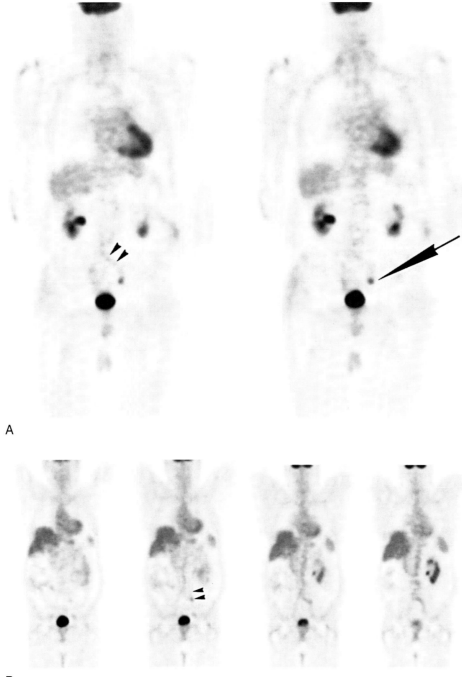

FIGURE 9. Focal ureteral activity; physiologic. **A,** Coronal PET images show a tiny, punctate focus of activity at the left distal ureteral level *(arrow)*, probably representing excreted ureteral FDG, hanging up at the iliac vessel crossing level. The iliac artery is faintly identifiable *(arrowheads)*. **B,** Another example of focal ureteral activity in a different patient. This series of coronal images shows a tiny punctate focus of activity in the mid-distal left ureter *(arrowheads)*, which can be traced to fainter more proximal ureteral activity. This example also shows the abdominal aorta to greater advantage, demonstrating the ureteral crossing level.

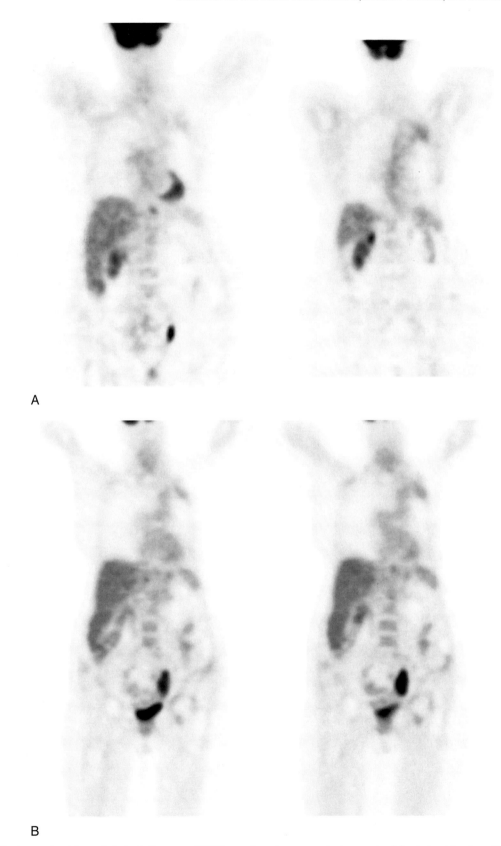

FIGURE 10. Focal ureteral activity; pathologic. **A,** Two coronal PET images from the same study show modest left apical activity, the residua of radiation therapy for lung cancer. A focus of intense left hemipelvic activity along the course of the left ureter was not recognized prospectively to be pathologic. Two clues to the abnormal nature of this activity, which might have distinguished it from ureteral excreted FDG, are the paucity of activity in the bladder and the asymmetry of activity in the intrarenal collecting systems. Correlation with a CT or other relevant imaging study would also have been helpful in avoiding this interpretive error. **B,** A follow-up study, 6 months later, shows progressive growth of the hypermetabolic mass at the left distal ureteral level, which proved to be a transitional cell carcinoma.   *Continued*

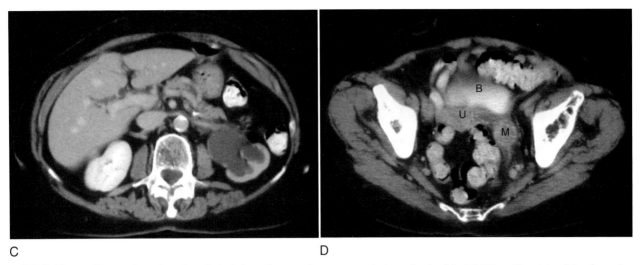

C   D

FIGURE 10. cont'd C, Enhanced CT through the kidneys shows moderate-to-severe hydronephrosis of the left kidney. Chronicity of the obstruction is indicated by cortical thinning. Renal parenchymal enhancement is also depressed, in contrast to the normal right kidney. **D,** The responsible obstructing soft tissue density transitional cell carcinoma mass at the level of the left distal ureter is demonstrated on CT through the pelvis. B, bladder; M, mass; U, uterus.

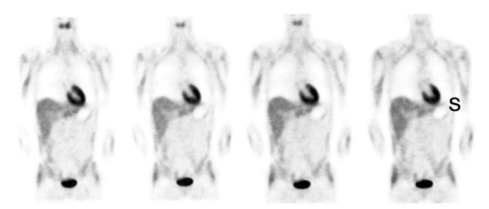

FIGURE 11. Non-NPO patient. Contiguous coronal PET images in a patient who had a full lunch before this study show intense myocardial activity and diffusely increased muscular activity, simulating a diabetic patient study. Note also the full stomach (S), manifested as a photopenic LUQ structure.

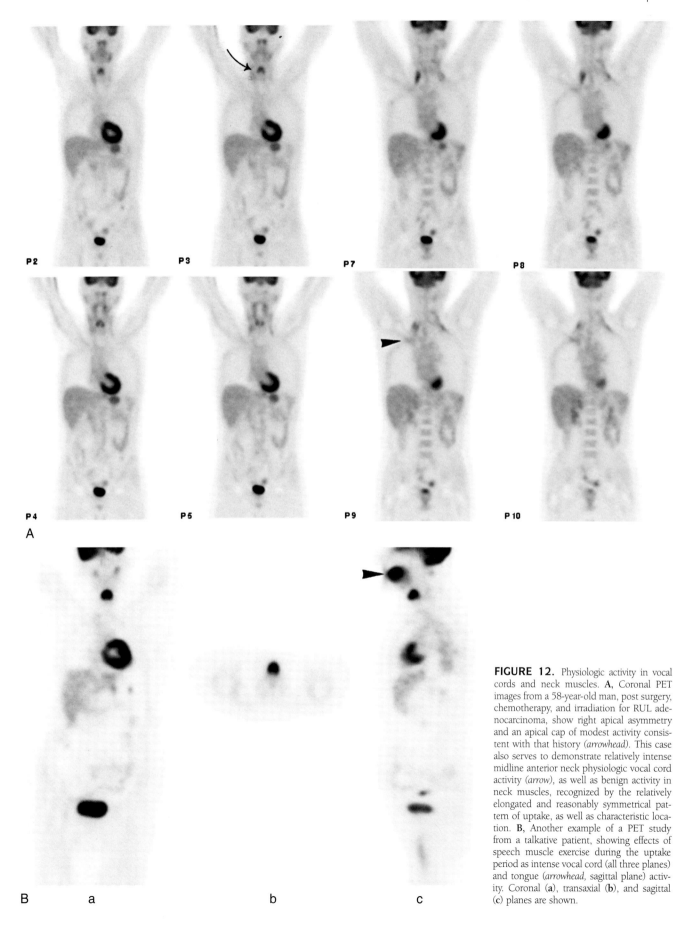

FIGURE 12. Physiologic activity in vocal cords and neck muscles. **A,** Coronal PET images from a 58-year-old man, post surgery, chemotherapy, and irradiation for RUL adenocarcinoma, show right apical asymmetry and an apical cap of modest activity consistent with that history (*arrowhead*). This case also serves to demonstrate relatively intense midline anterior neck physiologic vocal cord activity (*arrow*), as well as benign activity in neck muscles, recognized by the relatively elongated and reasonably symmetrical pattern of uptake, as well as characteristic location. **B,** Another example of a PET study from a talkative patient, showing effects of speech muscle exercise during the uptake period as intense vocal cord (all three planes) and tongue (*arrowhead, sagittal plane*) activity. Coronal (**a**), transaxial (**b**), and sagittal (**c**) planes are shown.

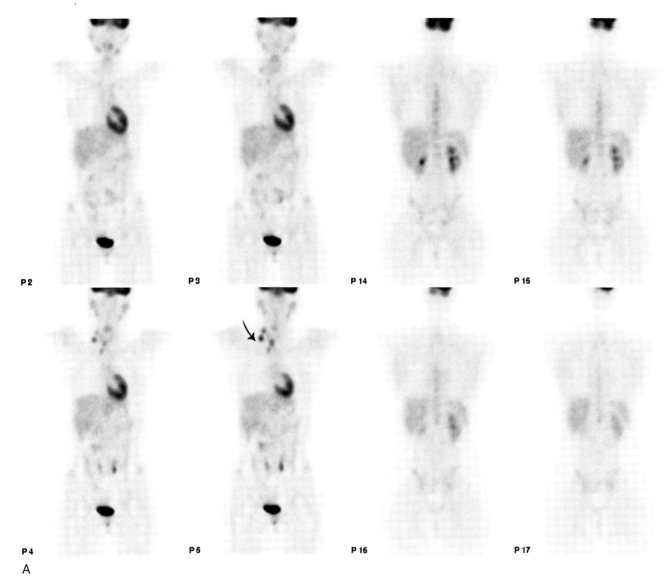

P 2 P 3 P 14 P 15

P 4 P 5 P 16 P 17

A

FIGURE 13. Differentiating cervical muscular activity from pathologic lymph node activity: 15-year-old girl with Hodgkin's disease (HD). **A,** Coronal PET images show four distinct small foci of activity in the low anterior right neck and thoracic inlet, consistent with persistently active disease (*arrow*). This was an unexpected result. Although the patient's disease was initially detected in the right neck as a large mass, this had clinically resolved after chemotherapy. PET scanning was performed to assess disease activity in the mediastinum, where CT showed a residual mass after chemotherapy, and in the splenic hilus. Both of these sites were negative on PET.

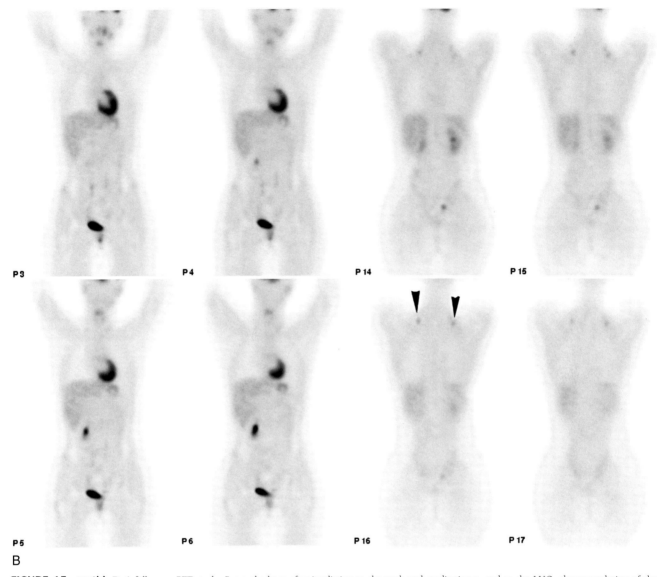

B

FIGURE 13. cont'd B, A follow-up PET study, 5 months later, after irradiation to the neck and mediastinum, and to the LUQ, shows resolution of the previously noted HD activity. New, fairly symmetrical posterior neck activity is now noted but seems most consistent with muscular activity *(arrowheads)*.

Continued

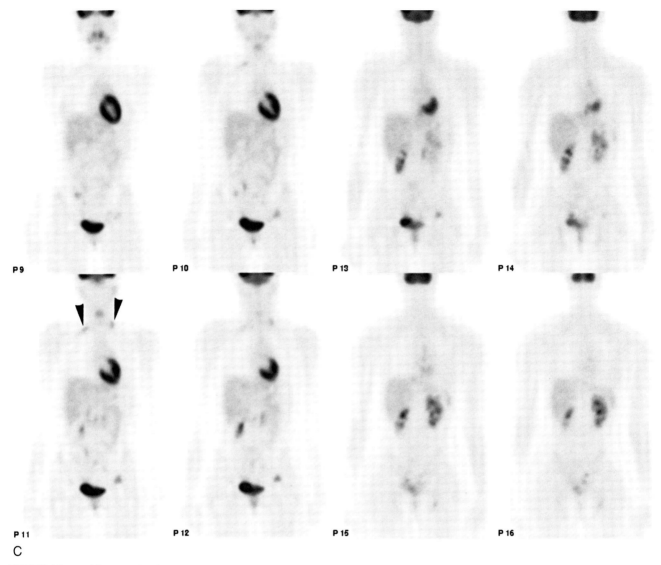

C

FIGURE 13. cont'd C, A further follow-up study, 3 months later, obtained because of increased erythrocyte sedimentation rate, shows findings suggestive of recurrent disease. New, relatively focal and asymmetrical low anterior neck activity is noted bilaterally *(arrowheads)*. In addition, there is new activity at the level of the left acetabulum, as well as a left inguinal node *(not shown)*. The posterior neck activity noted previously is not present, confirming the impression that it was muscular.

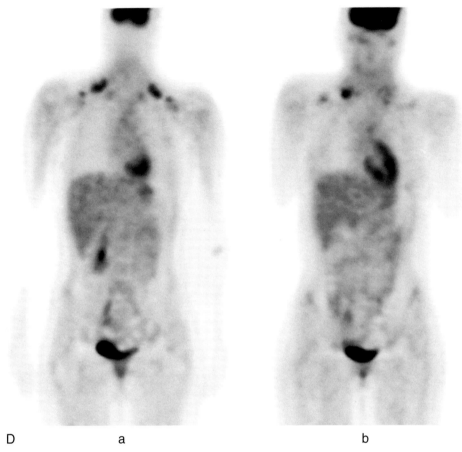

D   a   b

FIGURE 13. cont'd D, Importance of symmetry: Another, later PET study in the same patient, shows symmetric supraclavicular activity, which may be muscular or brown fat (**a**). A more anterior PET section (**b**) shows a focal, intense, asymmetrical site of activity in the right supraclavicular region, suggestive of recurrent HD. This was subsequently confirmed pathologically. Even with pronounced neck muscular or brown fat activity, careful image review and analysis of symmetry frequently enables one to "read around" inconvenient artifacts.

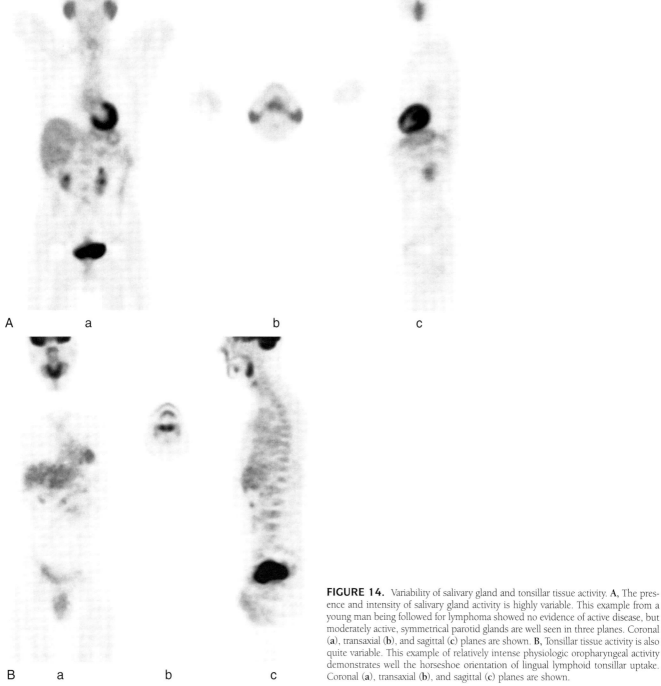

A   a   b   c

B   a   b   c

FIGURE 14. Variability of salivary gland and tonsillar tissue activity. **A,** The presence and intensity of salivary gland activity is highly variable. This example from a young man being followed for lymphoma showed no evidence of active disease, but moderately active, symmetrical parotid glands are well seen in three planes. Coronal (**a**), transaxial (**b**), and sagittal (**c**) planes are shown. **B,** Tonsillar tissue activity is also quite variable. This example of relatively intense physiologic oropharyngeal activity demonstrates well the horseshoe orientation of lingual lymphoid tonsillar uptake. Coronal (**a**), transaxial (**b**), and sagittal (**c**) planes are shown.

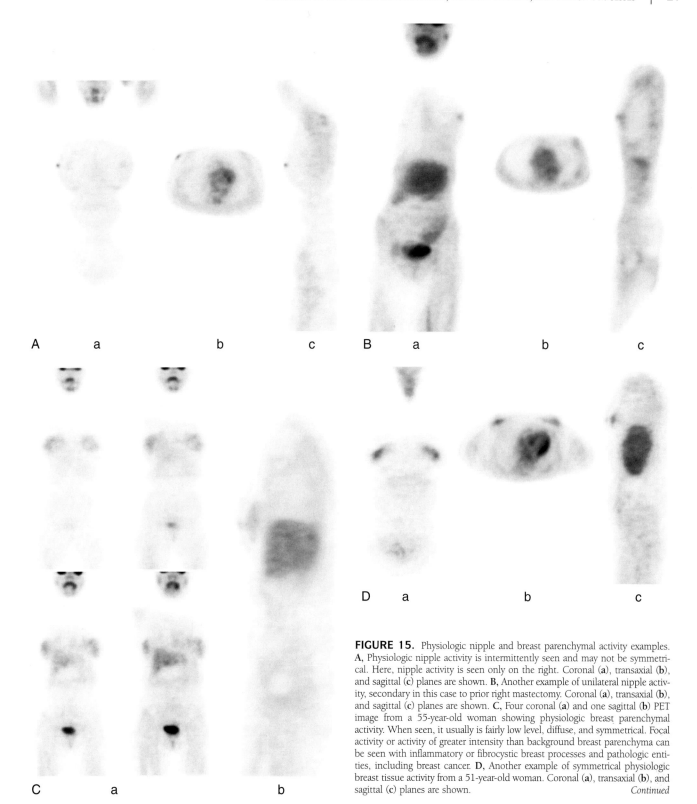

FIGURE 15. Physiologic nipple and breast parenchymal activity examples. **A,** Physiologic nipple activity is intermittently seen and may not be symmetrical. Here, nipple activity is seen only on the right. Coronal (**a**), transaxial (**b**), and sagittal (**c**) planes are shown. **B,** Another example of unilateral nipple activity, secondary in this case to prior right mastectomy. Coronal (**a**), transaxial (**b**), and sagittal (**c**) planes are shown. **C,** Four coronal (**a**) and one sagittal (**b**) PET image from a 55-year-old woman showing physiologic breast parenchymal activity. When seen, it usually is fairly low level, diffuse, and symmetrical. Focal activity or activity of greater intensity than background breast parenchyma can be seen with inflammatory or fibrocystic breast processes and pathologic entities, including breast cancer. **D,** Another example of symmetrical physiologic breast tissue activity from a 51-year-old woman. Coronal (**a**), transaxial (**b**), and sagittal (**c**) planes are shown. *Continued*

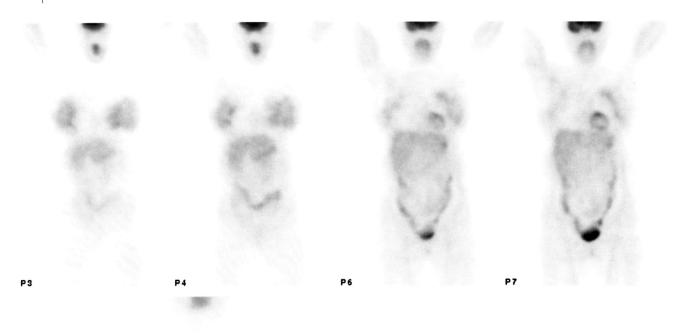

P3   P4   P6   P7

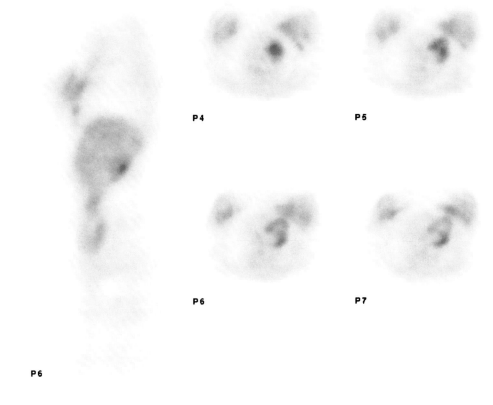

P4   P5

P6   P7

P6

E

FIGURE 15. cont'd E, Silicone injections: 62-year-old woman with a question of a breast lump, with difficult to interpret mammography because of marked increased density from prior silicone injections. PET images show a diffuse increase in breast tissue activity, without focality.

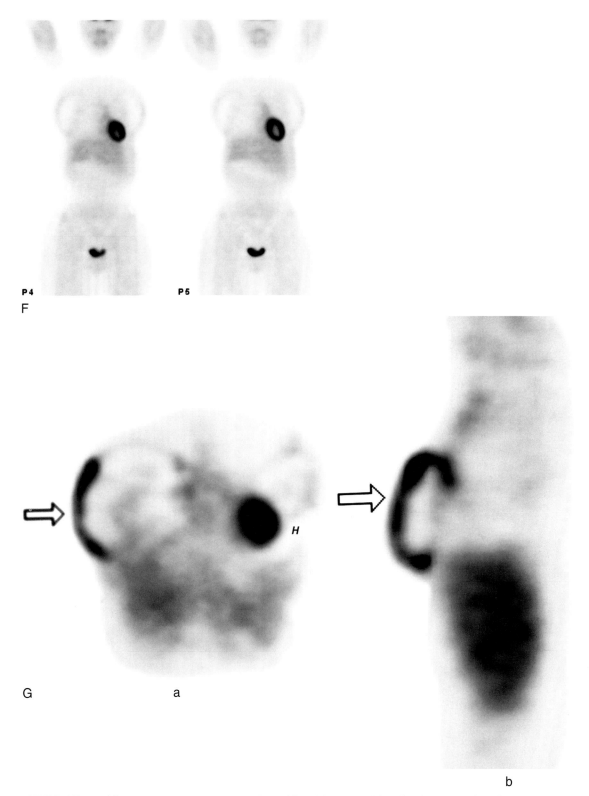

FIGURE 15. cont'd F, Implants: 44-year-old woman being followed for non-Hodgkin's lymphoma. PET showed no active disease. Typical appearance of breast implants demonstrating photopenia. **G**, Dramatic peri-implant inflammatory reaction (*arrow*) is noted in another patient in coronal (**a**) and sagittal (**b**) planes (H, heart).

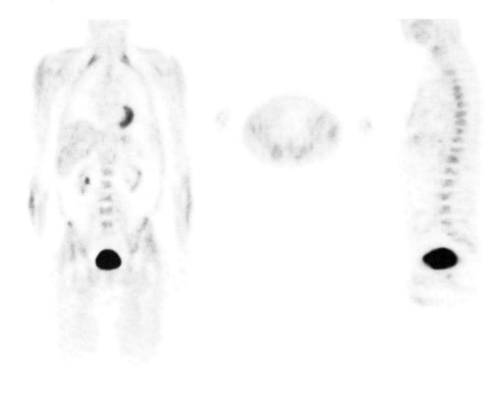

A   a   b   c

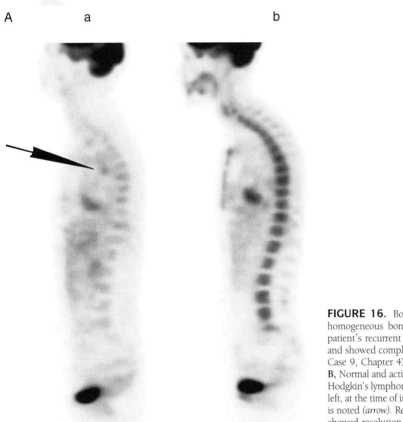

B

FIGURE 16. Bone marrow (normal and activated). **A,** Normal low-level, fairly homogeneous bone marrow activity on a follow-up PET scan. This lymphoma patient's recurrent disease was exclusively in bone marrow on his prior PET scan and showed complete clearance on this study after chemotherapy (same patient as Case 9, Chapter 4). Coronal (**a**), transaxial (**b**), and sagittal (**c**) planes are shown. **B,** Normal and activated marrow: 50-year-old woman with follicular, large cell non-Hodgkin's lymphoma (NHL), treated with chemotherapy. Sagittal PET image on the left, at the time of initial staging, shows normal marrow. A mediastinal focus of NHL is noted (*arrow*). Repeat PET scan, 3 months and four cycles of chemotherapy later, showed resolution of all NHL disease activity but development of diffuse marrow hyperintensity, well seen in both spine and sternum. Findings and clinical scenario are typical for activated marrow.

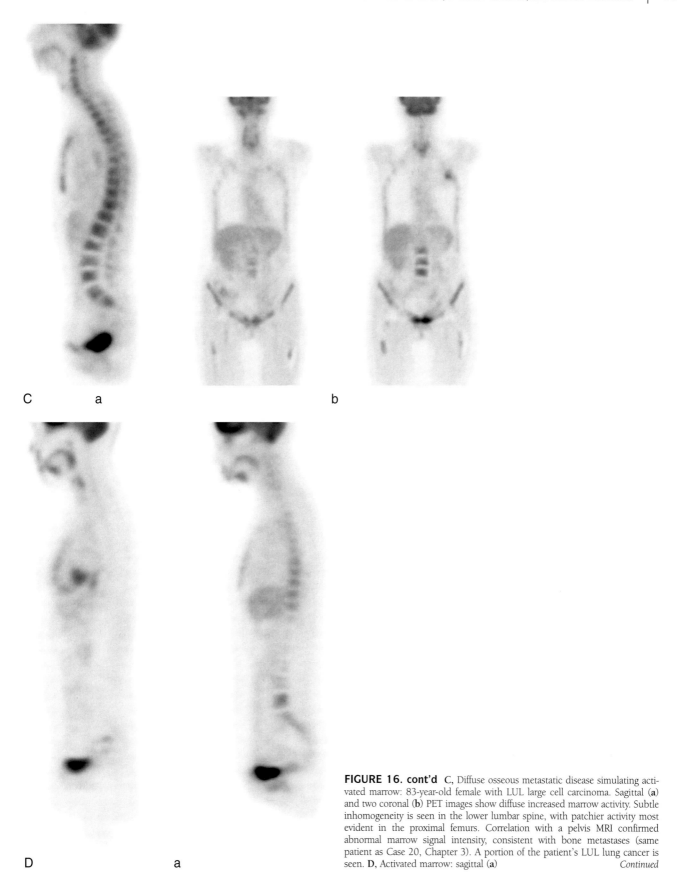

FIGURE 16. cont'd C, Diffuse osseous metastatic disease simulating activated marrow: 83-year-old female with LUL large cell carcinoma. Sagittal (**a**) and two coronal (**b**) PET images show diffuse increased marrow activity. Subtle inhomogeneity is seen in the lower lumbar spine, with patchier activity most evident in the proximal femurs. Correlation with a pelvis MRI confirmed abnormal marrow signal intensity, consistent with bone metastases (same patient as Case 20, Chapter 3). A portion of the patient's LUL lung cancer is seen. **D,** Activated marrow: sagittal (**a**) *Continued*

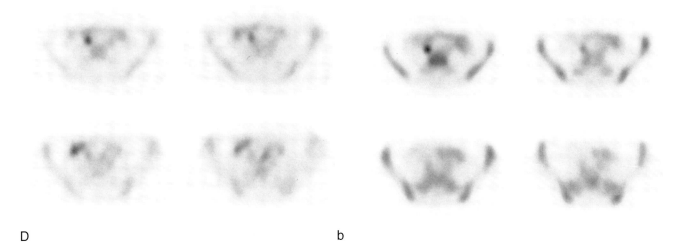

D   b

FIGURE 16. cont'd and axial (**b**) PET images are from two different studies (images on the right of each panel are 2.5 months after images on the left of each panel) in a 15-year-old girl with Hodgkin's disease being treated with chemotherapy (same patient as in Figure 13). The later study shows a marked increase in intensity of bone marrow activity, demonstrated on the sagittal view in the spine and sternum, and on the axials in the pelvis. The increased marrow activity is homogeneous and diffuse and typical of marrow activation. The multilevel sparing of the thoracolumbar spine is attributable to radiation therapy effect (the patient had previously been irradiated for splenic hilar disease).

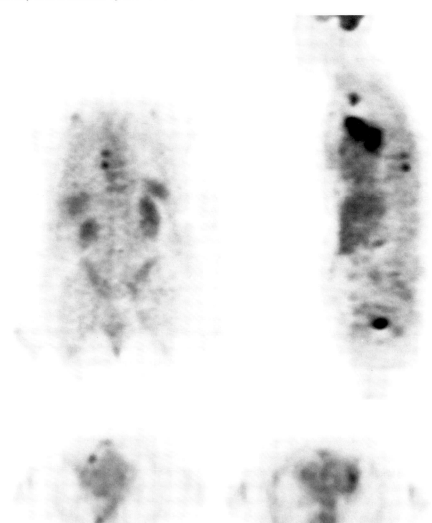

A

FIGURE 17. Importance of imaging correlation to accurately localize disease. **A,** Pleural metastases mimicking rib trauma: 82-year-old woman with recently diagnosed lung carcinoma. Characteristic patterns of activity can suggest particular causes, as adjacent foci of activity suggest rib fractures on bone scan or PET. In this case, in addition to very extensive findings of stage IV lung carcinoma, two adjacent foci of activity are seen on PET at the right costovertebral level. The pattern of activity suggests trauma.

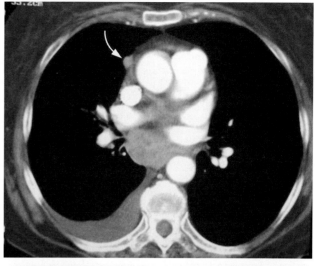

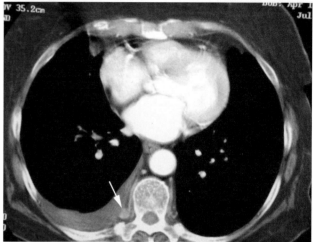

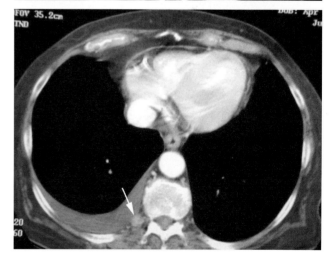

FIGURE 17. cont'd However, correlation with the chest CT shows that these foci actually represent adjacent pleural tumor nodules, indicating that the accompanying effusion is malignant (**B**). An additional pleural tumor nodule accounts for a focus of activity projecting on the surface of the heart (*curved arrow*). The two foci identified on PET (Figure 17-A) are shown on separate CT views (*straight arrows*). **B**

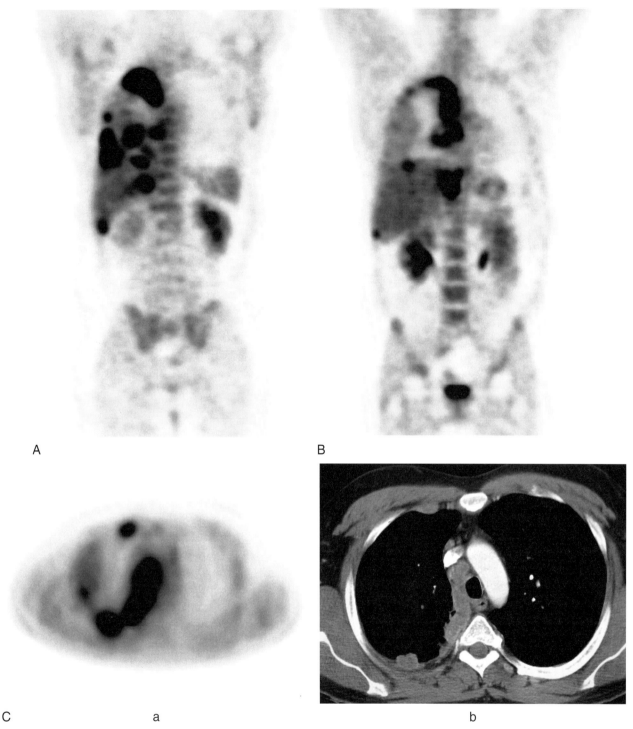

A

B

C   a   b

FIGURE 18. Importance of imaging correlation to accurately localize disease. **A,** A 41-year-old man presented with right pleural adenocarcinoma: PET scan shows extensive right hemithoracic disease. It is difficult based on this to determine the distribution of disease between lung parenchyma and pleural cavity. Review of these findings in the axial plane and correlation with CT demonstrate that essentially all of these foci are pleural in location, including at the inferior tip of the liver. Without imaging correlation, a lesion in this location would be difficult to differentiate from a serosal implant (e.g., from ovarian carcinoma) or even a peripheral liver lesion. **B,** A more anterior coronal PET section from the same study shows a peripheral curvilinear rind of hypermetabolic pleural neoplasia at the medial lung apex. Foci projecting at the dome of the liver, at the level of the left hepatic lobe, and at the inferior right hepatic lobe are harder to precisely localize. Correlation with CT shows that this is all part of the extensive pleural neoplasm, involving diaphragmatic pleura, and medial and lateral inferior costodiaphragmatic recesses. **C,** Corresponding axial PET (**a**) and CT image (**b**) pairs show near-perfect correlation, with confluent and localized nodular foci of pleural neoplasia showing intense hypermetabolism. Note disease involvement of right paratracheal region, which could be nodal (in the mediastinum) or pleural (pleural implant invaginating into a pleural reflection).

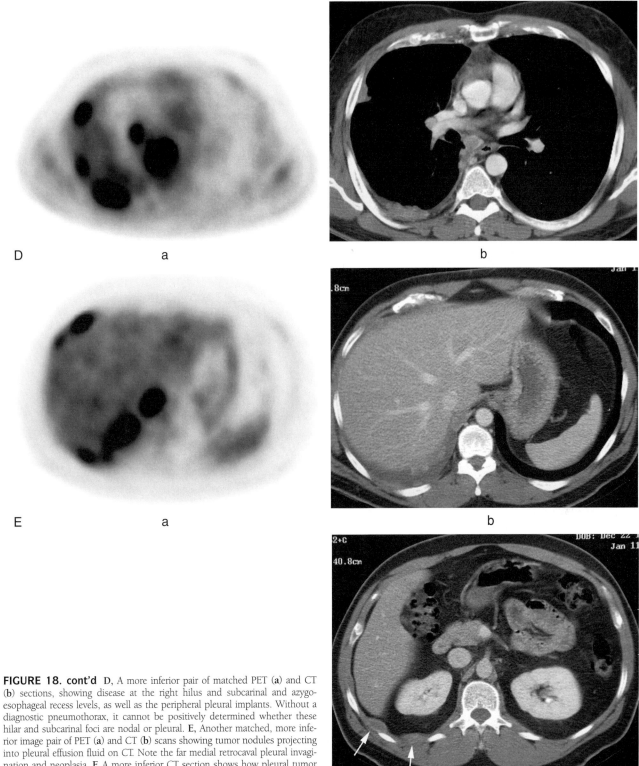

FIGURE 18. cont'd D, A more inferior pair of matched PET (**a**) and CT (**b**) sections, showing disease at the right hilus and subcarinal and azygo-esophageal recess levels, as well as the peripheral pleural implants. Without a diagnostic pneumothorax, it cannot be positively determined whether these hilar and subcarinal foci are nodal or pleural. **E,** Another matched, more inferior image pair of PET (**a**) and CT (**b**) scans showing tumor nodules projecting into pleural effusion fluid on CT. Note the far medial retrocaval pleural invagination and neoplasia. **F,** A more inferior CT section shows how pleural tumor nodules can extend inferiorly in costodiaphragmatic recesses, down to the inferior tip of the liver and level of the kidneys (*arrows*).   *Continued*

FIGURE 18. cont'd G, A 57-year-old woman presented with recurrent ovarian carcinoma: coronal (**a**) and axial (**b**) PET images show a disease distribution that resembles the prior case, with hypermetabolic tumor implants projecting on the surface of the liver, juxtasplenic, and in the right flank at the inferior tip of the right hepatic lobe. However, these disease foci are on serosal surfaces of the viscera and thus are below the diaphragm. **H**, A 63-year-old woman presented with right pyriformis colon cancer metastasis: The patient was 3 years post preoperative irradiation, surgery, and postoperative chemotherapy for colon cancer when she developed right posterior thigh pain. No definite abnormality was seen on CT prospectively. Coronal (**a**) and axial (**b**) PET images show an intensely active focus in the right sciatic notch region, which on correlation with CT (**c**) corresponds with a subtle enhancing lesion at the level of the right pyriformis muscle (*arrow*).

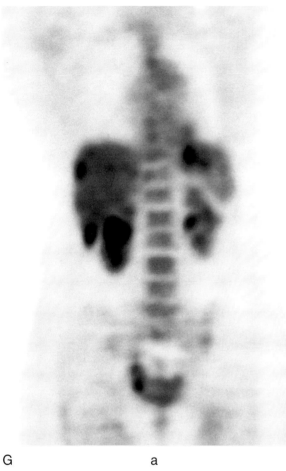

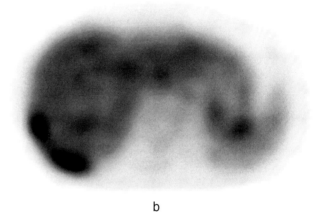

G　　　　a

b

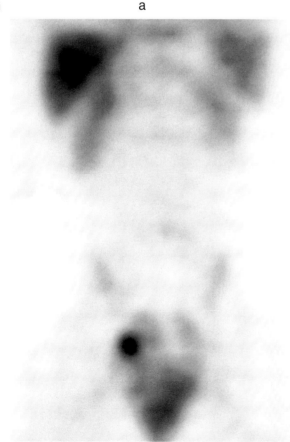

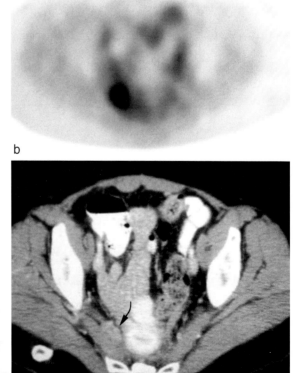

b

H　　　　a

c

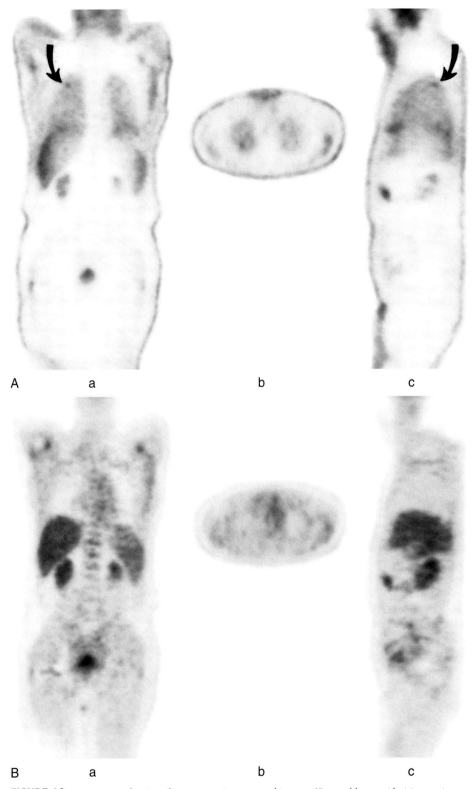

A   a   b   c

B   a   b   c

FIGURE 19. Importance of review of non-attenuation corrected images: 65-year-old man with rising carcinoembryonic antigen (CEA) level and suspected recurrent colorectal carcinoma. **A** and **B**, Non-attenuation corrected images (A) show a tiny posterior right upper lobe nodule, which is only faintly demonstrated on attenuation corrected images (B) and could easily have been overlooked. This was the only etiology for the increasing CEA level found on this PET study. Coronal (**a**), transaxial (**b**), and sagittal (**c**) views are shown. *Continued*

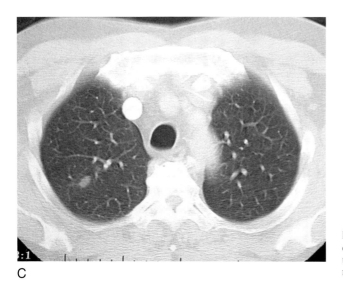

C

FIGURE 19. cont'd A subsequent chest CT study (**C**) identified a corresponding 5 × 10-mm new right upper lobe lung nodule, consistent with a lung metastasis. An additional, smaller new left upper lobe nodule was noted as well that was not seen on the PET study.

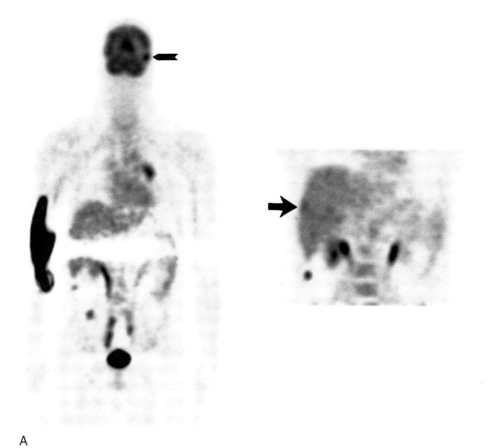

A

FIGURE 20. PET imaging artifacts. **A,** Dose extravasation reconstruction artifact masking liver metastasis: 49-year-old man, 3 years post right subtotal mastectomy for a chest wall melanoma, presented with seizure due to an intracranial hemorrhage. Metastatic melanoma was suspected, and he was referred for restaging. Multiple metabolically active foci were identified, including in the left parietal brain (*arrowhead*), left hilus, right flank, and mid-abdomen. Injection was through an existing intravenous line, and significant extravasation is evident. The marked intensity of the extravasated activity generates an artifact that traverses a portion of the liver. Re-imaging, with the arms overhead, shows a focal liver metastasis, which was obscured (*arrow*).

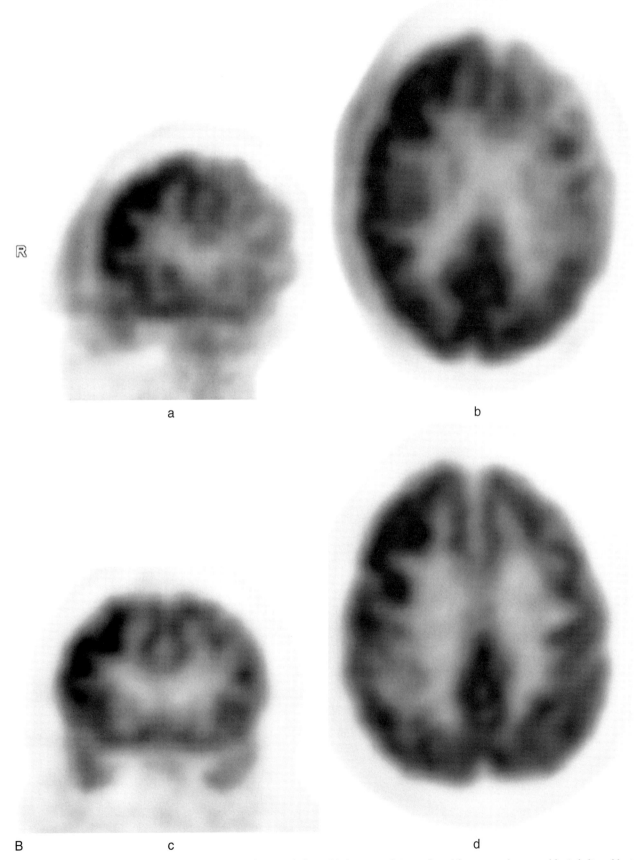

a

b

B   c   d

FIGURE 20. cont'd B, Motion artifact simulating brain hypometabolism: elderly woman, being evaluated for memory loss. **a** and **b**, A dedicated brain PET shows a large left frontal region of apparent hypometabolism. Careful evaluation of the coronal section (**a**) suggests a ghostly "double exposure" on the right, suggesting motion artifact. **c** and **d**, Repeat study, without motion, is more normal.

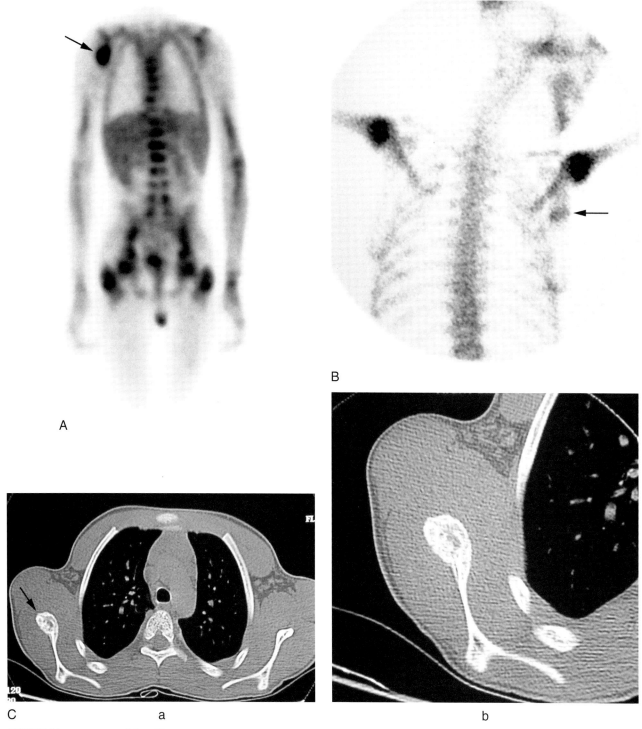

A

B

C   a   b

FIGURE 21. Importance of clinical history to PET scan interpretation. A 12-year-old boy status post irradiation and chemotherapy for left sacral Ewing's sarcoma. **A,** A routine PET surveillance scan obtained 16 months after completion of therapy showed a new and concerning change, with development of an intense hypermetabolic focus of the right scapula (*arrow*). Because there were no recent imaging studies of the area in question, a workup was recommended. No history of trauma had been elicited. A relevant injury had so completely resolved symptomatically that it had been forgotten by the time of imaging. **B,** Posterior thoracic bone scan image shows a new asymmetrical focus of increased activity at the right scapular level (*arrow*). **C,** Chest CT (**a**) through the scapulae, with bone windows, shows a proliferative bony lesion of the right lateral scapula (*arrow*). Detail (**b**) better shows Codman's triangle-like extension of periosteal new bone from the lesion onto the scapula.

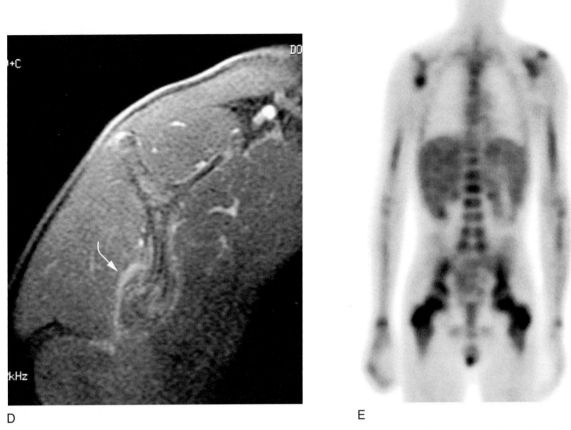

D   E

FIGURE 21. cont'd D, Fat-saturated, enhanced FSPGR sagittal MR sequence also shows nonspecific findings. The proliferative bony lesion is of the same signal intensity as the rest of the scapula, with an enhancing surrounding rim (*arrow*). Based on the history of direct trauma to this region, a healing fracture with callus is suspected. Biopsy of the lesion was entertained, but discouraged, owing to the potential for misleading pathologic results with healing osseous lesions. A repeat PET scan was suggested, with comparison of standardized uptake values, to confirm the impression of a healing fracture. It emerged that about 2 weeks before the PET scan, the patient had been dropped by a roughhousing sibling from a bed onto the floor, striking his shoulder. Although he cried initially and complained of pain with abduction, within 2 days his symptoms had largely resolved. The incident had been forgotten by the time he presented for PET scanning. The repeat PET scan, obtained just over a month later without interval therapy, showed improvement (**E**). The right scapular focus was smaller and less intense, consistent with a healing fracture.

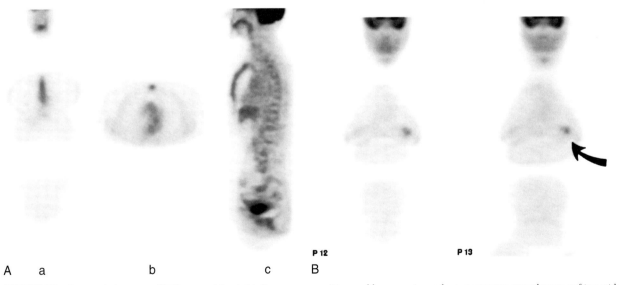

A   a   b   c   B

FIGURE 22. Post-surgical sources of PET scan activity. **A,** Median sternotomy: 71-year-old woman, 4 months post coronary artery bypass grafting, with intense linear sternal activity, consistent with recent time course and ongoing healing. Coronal (**a**), transaxial (**b**), and sagittal (**c**) views are shown. **B,** Breast biopsy: 93-year-old woman, 1 month post left surgical excisional breast biopsy, with mild activity at medial biopsy site (*arrow*). Biopsy results prompted evaluation for systemic lymphoma, which was negative. *Continued*

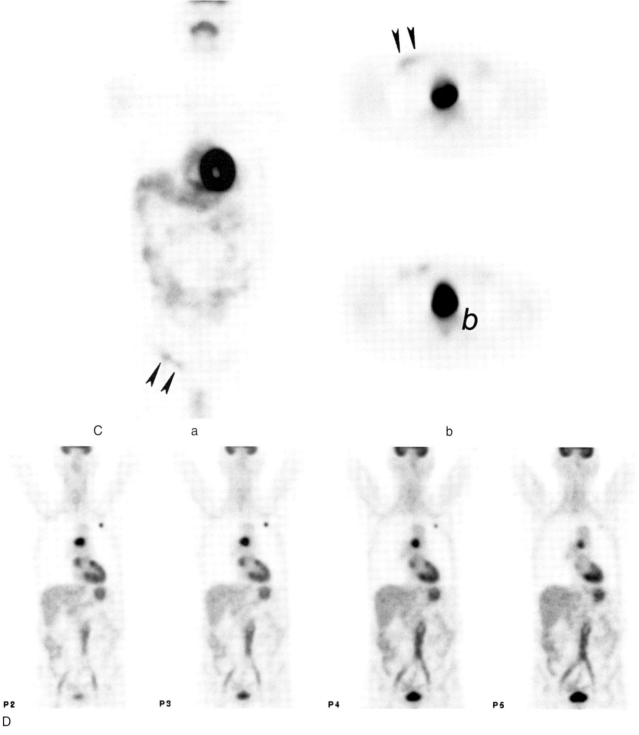

FIGURE 22. cont'd C, Herniorrhaphy. Coronal (**a**) and two corresponding, adjacent axial (**b**) PET images show mild, linear right groin activity in a 75-year-old man (*arrowheads*). Superficial location of the activity is apparent on the axial views (b, bladder). Patient had a prior history of hernia repair on this side. **D,** Abdominal aortic aneurysm repair: 71-year-old man, under investigation for recurrent lung cancer, was 1 year post surgical repair of an abdominal aortic aneurysm. Although vessels can be seen faintly as a normal variant and increased vascular wall activity may correlate with atherosclerosis, the aortoiliac activity displayed here is much more intense than usual and consistent with the prior repair history. Recurrent lung cancer was confirmed on this study, with activity in LUL pulmonary nodule, as well as in the subcarinal mediastinum.

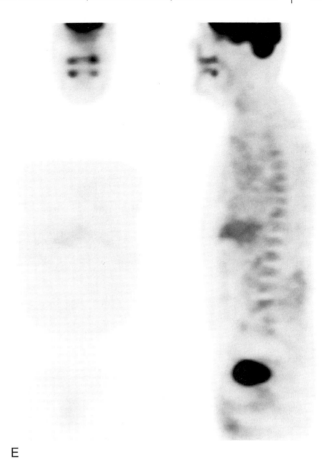

FIGURE 22. cont'd E, Dental work: Foci of increased uptake in both maxilla and mandible are consistent with dental sources of activity, most commonly from recent extraction or restoration.

E

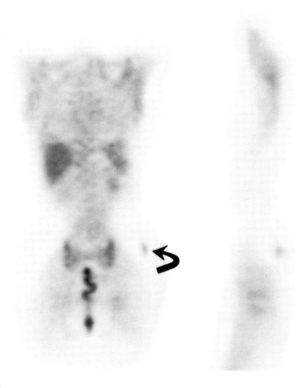

FIGURE 23. Additional iatrogenic sources of benign PET scan activity. **A,** Buttock injection site: 57-year-old woman on investigational vaccine therapy for inflammatory breast carcinoma with lung metastases *(arrow).* *Continued*

A

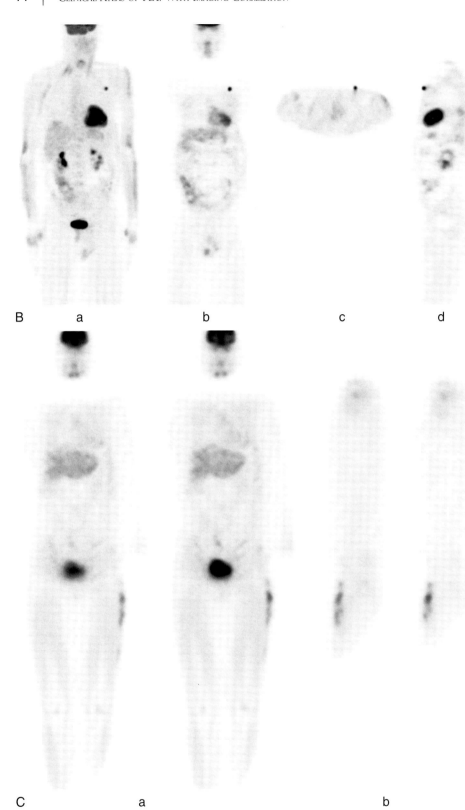

B   a   b   c   d

C   a   b

FIGURE 23. cont'd **B,** Port injection site: 52-year-old man undergoing chemotherapy for recurrent non-Hodgkin's lymphoma in bone marrow (same patient as Case 9 in Chapter 4). Projection image (**a**) suggests at first glance a left chest hypermetabolic nodule. Coronal (**b**), axial (**c**) and sagittal (**d**) corresponding planes show the activity to be superficial to the skin surface and consistent with the port injection site. **C,** Vaccine therapy: 43-year-old woman with melanoma, on long-term vaccine injection therapy. Coronal (**a**) and sagittal (**b**) PET scan images show linear left lateral thigh hypermetabolic activity, punctuated by foci of higher intensity. This appearance remained stable on follow-up studies and correlated with the location of the patient's vaccine injections. Her prior melanoma was in the right lower extremity.

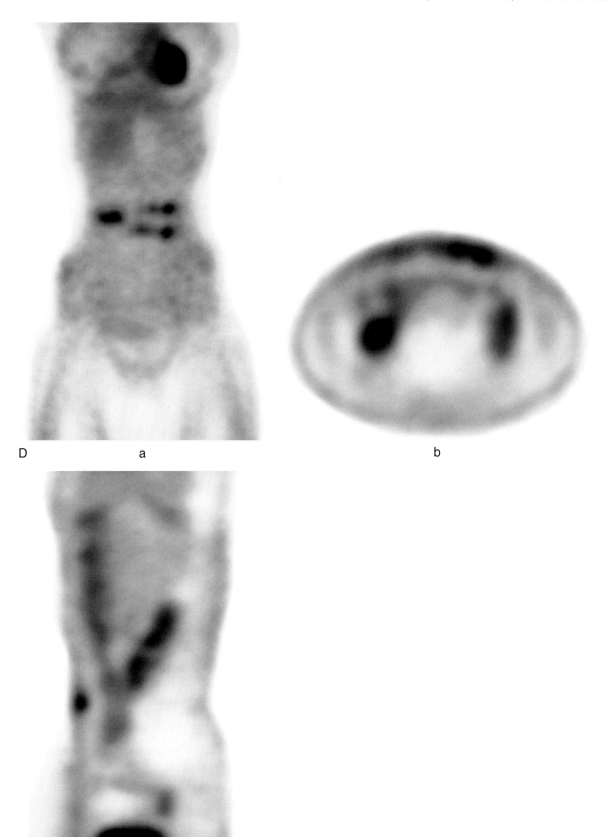

D

a

b

c

FIGURE 23. cont'd D, Immunotherapy: 16-year-old patient with relapsed Hodgkin's disease, with multiple anterior abdominal wall foci of activity from injection sites. Corona (a), axial (b) and sagittal (c) planes are shown.

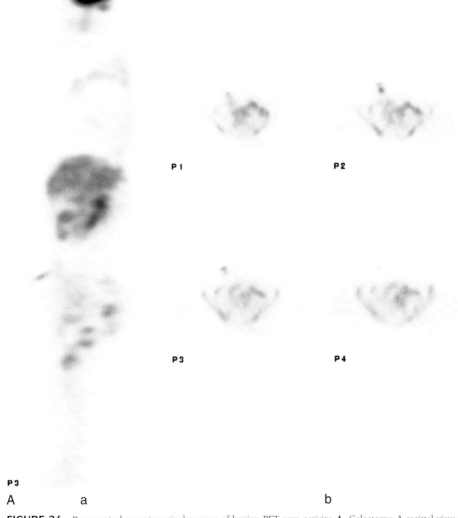

P1　　P2

P3　　P4

P3

A　　　a　　　　　　　　　　　　b

FIGURE 24. Post-surgical gastrointestinal sources of benign PET scan activity. **A,** Colostomy. A sagittal view (**a**) and corresponding contiguous transaxial sections (**b**) show linear, subcutaneous activity in a RLQ anterior abdominal wall colostomy of a colon cancer patient, being evaluated for increased level of carcinoembryonic antigen. This study showed bone metastases to be the cause (*not shown*).

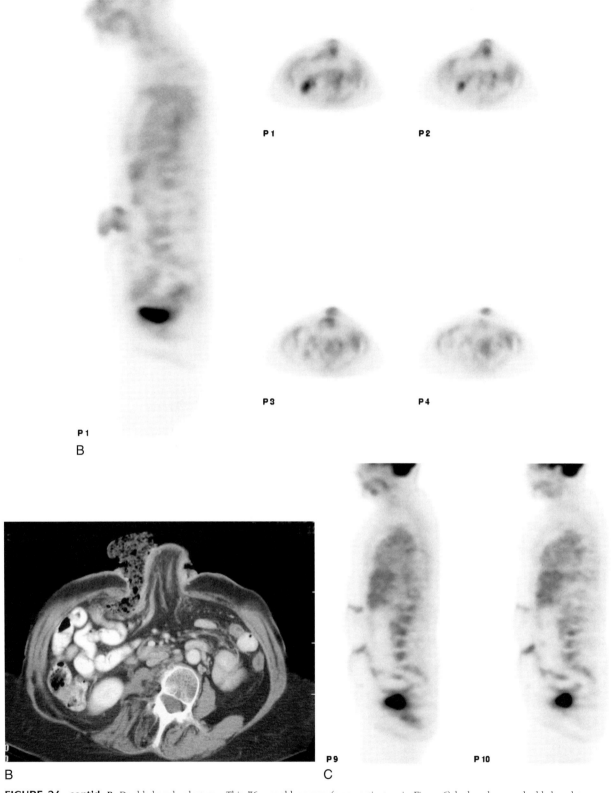

FIGURE 24. cont'd B, Double-barrel colostomy. This 76-year-old woman (same patient as in Figure 6) had undergone double-barrel tranverse colostomy after presenting with an obstructing omental mass, thought to be ovarian cancer (CA-125 was markedly elevated and declined in response to ovarian carcinoma chemotherapy). C, Laparoscopic cholecystectomy portals are well seen as linear subcutaneous anterior abdominal wall tracts in a 52-year-old woman, 2 weeks post laparoscopic cholecystectomy, at which gallbladder carcinoma was found.

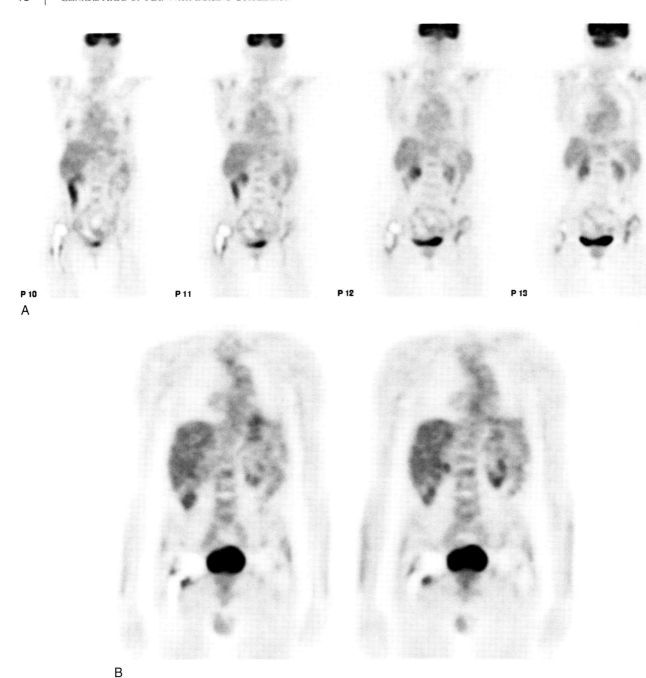

FIGURE 25. Orthopedic sources of benign activity (periprosthetic). **A,** A 74-year-old woman was evaluated with PET because of an abnormal CXR, obtained as a preoperative study before planned redo of symptomatic right total hip replacement (THR). A portion of a modestly active right lung process, thought to be inflammatory, is included. The right hip prosthesis is seen as a photopenic defect. A metabolically active rim surrounds the prosthesis. This activity is greatest along the shaft of the prosthesis, at the bone-prosthesis interface. Data presented at the Academy of Molecular Imaging/Institute of Clinical PET meeting, October 2002 (A. Alavi, University of Pennsylvania) indicated this distribution of activity as more specific for infection than activity at the femoral neck level, which may relate to loosening. Even in the first year post hip replacement, activity is not normally seen at the bone-prosthesis interface, although it can be seen normally at the femoral neck level postoperatively. Joint-centered activity is also noted here at the native left hip level, which was also symptomatic, from arthritis. **B,** An 80-year-old man was PET scanned for head and neck carcinoma follow-up, with right hip periprosthetic activity, correlating with a painful THR. This femoral neck distribution of activity is more suggestive of loosening.

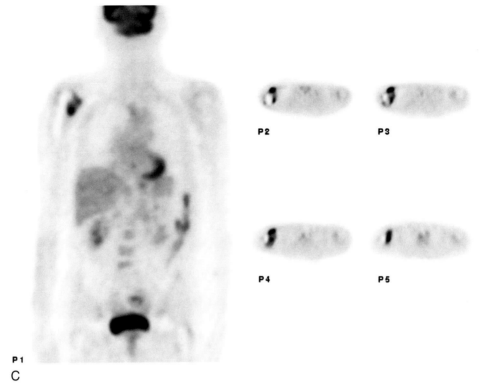

FIGURE 25. cont'd C, A 79-year-old man with intense activity at the level of his replaced right shoulder was plagued by recurrent dislocations.

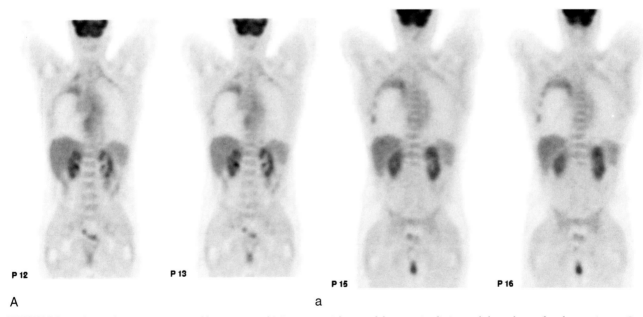

FIGURE 26. Radiation therapy. **A,** A 57-year-old man presented 2.5 years post right upper lobectomy, irradiation, and chemotherapy for adenocarcinoma. Coronal PET images (**a**) show a right apical cap of modest activity, *Continued*

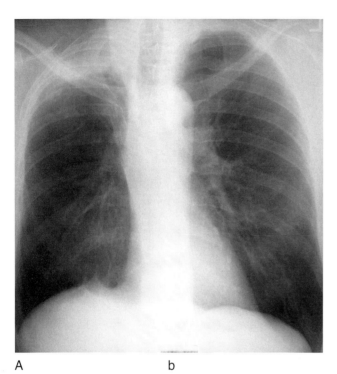

A   b

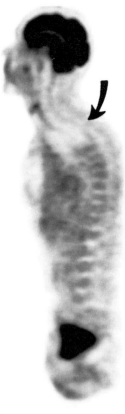

B

FIGURE 26. cont'd corresponding to CXR findings (**b**) of right apical pleural thickening from prior surgery and irradiation. **B,** Radiation therapy effects on the cervicothoracic spine: 68-year-old male with head and neck squamous cell carcinoma, status post bilateral neck irradiation for nodal involvement. PET shows photopenia of the cervicothoracic spine, analogous to radiation therapy changes seen on bone scans (*arrow*). **C,** Radiation changes of the lumbar spine: 42-year-old man, status post pelvic irradiation for seminoma. Relative photopenia is seen of the sacrum and lumbar spine, in contrast to the activated marrow seen in the rest of the spine and in the sternum. The patient had just concluded chemotherapy.

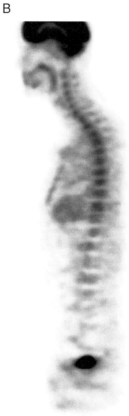

C

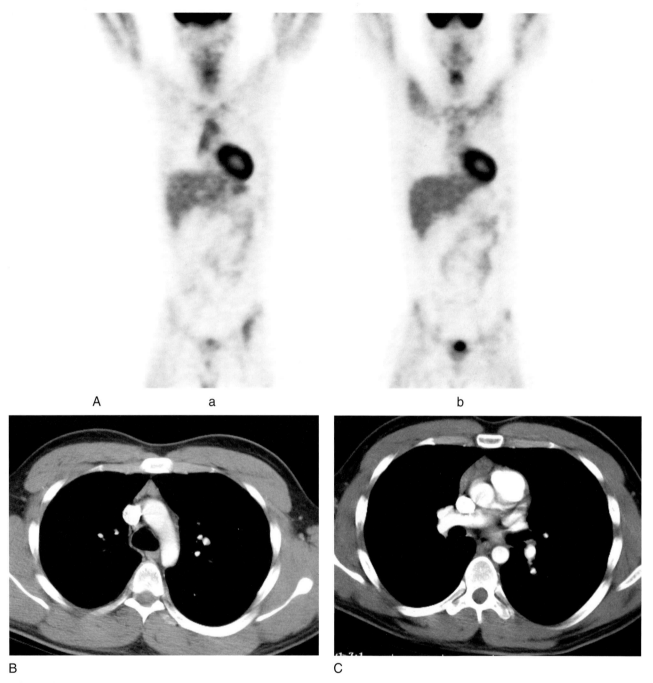

FIGURE 27. Thymic rebound. A 20-year-old man presented post surgical decompression and chemotherapy for intraspinal high-grade diffuse B cell lymphoma. **A,** PET scan showed new prevascular, anterior mediastinal activity (**a**), consistent with thymic rebound, compared with a PET scan 2 months before (**b**). The patient's chemotherapy had concluded approximately 6 weeks before the first PET scan. Correlation with contrast medium–enhanced chest CT (**B** and **C**) confirms the presence of prevascular, anterior mediastinal soft tissue, in characteristic triangular thymic shape.

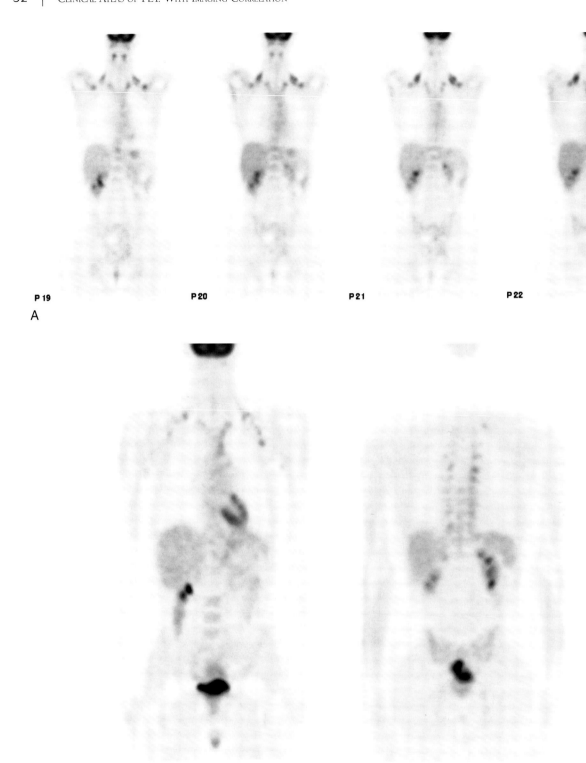

P 19
P 20
P 21
P 22

A

B

FIGURE 28. Benign musculoskeletal sources of activity. **A,** Benign muscular vs. brown fat activity: 44-year-old woman with non-Hodgkin's disease presented for follow-up. PET showed no active disease. Symmetrical activity at the thoracic inlet and upper paraspinous regions is incidentally noted. This activity pattern was thought until recently to be muscular, and in some patients, may be. The recent advent of image fusion and PET/CT shows this activity frequently localizes to so-called "brown fat". Brown fat appears to be activated by shivering. **B,** Benign muscular activity: 34-year-old man with metabolically active drop metastasis to pelvis from recurrent cholangiocarcinoma. PET scan shows a similar pattern of benign muscular activity, here more evident at thoracic paraspinous levels than at the thoracic inlet.

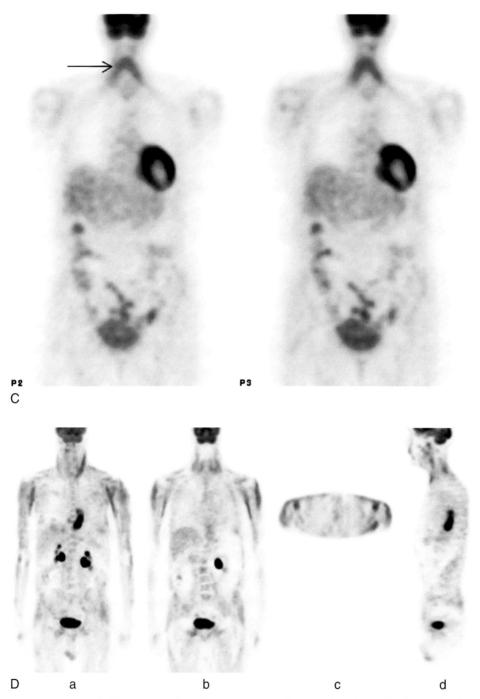

FIGURE 28. cont'd C, Benign muscular activity: trapezius muscular activity (*arrow*) is incidentally noted on this otherwise negative PET scan of a 93-year-old woman being evaluated for systemic lymphoma based on results from a recent breast biopsy. **D,** Proximal muscle activity, attributable to known dermatomyositis in a 74-year-old man, on steroids, recently diagnosed with esophageal carcinoma. Coronally oriented projection image (**a**) shows tubular hypermetabolic distal esophageal activity at the site of the in situ esophageal carcinoma. Muscular activity is pronounced at the shoulder girdles and sternocleidomastoid muscles of the neck, with less intense hip girdle muscular activity. Coronal (**b**), transaxial (**c**), and sagittal (**d**) images are also shown. *Continued*

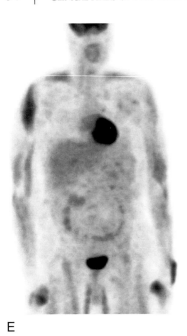

E

FIGURE 28. cont'd E, Upper extremity muscular activity in wheelchair-bound patient: coronally oriented projection image shows a 40-year-old man, for nodular sclerosing Hodgkin's disease follow-up, who is chronically disabled secondary to viral meningitis 3 years before. No evidence of recurrent or active Hodgkin's was seen. F, Respiratory muscle activity in a 78-year-old oxygen-dependent male with chronic interstitial lung disease and 40 pack-year smoking history, being evaluated for non–small cell lung cancer (*not shown*). In addition to the intensely active lower thoracic intercostal musculature, even the diaphragmatic crura are visualized.

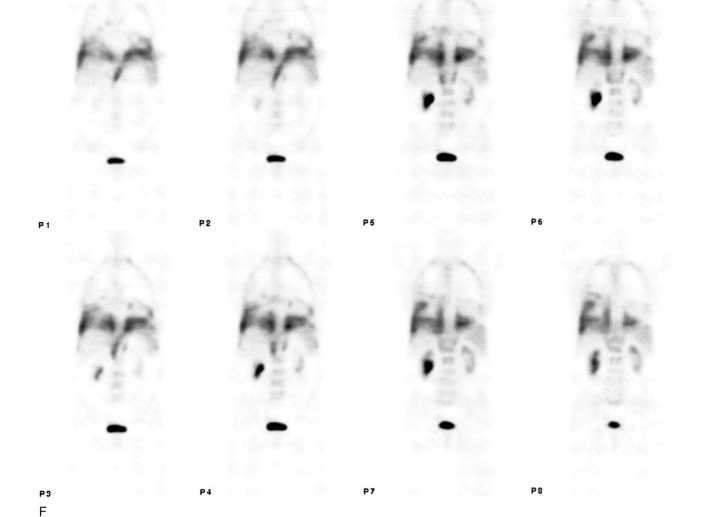

F

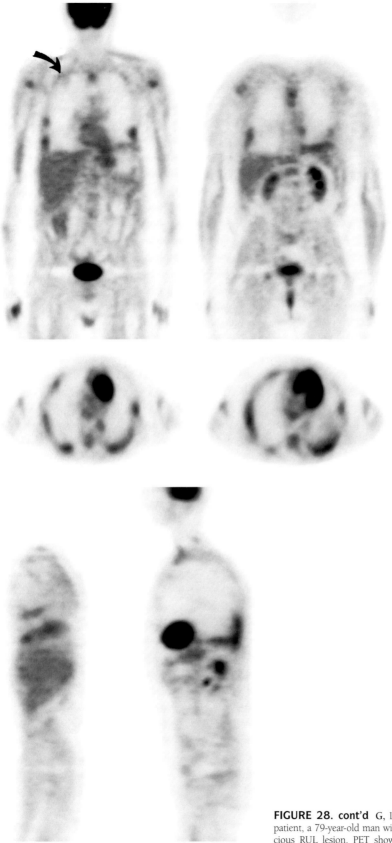

FIGURE 28. cont'd G, Less florid example of respiratory muscle activity in a different patient, a 79-year-old man with emphysema and 40 pack-year smoking history, with a suspicious RUL lesion. PET shows only mild activity of the RUL lesion, suggesting a benign etiology (*arrow*).   *Continued*

G

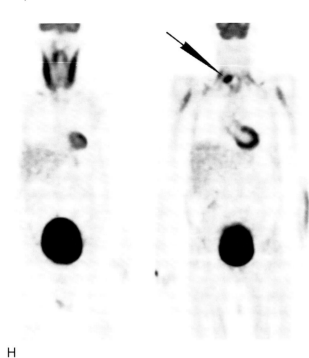

FIGURE 28. cont'd **H,** A 61-year-old man presented with intense neck muscular activity 3 days after anterior decompression with C7 corpectomy for cord compressing lung adenocarcinoma metastasis and pathologic fracture. The more anterior section (*left*) shows symmetrical, markedly increased neck muscular activity, especially of the sternocleidomastoid muscles, presumably from retraction during surgery. The more posterior section (*right*) shows a photopenic defect at the operative level, with a surrounding metabolically active rim. The asymmetrical, intensely active focus to the right of the post-surgical changes represents residual tumor (*arrow*). **I,** A 12-year-old boy with Ewing's sarcoma of the sacrum presented with sciatica, which affected his gait. After tiptoeing for months, he developed chronically shortened Achilles tendons. PET study was obtained to evaluate minimal residual MR signal intensity abnormality of the sacrum after completion of therapy and showed no finding to suggest active sarcoma. The patient had undergone tendon release procedure on the left 2 months before but had not yet undergone the procedure on the right side. Note linear, modest intensity gastrocnemius level activity and normal foot position on the operated side and plantarflexed position of the unoperated side. Projection image (**a**) and left (**b**) and right (**c**) leg images are shown.

H

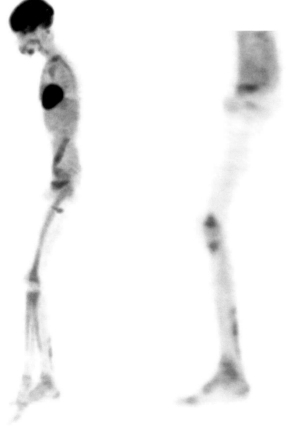

I a   b   c

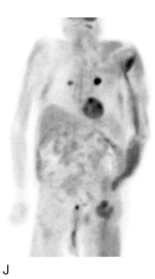

J

FIGURE 28. cont'd J, A 71-year-old man, with chronic right hemiparesis, 7 years post hemorrhagic stroke, under evaluation for recurrent squamous cell lung carcinoma. PET projection image, displayed coronally, shows bilateral hilar activity from known squamous cell carcinoma and diffuse increased muscular activity on the left. Presumably, this is secondary to the prior stroke and compensatory increased muscular usage and reliance on the left side of the body. **K**, Bone graft harvest site: 75-year-old man with stage III diffuse large B cell lymphoma with a history of lumbar spine fusion surgery 3.5 years before. Modest linear increased activity is seen on PET at the right iliac level on coronal (**a**) and axial (**b**) views (*arrows*). A portion of the bladder is included on the axial view. Correlation with a pelvis CT (**c**) shows an osseous defect at the iliac activity level, corresponding to a bone graft harvest site. *Continued*

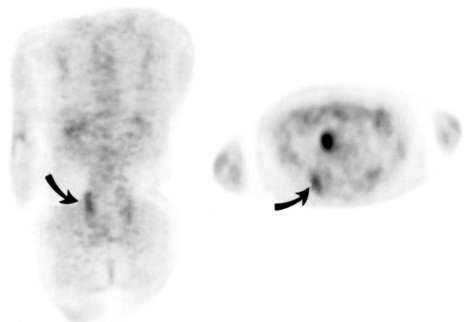

a   b

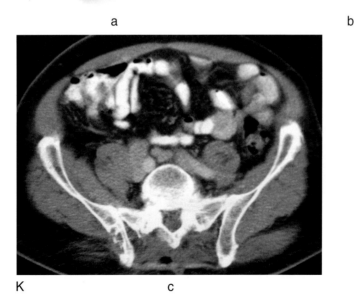

K   c

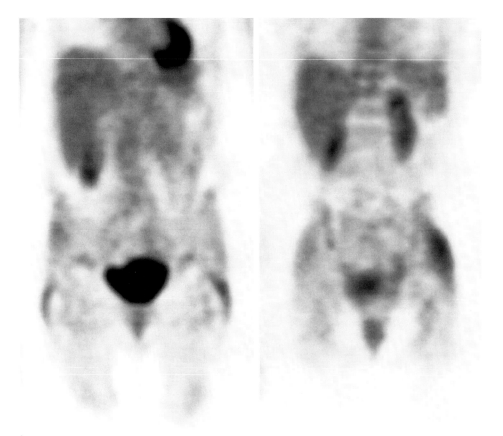

L

FIGURE 28. cont'd L, Bilateral trochanteric bursitis: 74-year-old woman, being evaluated for a nodular right upper lobe process. She was symptomatic with bilateral hip bursitis. Coronal PET images show linear increased activity at both hip greater trochanters, associated with increased gluteal muscular activity, particularly on the left.

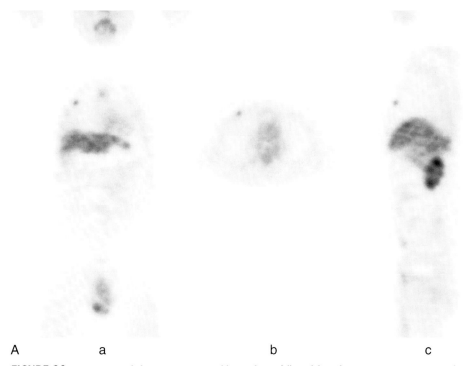

A   a   b   c

FIGURE 29. Trauma. **A**, Rib fracture. A 57-year-old man, being followed for colon carcinoma metastasis to liver undergoing radiofrequency ablation, was noted to have a new right anterior rib focus on PET. This was initially interpreted as suggestive of a bone metastasis. It resolved on a follow-up PET scan, and the history of trauma was subsequently elicited from the patient. Coronal (**a**), transaxial (**b**), and sagittal (**c**) views are shown.

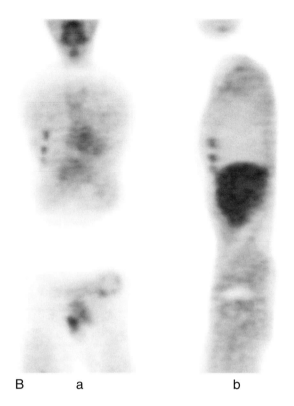

B a   b

FIGURE 29. cont'd B, Rib fractures. This 35-year-old man, with recent diagnosis of metastatic melanoma made from left inguinal lymphadenectomy, had an additional history of a recent surfboard injury. PET scan (coronal [a] and sagittal [b]) shows multiple adjacent right anterior rib foci of activity, consistent with fractures. Rib findings are analogous to traumatic rib findings on bone scan. Note also left inguinal findings from recent surgery, with large postoperative hematoma.

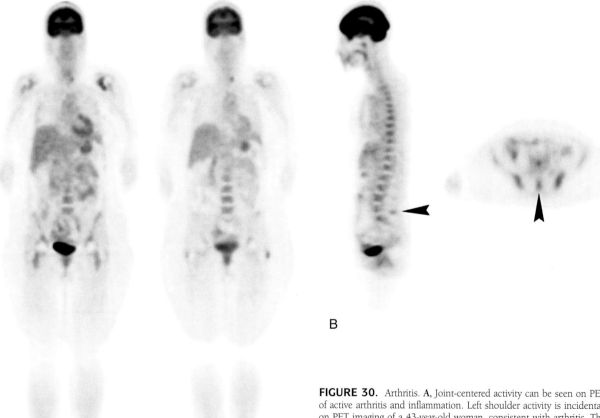

B

P8   P9

A

FIGURE 30. Arthritis. **A,** Joint-centered activity can be seen on PET at sites of active arthritis and inflammation. Left shoulder activity is incidentally noted on PET imaging of a 43-year-old woman, consistent with arthritis. The patient was being evaluated for left great toe melanoma, metastatic to the left groin (not shown here; same patient as Case 2 in Chapter 5). The activity resolved on a follow-up PET months later. **B,** Baastrup's disease. Occasionally, joint-related activity can be seen at unexpected levels, reflecting infrequently recognized arthritic processes. This activity in the lower lumbar spine is at the spinous process interspace and is consistent with Baastrup's disease, in which there is abnormal contact of apposing spinous processes (*arrowheads*).

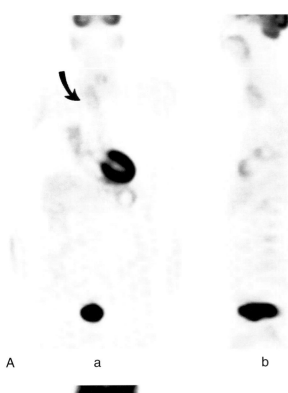

A   a   b

FIGURE 31. Thyroid sources of benign activity: variants (see also Figure 4). **A,** Goiter. Coronal (**a**) and sagittal (**b**) views from a PET scan of a 75-year-old man, being evaluated for recently diagnosed right lung adenocarcinoma (*not shown*). A mildly metabolically active ring at the right inferior neck level extends down into the right superior mediastinum, consistent with the patient's known substernal goiter (*arrow*). **B,** Thyroiditis. Coronal (**a**) and two axial (**b**) PET views of an 84-year-old woman being evaluated for gastric lymphoma. Intense activity in an enlarged thyroid gland such as this may be seen with Hashimoto's thyroiditis and Graves' disease.

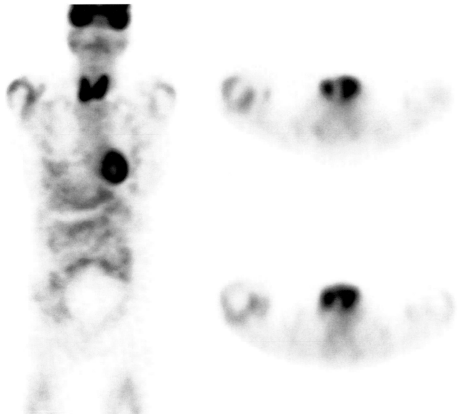

B   a   b

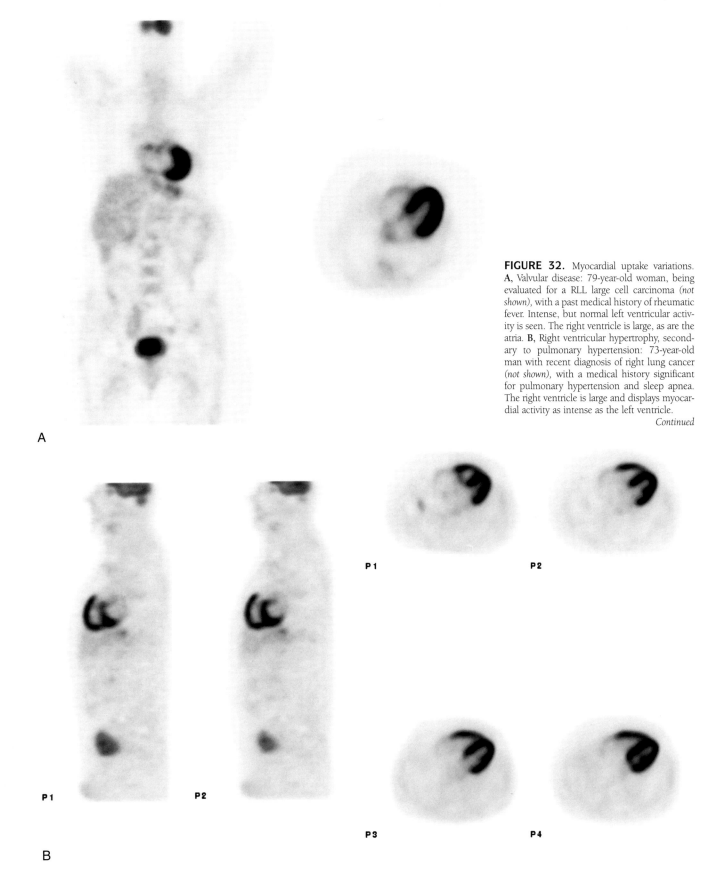

FIGURE 32. Myocardial uptake variations. **A,** Valvular disease: 79-year-old woman, being evaluated for a RLL large cell carcinoma *(not shown)*, with a past medical history of rheumatic fever. Intense, but normal left ventricular activity is seen. The right ventricle is large, as are the atria. **B,** Right ventricular hypertrophy, secondary to pulmonary hypertension: 73-year-old man with recent diagnosis of right lung cancer *(not shown)*, with a medical history significant for pulmonary hypertension and sleep apnea. The right ventricle is large and displays myocardial activity as intense as the left ventricle.

Continued

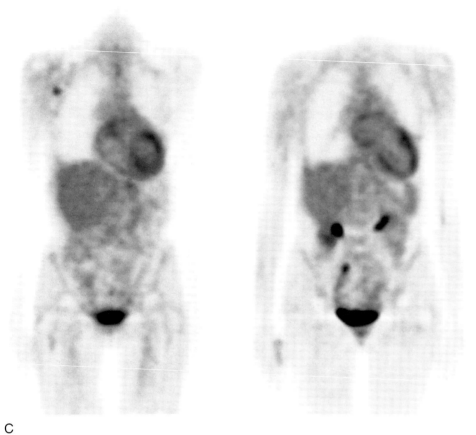

C

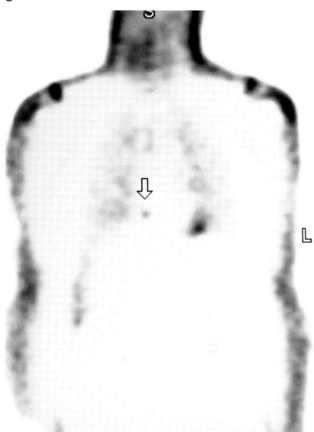

FIGURE 32. cont'd C, Cardiomyopathy: 62-year-old woman being imaged for right chest wall recurrence of breast cancer (note focus of hypermetabolism lateral chest wall, near axilla). She had also been recently diagnosed with a cardiomyopathy. Note enlargement of all chambers. D, Metastatic melanoma: A small focus of metabolic activity is noted on the coronal non-attenuation corrected PET image (a) at the atrial level (arrow). On a corresponding enhanced chest CT section (b), a small nodule is seen at the atrial septal level.

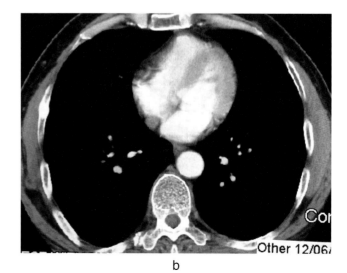

D   a   b

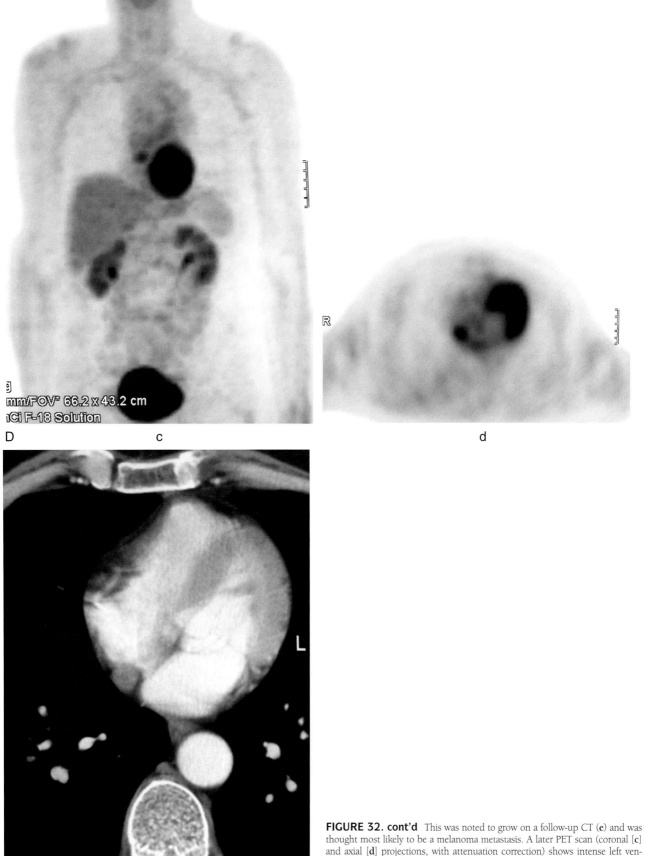

FIGURE 32. cont'd This was noted to grow on a follow-up CT (**e**) and was thought most likely to be a melanoma metastasis. A later PET scan (coronal [**c**] and axial [**d**] projections, with attenuation correction) shows intense left ventricular myocardial activity, which does not interfere with identification of the metabolically active growing metastasis to the atrial septum. *Continued*

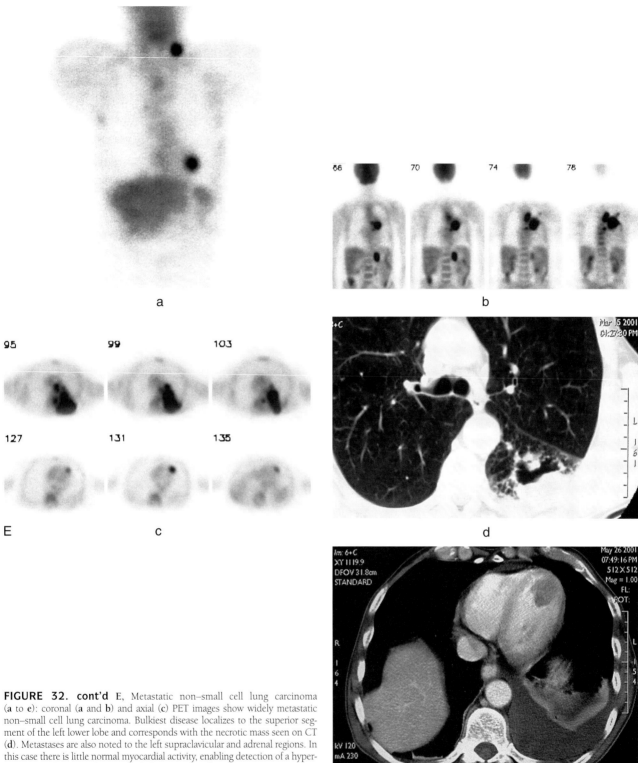

FIGURE 32. cont'd E, Metastatic non–small cell lung carcinoma (a to e): coronal (a and b) and axial (c) PET images show widely metastatic non–small cell lung carcinoma. Bulkiest disease localizes to the superior segment of the left lower lobe and corresponds with the necrotic mass seen on CT (d). Metastases are also noted to the left supraclavicular and adrenal regions. In this case there is little normal myocardial activity, enabling detection of a hypermetabolic left ventricular myocardial metastasis. The mass on corresponding CT image (e) occupies the left ventricular apex (Case courtesy of Gilbert Boswell, MD, San Diego, CA).

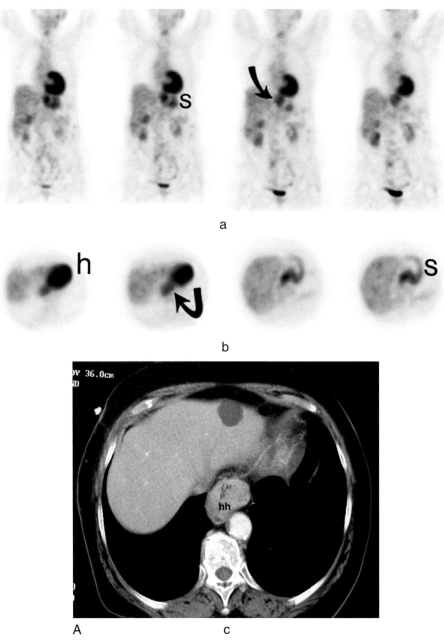

FIGURE 33. Gastrointestinal variant benign activity. **A,** Hiatal hernia. Coronal (**a**) and axial (**b**) PET images show gastric activity in the usual LUQ location (S, stomach). An additional focus of similar intensity is also noted, at the expected retrocardiac level of the gastroesophageal junction, consistent with a hiatal hernia (*arrows*) (h, heart). This is confirmed on a corresponding CT image (hh, hiatal hernia) (**c**). A liver cyst is noted on the CT image.

Continued

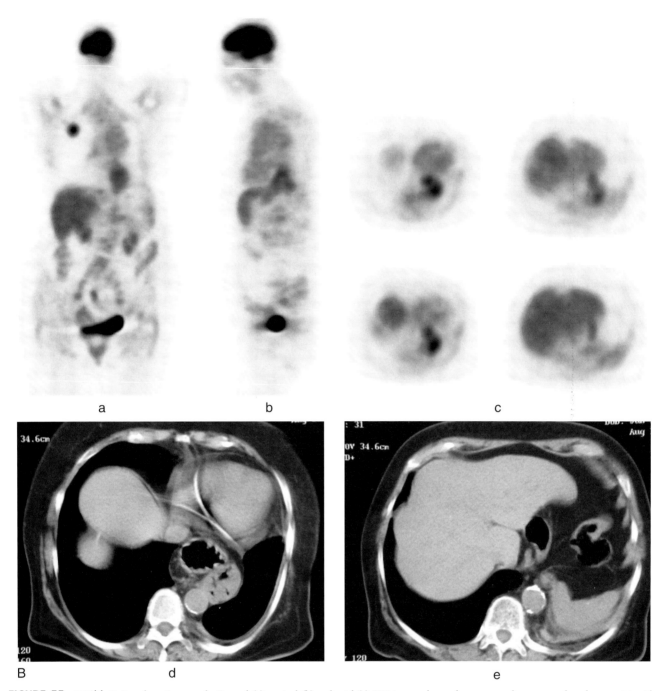

a b c

B d e

FIGURE 33. cont'd B, Intrathoracic stomach. Coronal (**a**), sagittal (**b**) and axial (**c**) PET images show a large retrocardiac source of moderate activity. The 79-year-old woman was undergoing lung cancer staging. A portion of the hyperintense right upper lobe poorly differentiated adenocarcinoma is visualized on the coronal section. Little gastric activity is visualized in the left upper quadrant. Correlation with CT (**d** and **e**) shows that the majority of this patient's stomach is intrathoracic and responsible for the retrocardiac activity on PET.

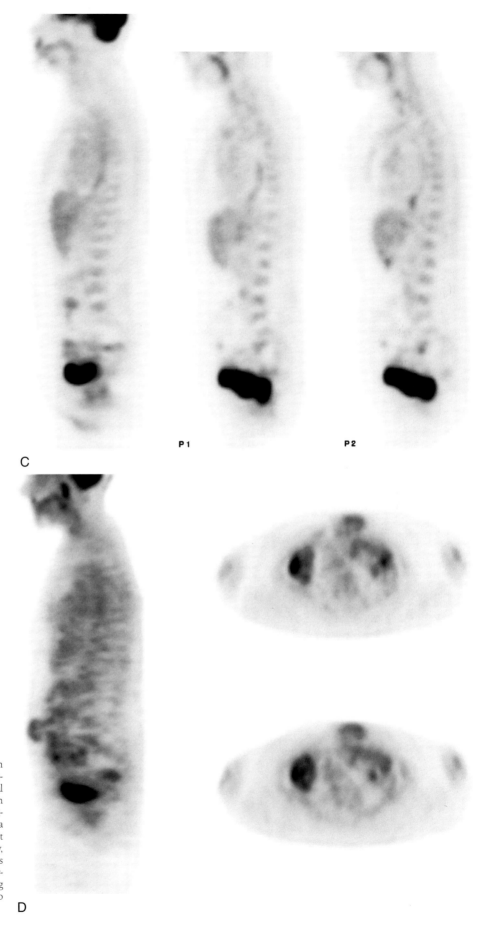

FIGURE 33. cont'd C, Examples from two different patients of benign, asymptomatic, low-level esophageal activity, a normal variant. Linear, retrocardiac, midline location allows ready recognition. **D,** Anterior abdominal wall hernia: 64-year-old woman with a past history of gastric carcinoma, 5 years post total gastrectomy and esophagojejunostomy, with no additional treatment. PET study was requested before planned repair of the hernia and shows bowel activity protruding through the anterior abdominal wall but no suspicious finding for gastric carcinoma.

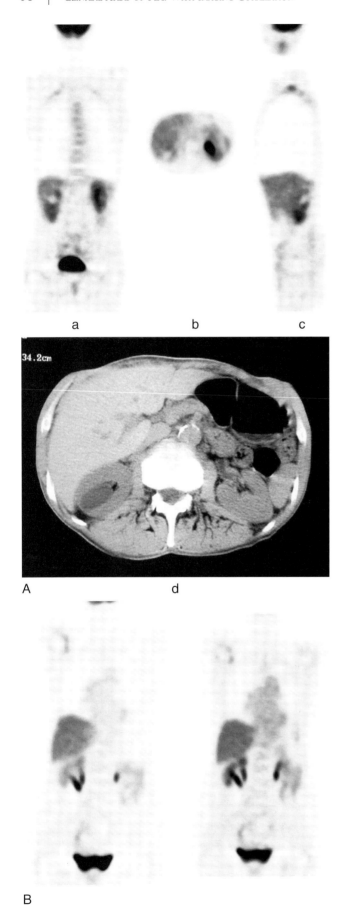

a   b   c

A   d

B

FIGURE 34. Renal and genitourinary variant benign activity. **A,** Renal cyst. Analogous to bone scans, renal cysts of sufficient size appear on PET as photopenic defects of the kidney and may produce distortion of renal shape if numerous. An intrarenal cyst of the right kidney of the mid to upper pole manifests on PET as a photopenic defect. Coronal (**a**), transaxial (**b**), and sagittal (**c**) views are shown. Unenhanced CT (**d**) shows corresponding near-water density right renal cyst. Liver cysts of sufficient size also can be visualized on PET regularly. **B,** Collecting system duplication. Partial collecting system duplication is noted on the right.

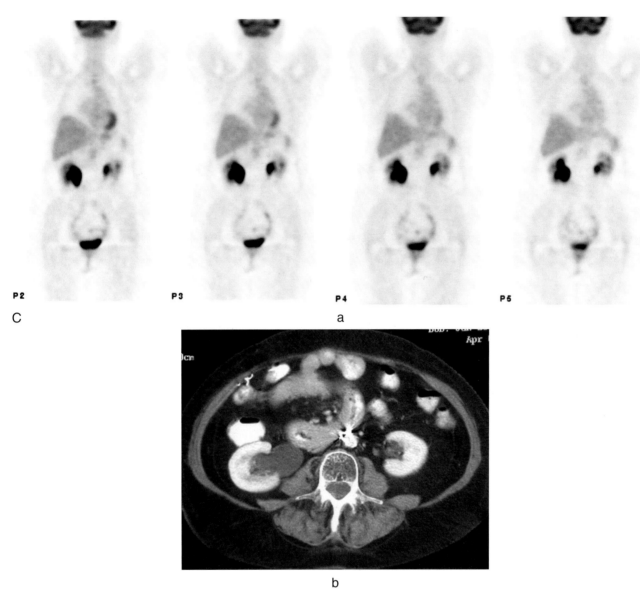

FIGURE 34. cont'd C, Ureteropelvic junction obstruction: Other congenital variations of the genitourinary system may be recognized on PET imaging (**a**), such as ureteropelvic junction disproportionation or obstruction. Here, the right renal pelvocaliceal system is asymmetrically distended without ureteral dilatation; **b**, Abdominal CT shows corresponding findings of a ureteropelvic junction obstruction. *Continued*

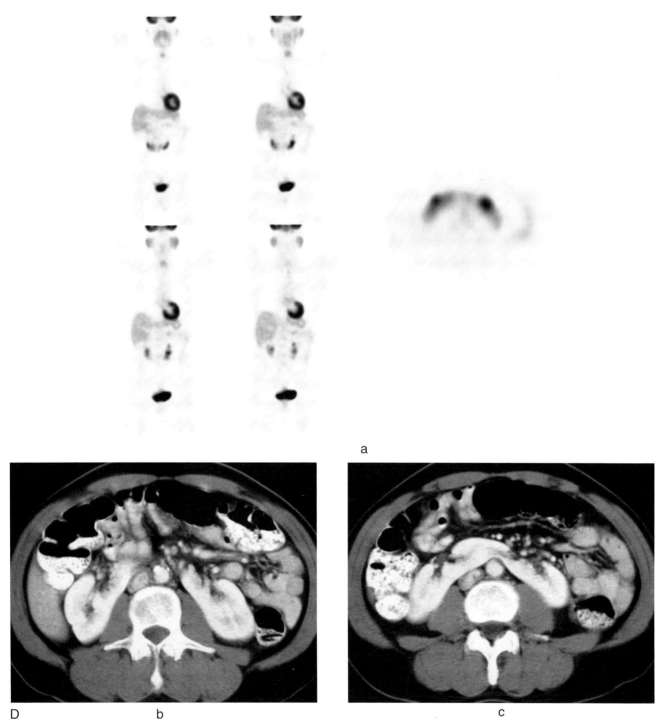

a

D   b   c

FIGURE 34. cont'd D, Horseshoe kidneys are recognized on PET (**a**) by the characteristic abnormal axis of the kidneys, with medially deviated and converging inferior poles. In this example, the horseshoe kidney is joined across the midline by functioning renal parenchyma, as demonstrated by the corresponding CT images (**b** and **c**).

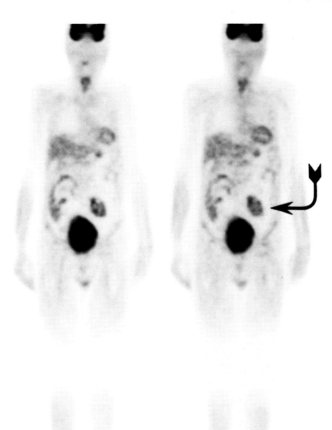

P 1   P 2

E

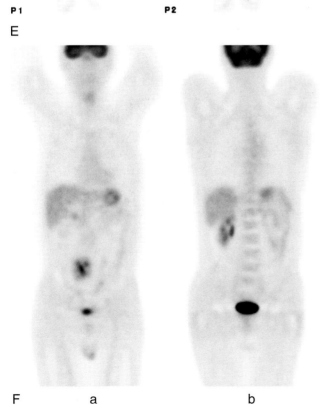

F   a   b

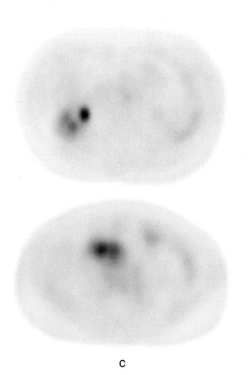

c

FIGURE 34. cont'd E, Pelvic kidney: ptotic or frankly ectopic positions of kidneys may be observed on PET imaging. An ectopic kidney, such as this LLQ pelvic kidney, potentially could be mistaken for a pathologic process if absence of a kidney from the expected position is not recognized (*arrow*). F, Ectopic kidney: 58-year-old man being staged for recent diagnosis of non-Hodgkin's lymphoma, surgically excised from left groin. *Continued*

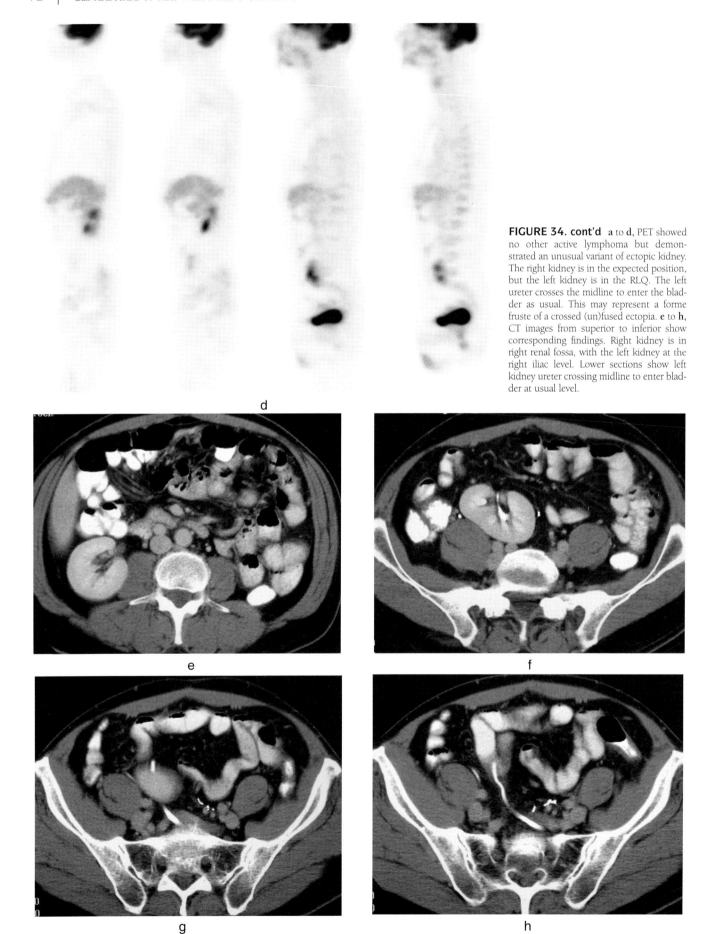

d

FIGURE 34. cont'd a to d, PET showed no other active lymphoma but demonstrated an unusual variant of ectopic kidney. The right kidney is in the expected position, but the left kidney is in the RLQ. The left ureter crosses the midline to enter the bladder as usual. This may represent a forme fruste of a crossed (un)fused ectopia. e to h, CT images from superior to inferior show corresponding findings. Right kidney is in right renal fossa, with the left kidney at the right iliac level. Lower sections show left kidney ureter crossing midline to enter bladder at usual level.

e

f

g

h

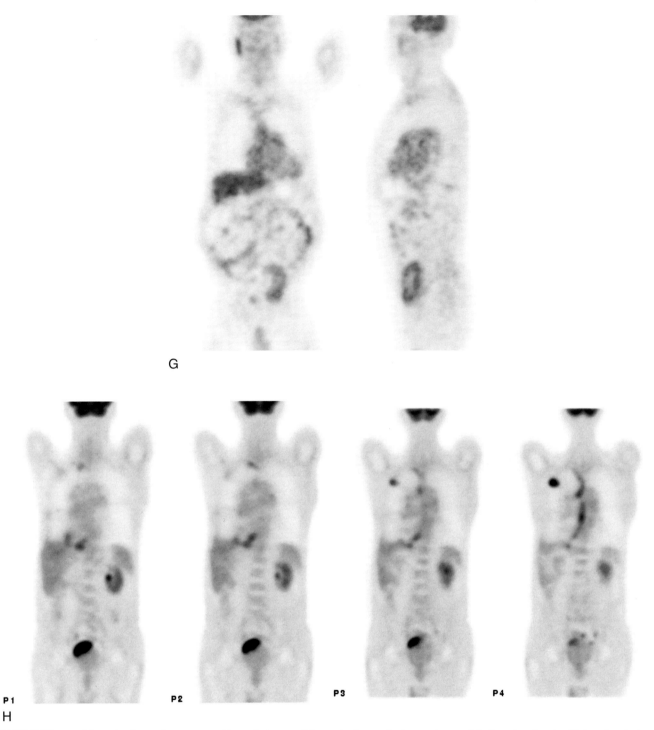

G

P 1   P 2   P 3   P 4

H

FIGURE 34. cont'd **G,** Renal transplant: 65 year old man being staged for newly diagnosed adenocarcinoma of the lung *(not shown),* with hypofunctioning 5-year-old transplanted kidney in LLQ. No intrarenal collecting system activity is evident. **H,** Benign prostatic hypertrophy: 85-year-old man status post radiation therapy for lung carcinoma, diagnosed 14 months before, with a new right apical nodule on CT. PET scan shows intense hypermetabolism of the new nodule in question, consistent with recurrent lung cancer, and right paramediastinal linear activity from radiation therapy. The markedly enlarged prostate gland is unusually well visualized, elevating the bladder base. *Continued*

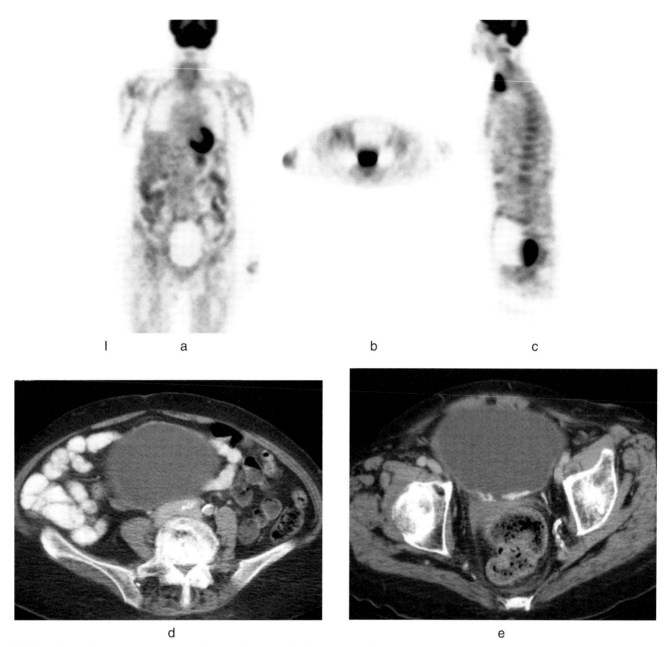

l   a   b   c

d   e

FIGURE 34. cont'd I, Neurogenic bladder: 84-year-old woman with diffuse large B cell gastric lymphoma. Coronal PET image (**a**) suggests there is a large photopenic or cystic pelvic mass. Correlation with axial (**b**) and sagittal images corroborate this impression, with the urinary bladder apparently posteriorly displaced by the mass. However, correlation with CT (**d** and **e**) shows no such mass, only the markedly distended and presumably neurogenic bladder extending above the iliac crest level. The PET appearance apparently represents dependently layering, unmixed FDG laden urine in the overdistended, mass-like urinary bladder. The sagittal PET image (**c**) also shows intensely increased anterior neck activity, corresponding to a markedly enlarged and hyperintense thyroid gland. This appearance is seen most commonly with Graves' disease or Hashimoto's thyroiditis.

Lung Cancer

Lung cancer is the most frequently diagnosed cancer worldwide. It is also the leading cause of cancer mortality, with an estimated 156,900 deaths in the United States in 2000. The overall 5-year survival is 13% to 14% and has not changed significantly over recent decades.[1] Although there is a trend toward reduction in U.S. lung cancer incidence and mortality rates, the American Cancer Society estimates more than 160,000 new cases in the year 2000. Despite the recognition that cigarette smoking is causally related to lung cancer, the worldwide incidence of lung cancer continues to increase. Unfortunately, gains made in reducing tobacco use among youth may be reversing and mortality rates in women have yet to demonstrate the decline seen in men (possibly due to a lag in smoking prevalence by about 2 decades). For these reasons, improved methods for diagnosis, staging, assessing recurrence, and monitoring patients are still needed. PET imaging has shown great potential in these areas.

DIAGNOSIS

Approximately 150,000 solitary pulmonary nodules (SPN) are discovered each year. Only one third of these will prove to be malignant.[2] The importance of separating a benign from a malignant nodule is related to the significantly higher survival rate (may be as high as 70%) in true stage I lung cancer. Also, a secure diagnosis of benignity reduces the need for invasive, expensive procedures. Noninvasive imaging studies such as chest radiography and CT are often inconclusive. Sensitivity and specificity for these methods vary considerably, and accuracy is closely related to nodule size. Generally accepted criteria of benignity by CT are (1) a benign pattern of calcification, (2) size stability over 2 years, and (3) a low probability of malignancy based on the patient's age and minimal exposure to tobacco smoke.[3] PET has consistently shown high sensitivity, specificity, positive predictive value (PPV), negative predictive value (NPV), and accuracy in the evaluation of SPN. The ability of PET to characterize a nodule as malignant depends on the degree of uptake of ^{18}F-fluorodeoxyglucose (FDG), the lesion size, and the absence of inflammation.[4] Sensitivity decreases

with nodules less than 1 cm and with low metabolic rate tumors (e.g., bronchoalveolar carcinoma, carcinoid). Specificity is reduced by high metabolic rate benign pulmonary lesions (e.g., granulomas, histiocytosis, coccidioidomycosis, tuberculosis, aspergillosis, blastomycosis, pneumonia).[5]

Interpretation of uptake in an SPN may be qualitative or quantitative. For qualitative assessment the reader compares nodular activity to the normal mediastinum. Uptake greater than mediastinum is generally reported as consistent with malignancy. As discussed in Chapter 1, uptake may theoretically be reduced in hyperglycemic patients owing to competitive inhibition. Quantitation is based on the standardized uptake value (SUV; see Chapter 1). The SUV is a quantification of the uptake of the tracer (e.g., FDG) by assigning a region of interest (ROI) surrounding the lesion ("hot spot") and calculating the ratio of this activity to that administered to the patient corrected for the patient's lean body mass.[6]

$$SUV = \frac{\text{Mean ROI activity (mCi / mL)}}{\text{Injected dose (mCi / body weight [kg])}}$$

Attenuation corrected images must be used and activities must be corrected for decay. The current recommendation is to use an SUV cutoff value of 2.5.

The use of PET in the evaluation of solitary pulmonary nodules has been shown to be cost effective, primarily by reducing the use of invasive procedures. An added benefit is the ability of PET to survey the entire body, providing an accurate staging examination in patients whose SPN proves to be malignant.

STAGING

The World Health Organization (WHO) classifies lung cancer as outlined in Table 1. Because small cell carcinoma is usually disseminated at the time of diagnosis, surgical resection is rarely indicated. PET is therefore most efficacious in staging non–small cell lung cancer (NSCLC). A recent revision of the International Staging System (ISS) proposed in 1997 is presented in Table 2.[7]

TABLE 1. WORLD HEALTH ORGANIZATION HISTOLOGIC CLASSIFICATION OF EPITHELIAL BRONCHOGENIC CARCINOMA

Classification				Feature
I				Benign
II				Dysplasia and carcinoma in situ
III				Malignant
	A			Squamous cell carcinoma (epidermoid) and spindle (squamous) carcinoma
	B			Small cell carcinoma
		1		Oat cell
		2		Intermediate cell
		3		Combined oat cell
	C			Adenocarcinoma
		1		Acinar
		2		Papillary
		3		Bronchoalveolar
		4		Mucus secreting
	D			Large cell carcinoma
		1		Giant cell
		2		Clear cell

From Abdulaziz A, Coleman RE: Applications of PET in lung cancer. Semin Nucl Med 1998;28(4):303-319.

TABLE 2. REVISED TNM CLASSIFICATION AND STAGING OF LUNG CANCER

PRIMARY TUMOR (T)

Tx	Tumor cannot be assessed, or malignant cells are in sputum or bronchial washings but not visualized by imaging or bronchoscopy
Tis	Carcinoma in situ
T0	No evidence of primary tumor
T1	Tumor < 3 cm, in a lobar bronchus or distal airways, and surrounded by lung or visceral pleura
T2	Tumor that is either > 3 cm, involving the main bronchus (>2 cm from the carina); invading the visceral pleura; or with atelectasis or obstructive pneumonitis that extends to the hilar region but does not involve the entire lung
T3	Tumor of any size that invades chest wall (including superior sulcus tumor), diaphragm, mediastinal pleura; parietal pericardium; or tumor in the main bronchus < 2 cm from, but not involving, the carina; or associated atelectasis or obstructive pneumonitis of the entire lung
T4	Tumor of any size that invades mediastinum, heart, great vessels, trachea, esophagus, vertebral body, carina; or presence of malignant pleural/pericardial effusion; or satellite tumor nodule within ipsilateral primary-tumor lobe of the lung

LYMPH NODES (N)

Nx	Regional lymph nodes cannot be assessed
N0	No regional lymph node metastasis
N1	Metastasis to ipsilateral peribronchial or ipsilateral hilar lymph nodes, and intrapulmonary nodes by direct extension
N2	Metastasis to ipsilateral mediastinal or subcarinal lymph nodes
N3	Metastasis to contralateral mediastinal, contralateral hilar, scalene, or supraclavicular lymph nodes

DISTANT METASTASIS (M)

Mx	Distant metastasis cannot be assessed
M1	No distant metastasis
M1	Distant metastasis present

STAGE	TNM SUBSETS		
O	Tis	N0	M0
IA	T1	N0	M0
IB	T2	N0	M0
IIA	T1	N1	M1
IIB	T2	N1	M1
	T3	N0	M0
IIIA	T3	N1	M0
	T1-3	N2	M0
IIIB	T4	N0-2	M0
	Any T	N3	M0
IV	Any T	Any N	M1

From Mountain CG: Revisions in the International System for Staging Lung Cancer. Chest 1997;111:1710-1717.

The importance of staging is reflected in the 5-year survival data (i.e., > 60% for stage IA and < 10% for stages III and IV). Accurate staging may be critical to patient management and extremely useful for research in lung cancer. In an analysis of more than 4000 patients, PET showed a sensitivity of 83%, specificity of 91%, PPV of 86%, NPV of 93%, and accuracy of 82% for staging.[8]

Within these numbers are important distinctions. PET is of limited value in the TNM system for staging tumor size and invasion (i.e., T). PET, like other nuclear studies, overestimates the size of lesions/nodules owing to the physical characteristics of radionuclides and detectors. Resolution of PET is suboptimal to assess invasion, which is more accurately depicted by CT. In the evaluation of nodal disease (N), PET has demonstrated clear superiority over CT and MR.[9-13] The diagnostic accuracy of PET for staging mediastinal nodal disease is in the range of 85% to 90% whereas that of CT is 60% to 75%. PET studies have confirmed the fact that lymph nodes larger than 1 cm may be benign and that nodes less than 1 cm may harbor metastatic disease. Based on the extremely high NPV of PET in the mediastinum, some authors now recommend proceeding to surgical resection with a negative PET study. However, because the PPV may only be 80% to 85%, mediastinoscopy is still indicated in a patient with a positive study to determine curability. A strategy utilizing PET and chest CT has been shown to be cost effective, with the major component of the savings due to the elimination of unnecessary mediastinoscopy and/or thoracotomy.[14,15]

With respect to metastatic disease (M), PET has proved to be of great value as a whole-body screen. Approximately 40% of newly diagnosed lung cancer patients have metastatic disease at the time of presentation. Even though the mediastinum is the most common site for metastases, a minimum of 10% of patients will show disease outside the chest. The whole-body screening capability of PET is without additional radiation and is especially helpful in the adrenals, where CT may be falsely positive.[1] Also, increased uptake in the pleura is strong evidence of pleural metastasis.[16] Patient management may be changed in a significant percentage of cases. In one series, the authors reported 29% of their patients were found to have unsuspected metastases and PET resulted in a change in management in 41% of the cases.[17]

ASSESSING RECURRENCE

The generally poor prognosis of lung cancer necessitates close follow-up of these patients. Tumor markers are rarely of benefit, and standard radiologic work-up, which relies on changes in size and shape of lesions, may be nondiagnostic. Patient symptoms may be due to a variety of factors, including recurrent disease, treatment-related complications, other medical conditions, or even psychological factors (e.g., depression, anxiety). PET provides an objective, highly accurate method to assess the entire body. Combined data on 337 patients showed a sensitivity of 98%, specificity of 92%, PPV of 93%, NPV of 97%, and overall accuracy of 96% in the evaluation of recurrence.[8] Changes on the PET scan may antedate anatomic changes by weeks to months, allowing earlier intervention.

RESPONSE TO THERAPY

Although this is a more recently established use for PET, the potential is enormous. Changes in FDG uptake during or after therapy hold great promise for assessing tumor response. Many quantitative parameters of glucose metabolism have been looked at, with the European Organization for Research and Treatment of Cancer recommending the standardized uptake value normalized for body surface area.[18] Should PET prove successful in predicting response of lung cancer to therapy, the potential benefits are clear: ineffective, expensive treatment may be curtailed or modified and alternate regimens initiated earlier. Issues that still need further evaluation include the best timing of PET imaging after irradiation, the frequency and duration of "flare phenomenon" (apparent worsening in a patient who is truly responding), and the reproducibility of PET measurements.

REFERENCES

1. Coleman RE: PET in lung cancer. J Nucl Med 1999;40:814-820.
2. Abdulaziz A, Coleman RE: Applications of PET in lung cancer. Semin Nucl Med 1998;28(4): 303-319.
3. Lowe VJ, Fletcher JW, Gobar L, et al: Prospective investigation of positron emission tomography in lung nodules. J Clin Oncol 1998;16:1075-1984.
4. Pieterman RM, van Putten JWG, Meuzelaar JJ, et al: Preoperative staging of non–small-cell lung cancer with positron-emission tomography. N Engl J Med 2000;343:254-261.
5. Bakheet SM, Saleem M, Powe J, et al: F-18 fluorodeoxyglucose chest uptake in lung inflammation and infection. Clin Nucl Med 2000;25(4):273-278.
6. Marom EM, McAdams HP, Erasmus JJ, et al: Staging non-small cell lung cancer with whole body PET. Radiology 1999;212:803-809.
7. Mountain CG: Revisions in the International System for Staging Lung Cancer. Chest 1997;111:1710-1717.
8. Gambhir SS, Czernin J, Schwimmer J, et al: A tabulated summary of the FDG PET literature. J Nucl Med 2001;42:2S-8S.
9. Dwamena BA, Sonnad SS, Angobaldo JO, et al: Metastases from non-small cell lung cancer: Mediastinal staging in the 1990s-meta-analytic comparison of PET and CT. Radiology 1999;213:530-536.
10. Graeber GM, Gupta NC, Murray GF: Positron emission tomographic imaging with fluorodeoxyglucose is efficacious in evaluating malignant pulmonary disease. J Thorac Cardiovasc Surg 1999;117:719-727.
11. Richter JA, Torre E, Garcia MJ, et al: PET-FDG in the preoperative evaluation of non–small cell lung cancer (NSCLC) staging: A comparison with CT scanning and MRI. Clin Positron Imag 1998;1(4):247.
12. Steinert HC, Hauser M, Allemann F, et al: Non-small cell lung cancer: Nodal staging with FDG PET versus CT with correlative lymph node mapping and sampling. Radiology 1997;202:441-446.
13. Gupta NC, Graeber GM, Rogers JS, et al: Comparative efficacy of positron emission tomography with FDG and computed tomographic scanning in preoperative staging of non–small cell lung cancer. Ann Surg 1999;229:286-291.
14. Dietlein M, Weber K, Gandjour A, et al: Cost-effectiveness of FDG-PET for management of potentially operable non–small cell lung cancer: Priority for a PET based strategy after nodal-negative CT results. Eur J Nucl Med 2000;27:1598-1609.
15. Gambhir SS, Hoh CK, Phelps ME, et al: Decision tree sensitivity analysis for cost-effectiveness of FDG-PET in the staging and management of non-small cell lung carcinoma. J Nucl Med 1996;37:1428-1436.
16. Erasmus JJ, McAdams HP, Rossi SE, et al: FDG PET of pleural effusions in patients with non-small cell lung cancer. AJR Am J Roentgenol 2000;175:245-249.
17. Lewis P, Griffin S, Marsden P, et al: Whole body F-18-fluorodeoxyglucose positron emission tomography in preoperative evaluation of lung cancer. Lancet 1994;344:1265-1266.
18. Young H: Measurement of clinical and subclinical tumor response using [18F]-fluorodeoxyglucose and positron emission tomography: Review and 1999 EORTC recommendations. Eur J Cancer 1999;35: 1773-1782.

CASE 1 | SPN, positive, no other disease sites (proven adenocarcinoma)

A 50-year-old woman with fever, chills, cough, malaise, and hemoptysis was evaluated with a CXR, which showed a mass in the posterior segment of the RUL. Review of systems was significant for painful swelling of the knees and ankles, with mild digital clubbing, thought to be hypertrophic pulmonary osteoarthropathy. Past medical history was significant for smoking 1.5 packs/day × 30 years. Chest CT showed the mass to be spiculated and noncalcified (Figure 1). Several liver lesions were seen, not all clearly cysts (Figure 2). PET scan showed the RUL lesion to be hypermetabolic, consistent with tumor, with no other evidence of disease (Figure 3). CT-guided biopsy established a diagnosis of large cell carcinoma. The patient was treated surgically with right upper lobectomy. Tumor was noted to cross the major fissure, requiring a segmental lobectomy of the superior segment of the RLL. Final pathology reported a 4-cm poorly differentiated adenocarcinoma, with no metastatic disease identified in 20 lymph nodes. The patient's recovery was uneventful, and she was without evidence of active disease at 7 months after surgery.

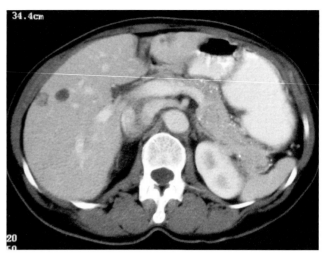

FIGURE 2. CT section through the upper abdomen shows two small liver lesions, one a cyst and the other indeterminate. Calcifications of the pancreas are consistent with chronic pancreatitis.

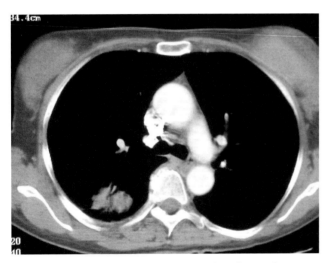

FIGURE 1. Enhanced chest CT shows an irregular, soft tissue density mass in the posterior RUL. Shotty precarinal lymph nodes are present, but no enlarged or suspicious nodes were seen.

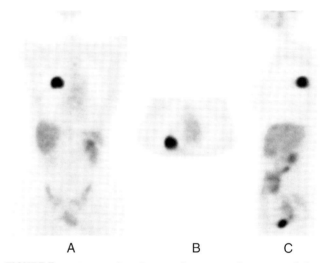

A   B   C

FIGURE 3. PET images show the intensely active RUL lesion. No pathologic findings are seen elsewhere, including in the liver. Coronal (**A**), transaxial (**B**), and sagittal (**C**) views are shown.

TEACHING POINTS

PET can be helpful in assessing the significance of focal liver lesions, but it may be limited by lesion size. Normal liver activity on PET is of low intensity, often with a diffusely mottled appearance, which can be disconcerting to the novice reader. True hepatic metastases generally stand out readily against the low background activity of the normal liver.

CASE 2 | *SPN, positive (proven adenocarcinoma)*

An 81-year-old woman, with a known but previously stable SPN of the RUL, was followed with serial CXRs. Four years after the nodule was initially detected and evaluated, it grew in size (Figure 1). Chest CT evaluation showed the nodule to be 2 cm, from 1.4 cm previously (Figure 2). Past medical history was significant for a right supraclavicular region melanoma 10 years before, as well as a right upper extremity melanoma 1 month prior. PET of the SPN was positive in the RUL, with no additional disease sites found (Figure 4). Correlation with chest CT suggested a primary lung carcinoma, with melanoma metastasis considered in the differential diagnosis. No enlarged mediastinal lymph nodes were seen on chest CT (Figure 3), and the mediastinum was also negative on PET.

The patient was treated with a right upper lobectomy. Pathology revealed a well-differentiated adenocarcinoma. Three of five lymph nodes showed metastatic adenocarcinoma (Figures 5 and 6; see color plates 1 and 2). These were micrometastases, with tumor foci ranging from 1 to 7 mm, which presumably contributed to the falsely negative PET mediastinal findings, even on retrospective review.

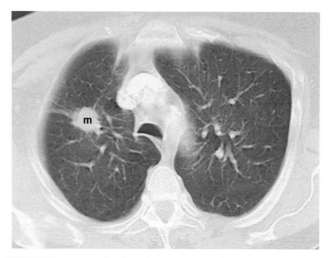

FIGURE 2. Lung window from chest CT confirms the RUL mass (m). Margin spiculation is a typical feature of lung cancer.

TEACHING POINTS

PET scan tumor activity is proportional to lesion size and metabolic activity level and is nonspecific with regard to tissue histology. PET cannot differentiate a primary lung tumor from a melanoma metastasis or any other metabolically active metastatic process.

PET may, as in this case, fail to identify microscopic foci of tumor in lymph nodes. However, it is capable of detecting metabolic activity and suggesting tumor involvement in lymph nodes, which are of normal size.

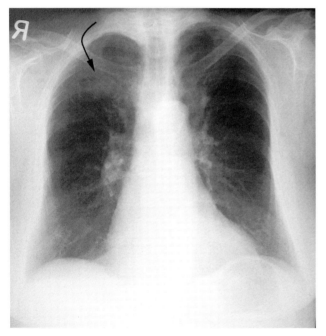

FIGURE 1. Posteroanterior CXR shows an asymmetrical nodular density at the level of the anterior end of the right first rib (*arrow*). Patient had a known SPN at this level, and comparison showed interval growth, prompting reevaluation with CT.

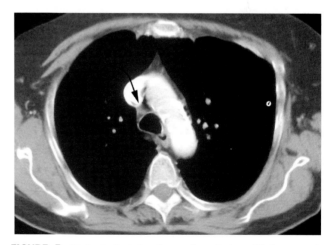

FIGURE 3. Mediastinal window from enhanced chest CT shows a sub-centimeter right paratracheal lymph node (*arrow*). No pathologically enlarged lymph nodes were seen.

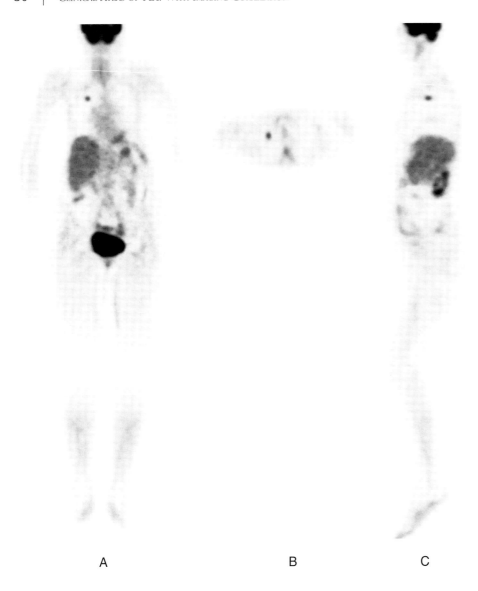

A   B   C

FIGURE 4. PET imaging (coronal [**A**], axial [**B**], and sagittal [**C**] planes) was performed of the whole body because of the patient's past history of melanoma. A small focus of hyper-intense metabolic activity in the RUL corresponds to the SPN. The mediastinum and remainder of the examination were negative.

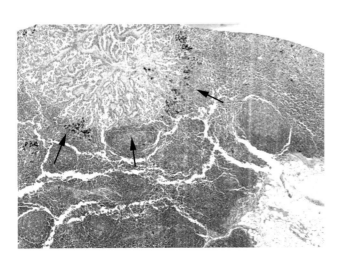

FIGURE 5. Low-power H & E stain of a lymph node showing a 1-mm focus of gland-forming metastatic adenocarcinoma (*arrows*). See color plate 1.

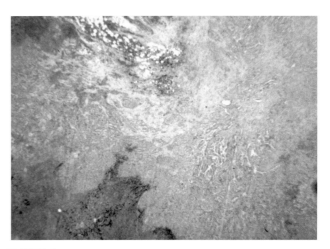

FIGURE 6. Low-power view of an H & E stain from another lymph node depicting the largest nodal focus (7 mm) of metastatic adenocarcinoma. Residual normal lymph node remains at lower left corner of image. See color plate 2. (Histopathology images courtesy of Gary Wilcox, MD, Tri City Medical Center, Oceanside, CA.) See color plate 2.

CASE 3 | *SPN, positive (proven recurrent squamous cell carcinoma)*

A 78-year-old woman was noted to develop a new peripheral LUL SPN. Her past medical history was notable for prior right lower lobectomy for a poorly differentiated 9 × 5 × 4.5-cm squamous cell carcinoma 6 years previous. Lymph nodes were negative. At the same time, a wedge resection of an additional 1.2-cm squamous cell carcinoma in the RUL had been performed. The new LUL SPN, identified on CXR (Figure 1), was confirmed on CT (Figures 2 and 3). Metachronous bronchogenic carcinoma was suspected. The patient's pulmonary function was marginal, with FEV$_1$ of 1 L. A "metabolic biopsy" was obtained with PET imaging, which confirmed the hypermetabolic nature of the LUL nodule (Figure 4). No nodal involvement was suggested on CT or PET. Because of the patient's pulmonary status, a wedge excision of the lesion was performed. At pathology,

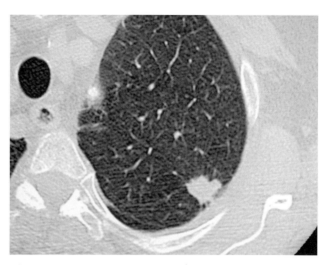

FIGURE 3. High-resolution thin-section chest CT image better shows characteristic findings of lung carcinoma, with lobular contours and marginal spiculations.

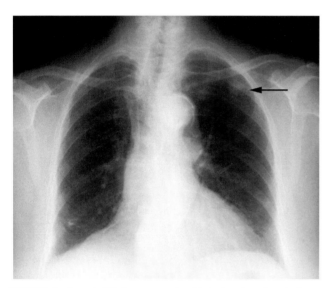

FIGURE 1. Frontal CXR shows a peripheral LUL SPN (*arrow*). Right hemothorax is smaller than left from prior lobectomy.

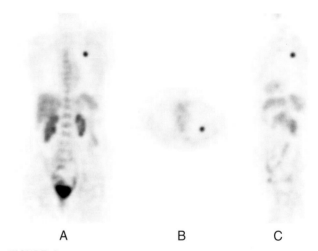

A   B   C

FIGURE 4. PET scan images in three planes show intense hypermetabolic activity in the small posterior LUL nodule. No additional abnormal sites of activity were found. Coronal (**A**), transaxial (**B**), and sagittal (**C**) views are shown.

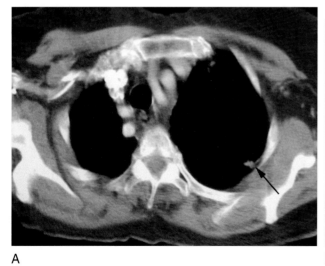

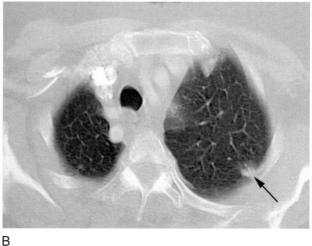

A   B

FIGURE 2. Mediastinal (**A**) and lung (**B**) windows from enhanced chest CT show small, peripheral, noncalcified lung nodule, focally abutting pleura (*arrows*).

a poorly differentiated 2-cm squamous cell carcinoma with negative margins and background chronic obstructive pulmonary disease was demonstrated.

TEACHING POINT

In this case, use of PET avoided potentially morbid diagnostic procedures, such as percutaneous biopsy, in an elderly patient with marginal pulmonary function. It also confirmed the CT impression of limited disease and guided the minimal therapy utilized.

CASE 4 | SPN, positive (proven large cell carcinoma)

A 68-year-old woman, establishing care with a new physician, had a CXR showing a lobulated peripheral mass in the RLL. This was evaluated with CT (Figure 1), which showed no pathologic adenopathy. PET confirmed intense hypermetabolic activity corresponding to the mass, but no indication of other disease sites (Figure 2). Subsequent CT-guided biopsy established a diagnosis of non–small cell carcinoma. Because of the patient's symptoms of "unusual chest sensations" and the peripheral, pleural-based location of the tumor, chest MRI was also performed, showing no evidence of chest wall invasion (Figures 3 and 4).

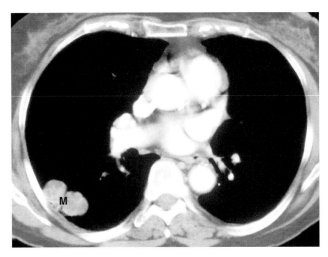

FIGURE 1. Mediastinal window of a contrast medium–enhanced chest CT shows a peripheral, bilobed superior segment RLL mass (M), with relatively smooth margins. Pleura is abutted. No suggestion of chest wall invasion is seen.

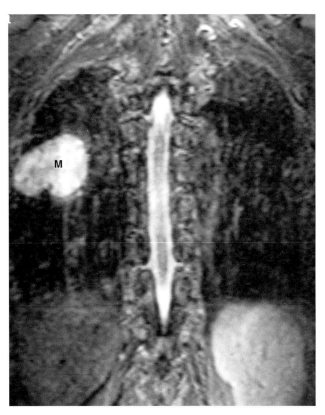

FIGURE 3. Coronal MRI image shows the bilobed, smoothly marginated, hyperintense mass (M) in the superior segment, RLL.

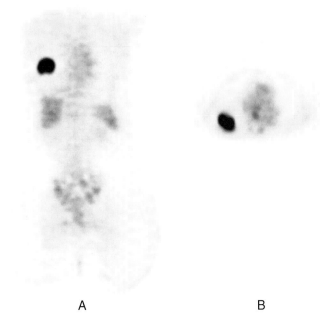

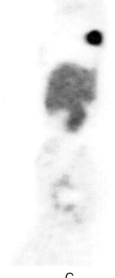

A   B   C

FIGURE 2. PET scan coronal (**A**), axial (**B**), and sagittal (**C**) images show corresponding morphology and intense hypermetabolic activity of the lesion, consistent with malignancy. Mediastinum and hila were negative, and no additional disease sites were found.

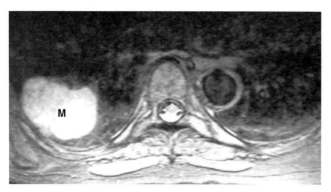

FIGURE 4. Axial MRI shows the mass (M) to broadly abut the posterior pleura without evidence of chest wall transgression.

The patient underwent right lower lobectomy with in-continuity hilar and mediastinal lymphadenectomy. Final pathologic diagnosis was large cell carcinoma with spindle cell component and focal squamous differentiation. Ten examined lymph nodes were negative for tumor.

TEACHING POINT

PET imaging in such a case serves both to guide further management of SPNs and, in those proving to be lung carcinomas, to noninvasively aid in staging them.

CASE 5 | *SPN, positive (proven squamous cell carcinoma)*

A 76-year-old woman was evaluated for shortness of breath. A CXR showed a mass-like infiltrate in the superior segment of the LLL (Figure 1). Chest CT confirmed a bilobed, cavitary left infrahilar mass, with spiculated margins (Figures 2 and 3). Bilateral adrenal gland enlargement was thought to be hyperplasia (Figure 4).

PET scanning demonstrated a corresponding, hypermetabolic, bilobed LLL focus of activity, correlating well with the CT findings (Figure 5). No additional sites of disease were found. The scintigraphic inactivity of the adrenal glands confirmed the CT impression of hyperplasia as the cause of the bilateral adrenal gland enlargement.

The patient underwent a left lower lobectomy with in-continuity hilar and mediastinal lymphadenectomy. Pathology revealed a poorly differentiated squamous cell carcinoma, 4 cm in maximal dimension, with margins negative and six negative lymph nodes. A separate sample of five interlobar LLL lymph nodes was also negative for metastatic carcinoma.

TEACHING POINTS

In this case, PET scanning indicated a malignant etiology of the suspicious LLL mass and effectively staged this squamous cell carcinoma in the same whole-body study. Any residual doubt about the benign etiology of the bilateral adrenal gland enlargement in this patient was allayed by the inactivity of the glands on PET scanning.

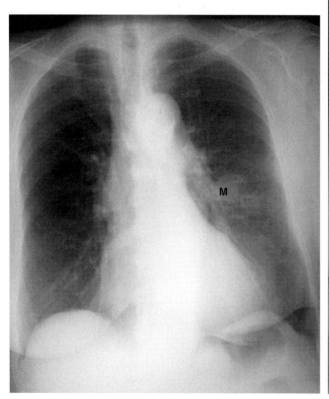

A

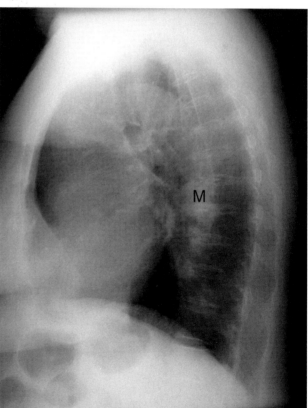

B

FIGURE 1. Posteroanterior (**A**) and lateral (**B**) CXR films show a mass (M) localizing to the superior segment of the LLL.

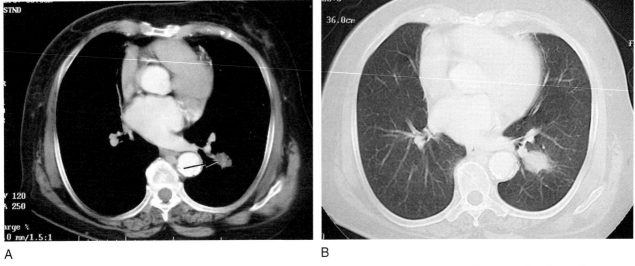

FIGURE 2. Contrast medium–enhanced chest CT (soft tissue [A] and lung [B] windows) confirms a mass (*arrow*) abutting LLL bronchovascular structures.

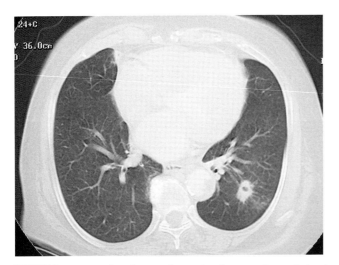

FIGURE 3. A more inferior lung window section shows a cavitary, spiculated inferior component of this bilobed mass.

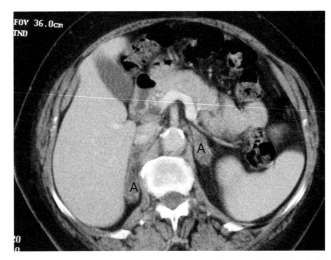

FIGURE 4. CT section through the abdomen at the level of the adrenals (A) show them to be enlarged (right larger than left) and lumpy. However, they maintain their adreniform shape, suggesting hyperplasia.

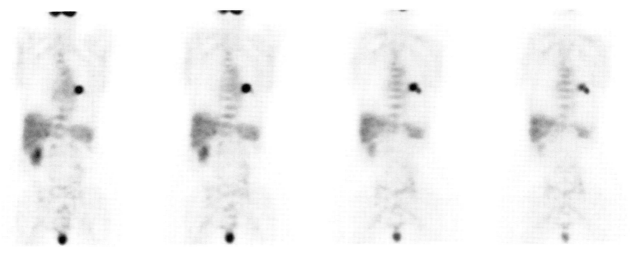

FIGURE 5. Coronal PET sections show two adjacent hypermetabolic foci in the left lung, corresponding to this lesion's bilobed configuration. No additional sites of pathologic activity were seen. Adrenal glands are scintigraphically inactive, confirming CT impression of bilateral hyperplasia.

CASE 6 | *SPN, negative, tuberculoma*

A 76-year-old man was evaluated for weight loss with a CXR (Figure 1) and found to have a new left lung nodule. Past medical history was significant for 70+ pack-year smoking history and severe bullous emphysema. Chest CT showed pulmonary parenchymal emphysema and a posterior LUL 2-cm mass with marginal spiculation, suggestive of lung cancer (Figure 2). A CT-guided fine-needle aspiration stain showing 4+ acid-fast bacilli was complicated by a large pneumothorax, requiring a chest tube. The patient was placed on antituberculous medications, although the cultures were ultimately negative. A repeat biopsy was performed bronchoscopically but was negative for malignancy and granulomas. He again required chest tube treatment for pneumothorax. PET scan showed minimal, barely discernible activity at the lesion site, consistent with a benign etiology (Figure 3). The patient's follow-up chest CTs show no change in the size or appearance of the nodule 1 year later.

TEACHING POINTS

This SPN displayed suspicious morphologic characteristics and occurred in a high-risk patient. Although the smear showed acid-fast bacilli, no specific organism was cultured. The patient suffered significant morbidity with biopsy efforts, developing two large (50% to 60%)

pneumothoraces requiring chest tube placement for treatment. With the PET scan suggesting a benign etiology, no further attempts were made to establish a firmer diagnosis. Other than symptoms related to the pneumothoraces, the patient was asymptomatic, with no clinical evidence of active tuberculosis. He was followed with periodic chest CTs, which showed stability of the lesion 1 year later.

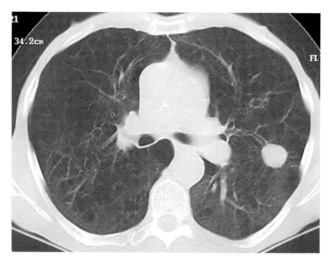

FIGURE 2. Chest CT lung window shows the mass to be fairly smoothly marginated, but there are fine spicules radiating from it. Chest CT findings suggest a bronchogenic carcinoma.

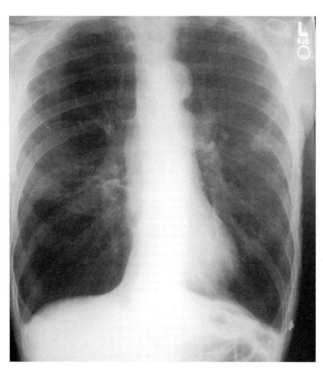

FIGURE 1. Frontal CXR shows stigmata of chronic obstructive pulmonary disease and emphysema, including marked hyperinflation, lung lucency, and flattened hemidiaphragms. A 2-cm solitary nodule is seen in the left mid lung.

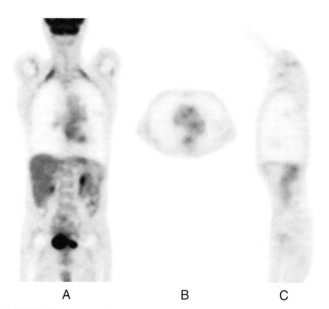

A   B   C

FIGURE 3. PET scan shows the nodule to be only faintly visible, suggesting a benign etiology, probably a granuloma. Coronal (**A**), transaxial (**B**), and sagittal (**C**) views are shown.

CASE 7 | *SPN, negative, aspergillosis*

An LUL abnormality was identified on CXR in a 65-year-old man. CT evaluation showed a thick-walled cavitary nodule, with adjacent, additional noncavitary nodules (Figures 1 to 3). Biopsy showed no evidence of malignancy. The patient was followed with repeat CT 4 months later, with minimal change. He was referred for PET imaging for further evaluation. On PET, the nodules in question were scintigraphically inactive, consistent with a benign etiology (Figure 4). Bronchoscopic evaluation with culture showed *Aspergillus*. Continued CT follow-up showed no change 1 year later.

TEACHING POINTS

After a negative biopsy, the normal PET scan provided further reassurance that these nodules were benign inflammatory/infectious lesions, enabling the patient to be followed noninvasively thereafter.

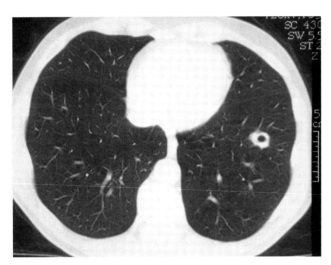

FIGURE 1. Chest CT shows a 2-cm, thick-walled cavity in the LLL.

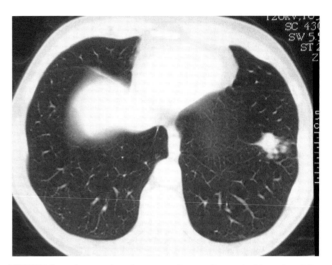

FIGURE 2. Inferior to this, there is an adjacent cluster of additional nodules.

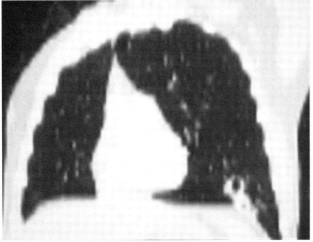
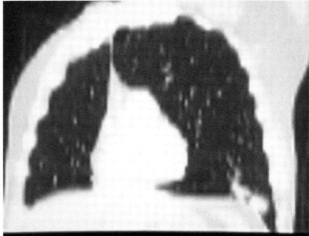

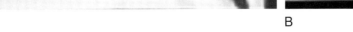
A   B

FIGURE 3. Two coronal (**A** and **B**) reconstructions show the clustering of these nodules at the lung base.

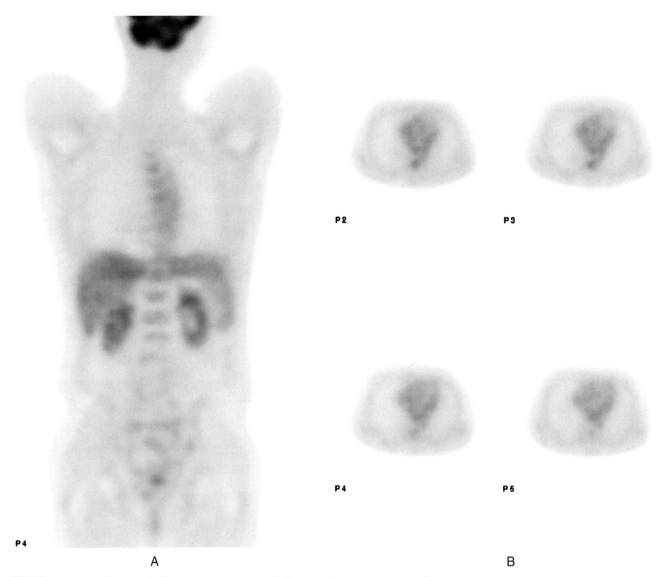

P2   P3

P4   P5

P4

A   B

FIGURE 4. Coronal (**A**) and axial (**B**) PET images are negative. No hypermetabolic activity is seen in the LLL.

CASE 8 | *SPN, negative, cocci granuloma*

A 52-year-old female heavy smoker had a preoperative CXR before a podiatric procedure and was found to have a right apical SPN. This was confirmed on chest CT, which showed a soft tissue density 1.5-cm noncalcified nodule in the apical segment of the RUL (Figures 1 and 2). Bronchoscopic evaluation was unrevealing. The lesion was inactive on PET imaging, consistent with a benign etiology (Figure 3). The patient underwent a thoracoscopic segmental resection of the apical and posterior segments. The specimen contained a 2.5- to 3-cm multilobated, firm, necrotic granuloma, with stainable fungal organisms compatible with *Coccidioides immitis* (Figures 4 and 5; see color plates 3 and 4).

TEACHING POINT

PET imaging can reliably differentiate between benign and malignant causes of lung nodules, as long as they are of sufficient size (≥1 cm and variably down to 6 mm). This provides an attractive, noninvasive, "metabolic biopsy" alternative to percutaneous biopsy. In the case of scintigraphically inactive, benign nodules (most commonly granulomas) this provides important information to guide further management. Note should be made that lesions less than a centimeter that are PET negative should continue to be followed for a reasonable interval, generally 2 years, with CXR or CT, because there is a threshold effect, based on size and metabolic activity, of nodule visibility on FDG PET.

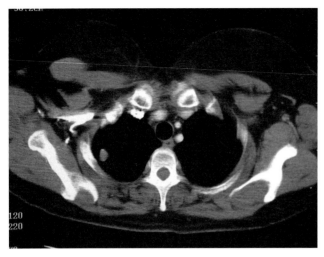

FIGURE 1. Contrast medum–enhanced chest CT demonstrates a noncalcified, indeterminate, soft tissue density right apical lung nodule.

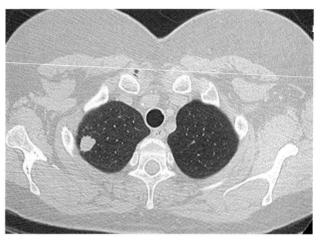

FIGURE 2. High-resolution lung window better displays microlobularity of margins of this indeterminate mass.

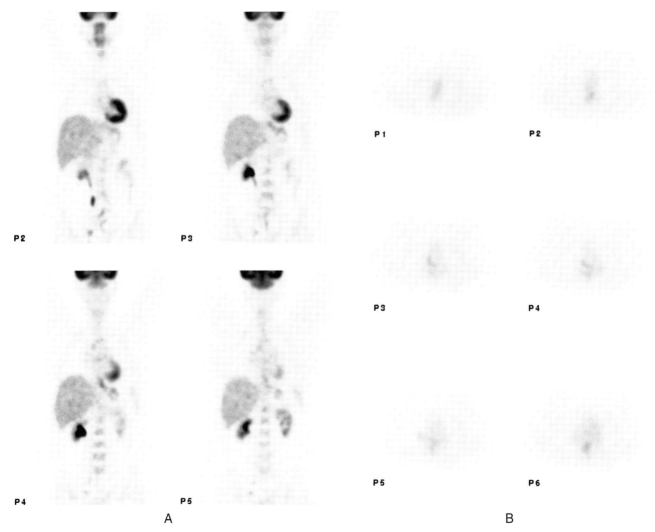

A

B

FIGURE 3. The nodule is inactive on PET images (coronal [**A**] and axial [**B**]), consistent with a benign etiology.

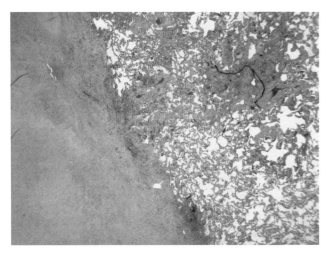

FIGURE 4. Low-power H & E–stained view from the surgical specimen showing lung to the right, and a portion of the necrotic granuloma to the left. The nodule margin is relatively smooth. See color plate 3.

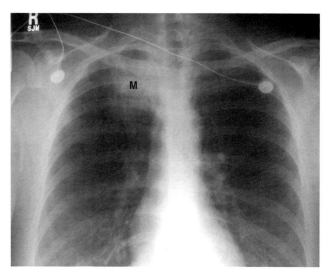

FIGURE 1. Frontal CXR demonstrates a RUL mass (M).

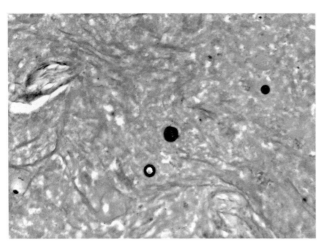

FIGURE 5. High-power view of the methenamine silver stain study of the nodule, showing stainable spherules, both empty and filled with endospores. The fungal organisms are compatible with *Coccidioides immitis* (Histopathology images courtesy of Gary Wilcox, MD, Tri City Medical Center, Oceanside, CA). See color plate 4.

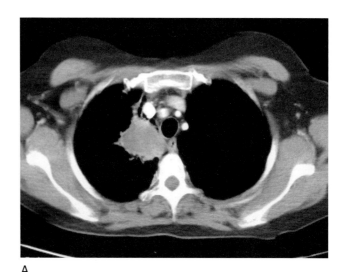

A

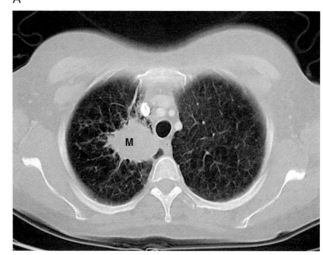

B

FIGURE 2. Enhanced chest CT images, mediastinal (**A**) and lung (**B**) windows, show the RUL mass to be low-density, irregularly marginated, and to focally abut the mediastinum at the posterior tracheal level (M). The mass arises in the setting of background lung disease.

CASE 9 | SPN, positive, with hilar and/or mediastinal disease (proven large cell carcinoma)

A 58-year-old woman complained of left rib pain. CXR identified an RUL mass (Figure 1). Chest CT confirmed a low-density RUL mass, focally abutting the mediastinum, as well as a borderline right paratracheal lymph node (Figures 2 and 3). Bronchoscopy was performed, but biopsies were negative. PET scan showed intense activity in the RUL mass, as well as small foci of lesser activity in the right paratracheal mediastinum and right hilus, suggesting stage IIIA disease (Figure 4). CT-guided biopsy of the mass established a diagnosis of large cell carcinoma. At the time of this procedure, 6 weeks after the

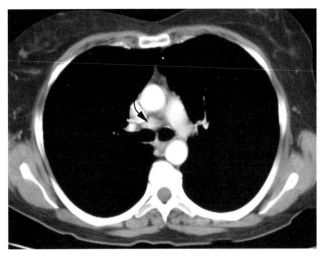

FIGURE 3. A more inferior chest CT section shows a borderline size right paratracheal lymph node (*arrow*).

first chest CT, interval growth was noted of the tumor, with infiltration posterior to the trachea, and a right hilar lymph node also grew. She was started on neoadjuvant chemotherapy, but CT follow-up showed progression of disease. Radiation therapy was also performed to the RUL and mediastinum. Toward the end of the course of radiation therapy, the patient developed back pain. Bone metastases were confirmed by bone scan and pelvic MRI. She died shortly thereafter, 7 months after the lung cancer was first identified.

TEACHING POINTS

The PET scan in this patient confirmed intense activity at the RUL site of suspected lung cancer. The small, less intense foci of activity in the mediastinum and hilus are less clearly pathologic, but of concern. If this patient had been considered for surgery with curative intent (precluded in this case by the rapid tumor growth and mediastinal involvement), mediastinoscopic evaluation would have been appropriate. False-positive PET scan activity can be seen in reactive lymph nodes (see Case 10). In this case, the rapid tumor growth and infiltration of the mediastinum observed during the course of the work-up confirmed the PET impression of nonoperable disease.

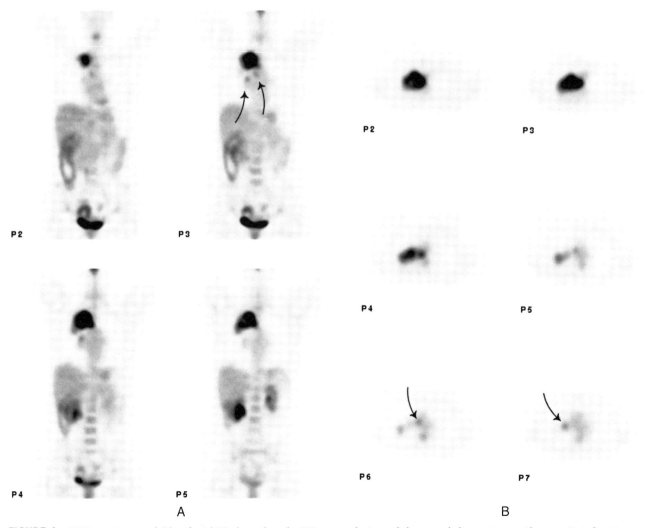

FIGURE 4. PET images in coronal (**A**) and axial (**B**) planes show the RUL mass to be intensely hypermetabolic, consistent with tumor. Foci of activity are also seen at the right paratracheal mediastinal and right hilar levels, suggesting stage IIIA disease (*arrows*). Tubular activity in the right abdomen on coronal sections is bowel.

CASE 10 | *SPN, positive, with false-positive mediastinal disease (proven squamous cell carcinoma)*

A 73-year-old woman, with a long smoking history and progressive chronic obstructive pulmonary disease, was found to have a 1-cm LUL lung nodule on CXR (Figure 1). Chest CT confirmed a lobulated, irregularly marginated solitary pulmonary nodule in the LUL, suggestive of a bronchogenic carcinoma (Figure 2). No pathologically enlarged mediastinal lymph nodes were identified, although 1-cm right paratracheal lymph nodes were noted (Figure 3). A "metabolic biopsy" with PET was performed for a suspected stage 1A lung cancer. This confirmed the suspected primary to be metabolically active (Figure 4) but also showed mild mediastinal activity, precluding exclusion of mediastinal involvement (Figure 5). The patient underwent mediastinoscopy, which was negative. She was treated with left upper lobectomy with in-continuity node resection for what proved to be a 1.5-cm stage 1A (T1N0M0) squamous cell carcinoma. Six hilar lymph nodes were negative for metastases.

TEACHING POINTS

Normal mediastinal activity is low level. Activity within the hila or mediastinum over this low background level is abnormal, but nonspecific. In this case of staging a presumed lung cancer with normal-size lymph nodes, the differential diagnosis for mediastinal activity includes metastases in nonenlarged nodes and benign causes of lymph node activity, such as from granulomatous disease or other inflammatory processes. The degree of PET scan activity within lymph node regions, in conjunction with imaging findings, can aid in assessing the likelihood of mediastinal involvement. The primary lesion itself serves to some degree as an internal control for metabolic activity of a disease process.

If a patient is otherwise a candidate for a potentially curative surgery, mediastinal involvement suggested by PET should be confirmed by tissue sampling before excluding a patient from consideration for a potentially curative surgery.

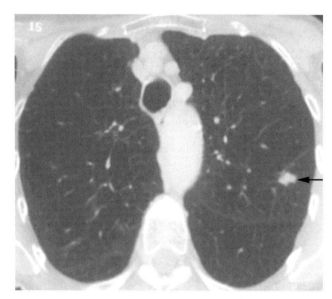

FIGURE 2. Lung window from chest CT shows an irregularly marginated, lobular nodule in the apical posterior LUL segment (*arrow*).

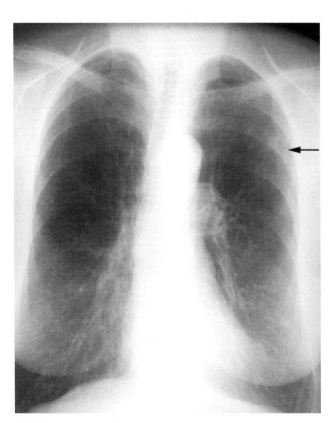

FIGURE 1. Frontal CXR shows stigmata of chronic obstructive pulmonary disease and emphysema, with marked hyperinflation, flattened hemidiaphragms, and attenuated pulmonary parenchymal markings. In the periphery of the LUL, an irregularly shaped solitary pulmonary nodule is seen (*arrow*).

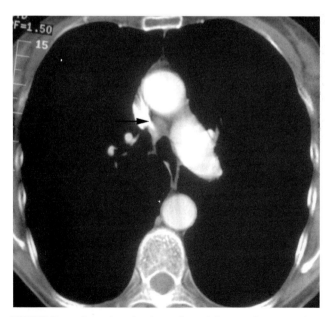

FIGURE 3. Mediastinal window from enhanced chest CT shows normal size (<1 cm) right paratracheal lymph node (*arrow*).

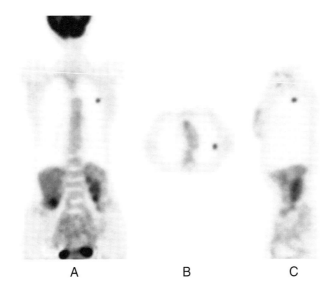

FIGURE 4. Coronal (**A**), axial (**B**), and sagittal (**C**) PET sections through the LUL show the small nodule to be intensely hypermetabolic, consistent with the impression of probable lung cancer. Note marked lung hyperinflation of COPD.

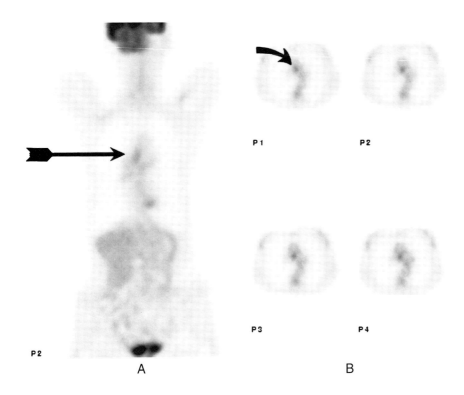

FIGURE 5. Coronal (**A**) and four contiguous, corresponding transaxial (**B**) PET images of the mediastinum show mild right paratracheal mediastinal activity, corresponding in location to the normal size lymph nodes on CT (*arrows*). Lymph node activity is assessed by comparison to background mediastinal activity, and so is abnormal by this standard, although the activity is faint.

CASE 11 | *SPN, positive, with hilar and/or mediastinal disease (advanced squamous cell carcinoma)*

A 77-year-old woman was admitted with syncope and was found on CXR to have a large RUL mass (Figure 1). She had a history 3 years before of mastectomy-treated breast cancer and was a heavy, life-long smoker.

Chest CT showed a large soft tissue density RUL mass, infiltrating the mediastinum posterior to the trachea (Figure 2). Suspicious, enlarged right paratracheal, right hilar and subcarinal lymph nodes were present (Figure 3). An additional nodular mass was noted in the LUL (Figure 4). A fine-needle aspiration of the RUL mass showed malignant squamous cell carcinoma. PET was requested for staging of newly diagnosed lung cancer (Figure 5). It showed the RUL dominant mass to be centrally necrotic, with metabolically active tissue peripherally.

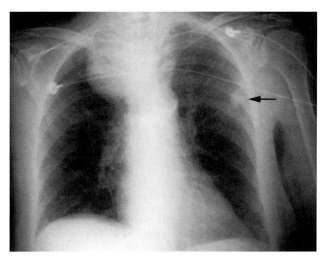

FIGURE 1. Frontal CXR shows marked widening of the mediastinum, particularly in the right paratracheal region, and a LUL mass-like opacity (*arrow*).

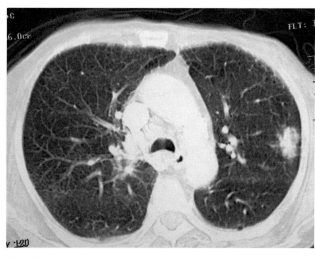

FIGURE 4. A separate spiculated pulmonary parenchymal mass is noted in the posterior LUL. Advanced changes of chronic obstructive pulmonary disease are noted on the lung parenchyma.

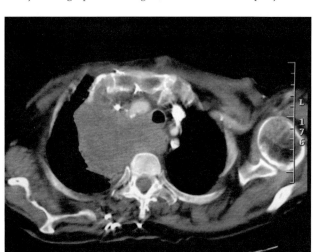

FIGURE 2. Contrast medium–enhanced chest CT confirms a large soft tissue density mass, infiltrating the mediastinum and bulging into the RUL. The mass displaces brachiocephalic vessels anteriorly and extends posterior to the trachea and laterally to the esophagus.

Increased activity was noted at multiple additional sites, including the separate LUL focus, the mediastinum, and the right hilum. The patient was discharged from the hospital to hospice and died 1 week later.

TEACHING POINTS

Advanced disease was suggested based on imaging staging. Demonstration of abnormal metabolic activity at these multiple sites on PET served to confirm this impression.

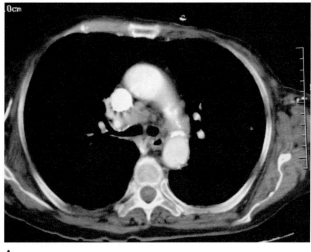
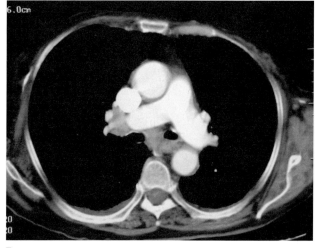

A   B

FIGURE 3. Chest CT images (two levels, **A** and **B**) show pathologically enlarged lymph nodes in the right paratracheal region, as well as at the right hilar and subcarinal levels.

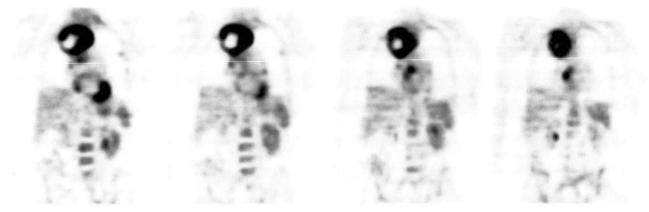

FIGURE 5. Coronal PET images show the dominant RUL mass to be centrally photopenic, indicating necrosis. Advanced disease was confirmed on PET, with increased metabolic activity seen at multiple additional sites, including at the levels of the suspicious nodes on CT and in the separate LUL lesion.

CASE 12 | Lung cancer staging, primary positive, no other disease (large cell undifferentiated carcinoma)

An 80-year-old man was evaluated with a CXR for right-sided back pain after a motor vehicle accident. A large RUL mass was identified (Figure 1) and further evaluated with CT, which also showed mild mediastinal adenopathy (Figures 2 and 3). Fine-needle aspiration showed non–small cell lung carcinoma. PET imaging showed the large RUL mass to be intensely hypermetabolic, but no mediastinal or other abnormal foci of activity were identified (Figure 4). Preoperative staging was T2N0M0. He was treated surgically with a right upper lobectomy, as well as segmental resection of the superior segment of the RLL because of tumor compromise. Dense adherence between the pleura

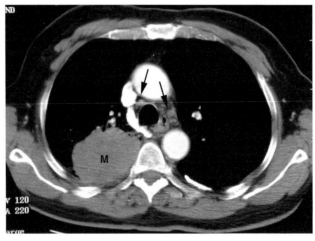

FIGURE 2. Contrast medium–enhanced chest CT section through the anteroposterior window shows corresponding, lobular, relatively smoothly marginated mass with a broad base of posteromedial pleural abutment (M). Subcentimeter right paratracheal and aortopulmonary window lymph nodes are also depicted (arrows).

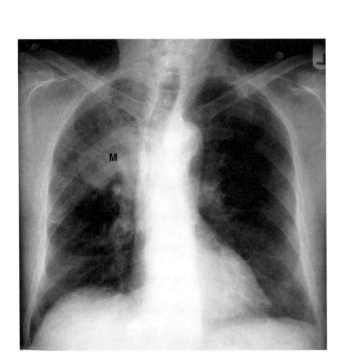

FIGURE 1. Posteroanterior CXR shows a large RUL lung mass (M). There is increased density of the RUL parenchyma peripheral to the mass, suggesting a postobstructive pneumonitis.

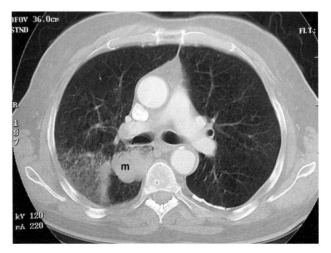

FIGURE 3. Lung window from a more inferior section, at the level of the carina, shows the inferior aspect of the mass (m), as well as postobstructive infiltrate peripheral to tumor.

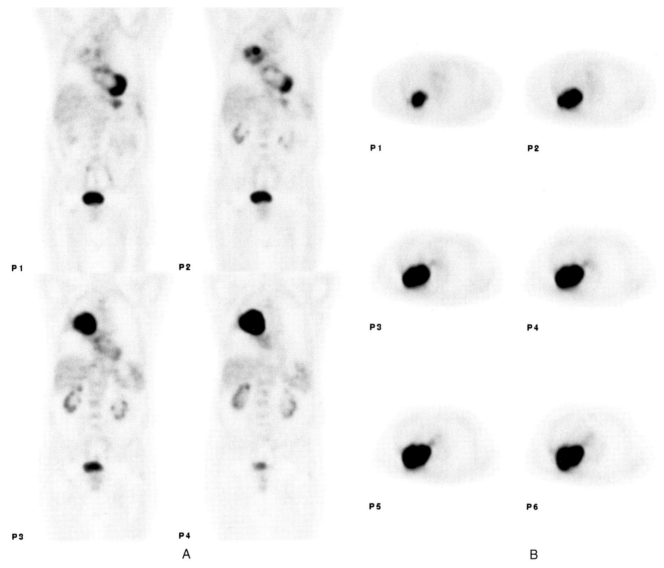

P1 P2

P3 P4

A

P1 P2

P3 P4

P5 P6

B

FIGURE 4. Coronal (**A**) and corresponding axial (**B**) PET images show marked hypermetabolism of this non–small cell lung carcinoma. Very faint lung parenchymal activity is noted peripheral to the mass, corresponding to the presumed postobstructive pneumonitis noted on CXR and CT. The remainder of the examination was negative.

and the posterior RUL was addressed with a partial pleurectomy. Hilar and mediastinal lymphadenectomy was performed in continuity with the resected specimen. Pathologic evaluation of the specimens showed a large cell undifferentiated carcinoma, with hilar and right paratracheal lymph nodes negative for tumor. Tumor did not invade the thickened and chronically inflamed pleura.

TEACHING POINT

FDG PET activity is noted in proportion to metabolic activity of disease processes, which generally is much greater in tumors than in inflammatory processes. In this example, the differential between the tumor activity and the faint activity seen in the peripheral pneumonitis is extreme and easily differentiated. However, there is overlap in metabolic activity levels between tumors and inflammatory lesions, and differentiation is not always so easily made. Fairly intense increased metabolic activity can be seen in non-neoplastic processes, such as

pulmonary infarction (see Case 39), and radiation therapy pneumonitis (see Case 32), but generally metabolic activity seen in non-neoplastic, inflammatory processes is modest compared with that seen in most cancers.

CASE 13 | Lung cancer staging, primary positive (proven adenocarcinoma)

A 79-year-old woman had an RUL mass noted on CXR, obtained because of a possible Horner's syndrome on physical examination (Figure 1). CT confirmed a spiculated mass (Figure 2). Diagnosis of a non–small cell lung carcinoma was made with CT-guided percutaneous biopsy. Only the tumor was positive on PET scanning, suggesting a stage I lesion (Figure 3). She underwent a right upper lobectomy with in-continuity mediastinal lymphadenectomy. Pathology showed

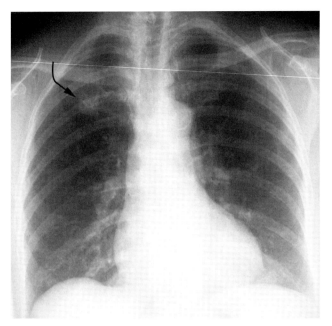

FIGURE 1. A frontal CXR shows an asymmetrical nodular density at the level of the anterior end of the right first rib, suggesting an underlying nodule (*arrow*).

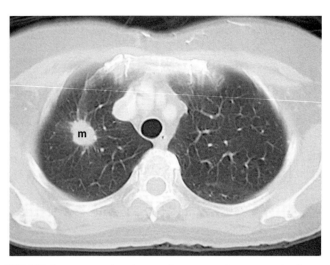

FIGURE 2. Lung window from a chest CT confirms a spiculated RUL mass (m), with a typical appearance of a bronchogenic carcinoma.

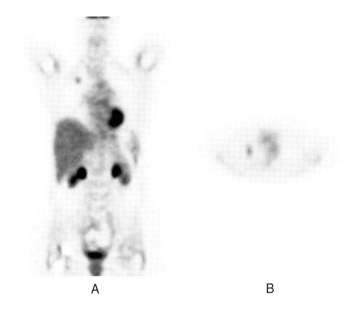

A

B

C

FIGURE 3. PET images (coronal [**A**], axial [**B**] and sagittal [**C**]) show the lesion to be metabolically active, although not as intense as other examples in this chapter. No additional disease was identified. PET did not suggest hilar or mediastinal involvement and thus underestimated the extent of disease found at surgery (one positive hilar lymph node). However, even if this disease site had been seen on PET that would not have changed the preoperative assessment of the lesion's resectability.

an invasive, poorly differentiated 2-cm adenocarcinoma, with one of six hilar lymph nodes positive for metastatic adenocarcinoma. Four right paratracheal lymph nodes were negative. Postoperative stage was stage IIA.

TEACHING POINTS

Preoperative nodal staging of lung carcinomas based on anatomic imaging alone is notoriously unreliable, relying as it does predominantly on lymph node size. Tumor involvement in normal size lymph nodes is missed, and nodal involvement is overestimated when there is coexisting benign or reactive lymph node enlargement. PET offers the ability to noninvasively assess nodal status and can identify tumor in normal size lymph nodes. FDG uptake is proportionate to tumor metabolic activity and extent of lymph node involvement. Accordingly, PET is likely to miss nodal micrometastases.

In lung cancer staging, it is important to recognize that ipsilateral hilar nodal metastatic disease does not generally preclude a patient from surgery. The important distinction is from contralateral hilar and/or mediastinal involvement, which generally indicates a patient is incurable by surgery.

CASE 14 | *Lung cancer staging, primary only positive (NSCLC), coexisting infiltrative lung disease*

A 69-year-old woman, a long-standing cigarette smoker with oxygen-dependent chronic obstructive pulmonary disease, developed worsening shortness of breath. A CXR showed diffuse changes of chronic infiltrative lung disease, with a mass in the superior segment of the RLL (Figure 1), which was confirmed on chest CT (Figure 2). Bronchoscopy showed no endobronchial lesions, and biopsies, washing, and brushings were negative for malignancy. A CT-guided biopsy

confirmed non–small cell carcinoma. PET imaging showed increased metabolic activity corresponding to the mass identified on chest CT. It also showed a diffuse, low-level rim of mild activity at the periphery of both lungs (Figure 4). Correlation with chest CT suggests this corresponds to the patient's peripheral changes of chronic infiltrative lung disease with honeycombing (Figure 3). No additional disease sites were suggested by PET, but the patient's pulmonary dysfunction excluded her from surgery.

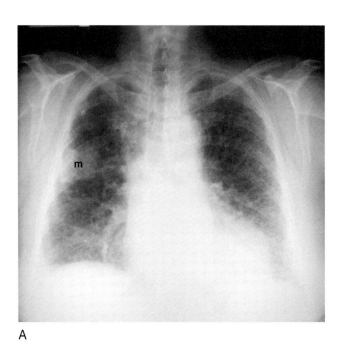

A

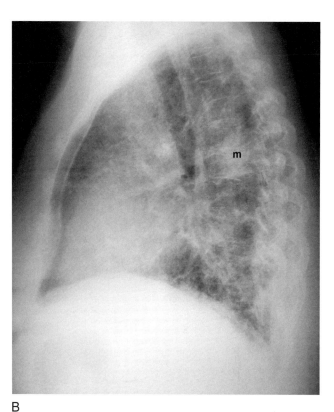

B

FIGURE 1. Posteroanterior (**A**) and lateral (**B**) views of the chest show advanced changes of chronic infiltrative lung disease, with coarsening of the pulmonary interstitium, particularly peripherally. A mass (m) localizes to the superior segment of the RLL.

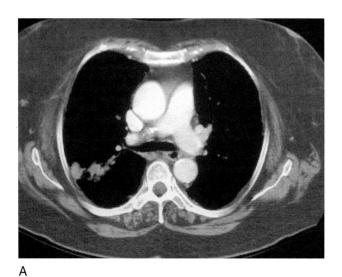

A

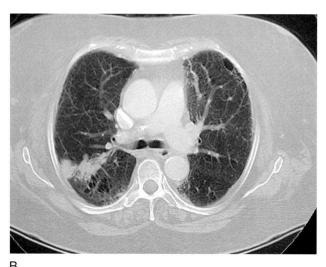

B

FIGURE 2. Mediastinal (**A**) and lung (**B**) windows from the enhanced chest CT show a bilobed, irregular, nodular abnormality in the superior segment of the RLL, corresponding to the CXR. This occurs in a background of lung disease, better demonstrated in Figure 3.

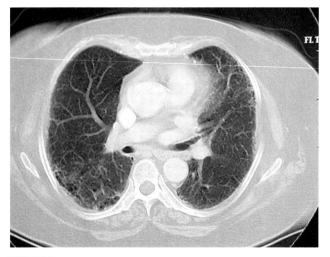

FIGURE 3. A more inferior lung window shows advanced changes of chronic infiltrative lung disease, with peripheral septal line thickening and cystic subpleural lung destruction, or honeycombing.

TEACHING POINTS

Coexisting benign and malignant pulmonary parenchymal processes usually display differential levels of metabolic activity on PET, aiding in the distinction between them. There is overlap, but typically, malignancies are markedly hypermetabolic, with benign processes displaying lower level, less intense metabolic activity. Examples include postobstructive pneumonitis (see Case 12) and collapse (see Case 26) and coexisting lung disease (as in this case with chronic infiltrative lung disease). There is some evidence that PET may have a role to play in the assessment of the activity of infiltrative and inflammatory lung diseases, because it may be more sensitive to disease activity than gallium.

Correlation with CT suggested that the rim of peripheral thoracic activity noted in this case was produced by the patient's advanced lung disease. A similar appearance can be produced by other causes, including pleural disease (effusion), intercostal muscle activity, and a long segment of activity in a rib. Correlation with CT should enable identification of peripheral lung disease and pleural abnormalities, whereas rib activity would be more isolated and localized than generalized intercostal muscle activity.

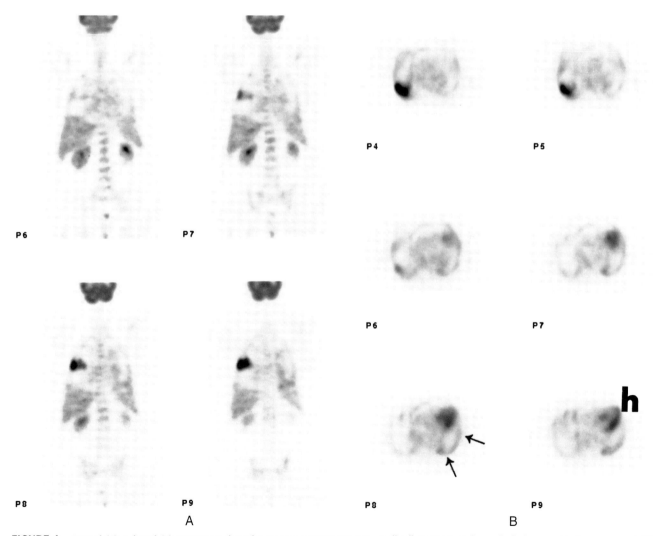

FIGURE 4. Coronal (**A**) and axial (**B**) PET images show the superior segment RLL non–small cell carcinoma to be markedly hypermetabolic, as expected. Note also the metabolically active outline of both lungs, best seen at the left base, correlating with the advanced chronic infiltrative lung disease on CT (*arrows*) (h = heart).

CASE 15 | Lung cancer staging, primary site only positive (proven squamous cell carcinoma)

A 58-year-old woman with asthma presented with hemoptysis. On CXR, a left suprahilar mass was suggested (Figure 1). On chest CT, this proved to be an LUL infiltrate (Figure 2). A small left hilar soft tissue density mass versus adenopathy was also identified (Figure 3). Bronchoscopy was performed for further evaluation. LUL biopsies returned poorly differentiated squamous cell carcinoma. Staging with PET imaging demonstrated a solitary left hilar focus of hypermetabolic activity, corresponding to the left hilar mass or adenopathy on CT, with no other abnormalities (Figure 4). The patient underwent a left upper lobectomy. Pathology showed a 2.1-cm, invasive, poorly differentiated

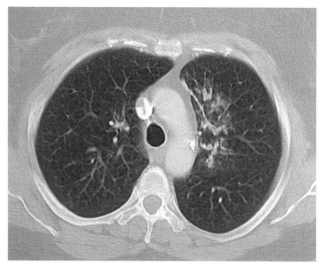

FIGURE 2. Chest CT shows CXR findings are produced by left suprahilar infiltrate.

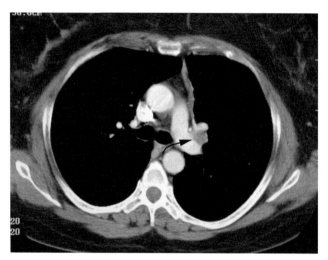

FIGURE 3. A more inferior section (soft tissue window) at the level of the left pulmonary artery shows a left hilar soft tissue density mass (arrow). Differential diagnosis includes a central primary bronchogenic carcinoma versus adenopathy, whether neoplastic or inflammatory.

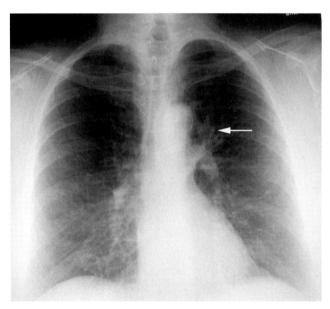

FIGURE 1. Frontal chest radiograph shows a left suprahilar opacity, possibly a mass (arrow).

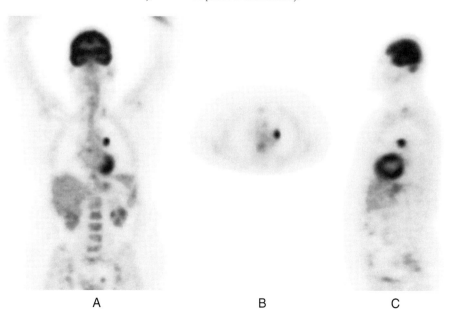

FIGURE 4. PET images demonstrate the marked hypermetabolism of the small left hilar mass noted on CT. No evidence of mediastinal involvement or remote disease was seen. Coronal (**A**), transaxial (**B**), and sagittal (**C**) views are shown.

A   B   C

squamous cell carcinoma at the hilus. Unfortunately, there was extensive involvement of the bronchial margin of resection. Seventeen examined lymph nodes showed no evidence of metastatic squamous cell carcinoma. However, two of the lymph nodes were involved by direct extension from the adjacent mass. The patient returned to surgery 2 weeks later, at which time a left pneumonectomy was completed. No residual tumor was identified in the specimen, with the previous bronchial resection margin showing fibrosis and giant cell reaction and the new bronchial and vascular margins negative for tumor. Six subcarinal lymph nodes from this specimen showed no metastatic disease. Twenty LLL lymph nodes were also negative.

TEACHING POINT

PET is a valuable aid in accurate staging of known lung cancer, with a high negative predictive value of approximately 95%. If the mediastinum is negative on PET imaging, a patient may be considered for curative surgery and obviate the need for mediastinoscopy.

CASE 16 | Lung cancer staging, with subtle mediastinal involvement (squamous cell carcinoma)

A 72-year-old man, followed for idiopathic pulmonary fibrosis (IPF), was found to have an LUL mass on CXR (Figure 1). Chest CT confirmed a 3.5-cm pleural-based mass (Figure 2). This was accompanied by lymph nodes on the order of 1 cm in the aortopulmonary window and left hilus (Figure 3). CT-guided biopsy confirmed moderate to poorly differentiated squamous cell carcinoma. PET scan showed intense hypermetabolism of the mass, with subtle increased activity in the left hilus (Figures 4 and 5). Mediastinoscopy was negative.

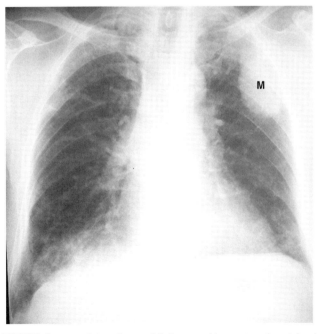

FIGURE 1. Frontal CXR shows a lobular, smoothly marginated, peripheral LUL mass (M). Diffuse coarsening of lung parenchymal markings is noted and best seen in periphery of right lung. The patient had a known diagnosis of idiopathic pulmonary fibrosis.

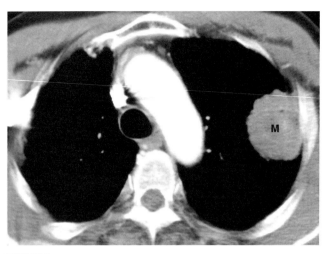

FIGURE 2. Contrast medium–enhanced chest CT confirms a lobular, soft tissue density LUL mass (M), with a broad base of pleural abutment. No frank chest wall transgression is evident here. A tiny prevascular lymph node is also noted.

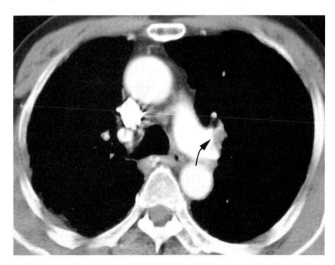

FIGURE 3. A more inferior chest CT section through the left pulmonary artery shows mild left hilar and aortopulmonary window adenopathy, on the order of 1 cm and not clearly pathologic (arrow).

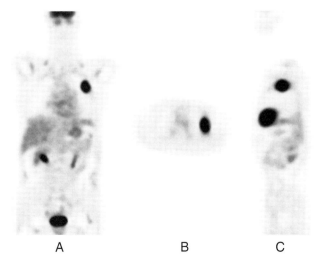

A   B   C

FIGURE 4. PET images through the LUL mass, showing marked hypermetabolism of the known squamous cell carcinoma. No comment can be made based on PET regarding the chest wall involvement suggested by the patient's symptoms and progressive chest CT findings (not shown). Coronal (**A**), transaxial (**B**), and sagittal (**C**) views are shown.

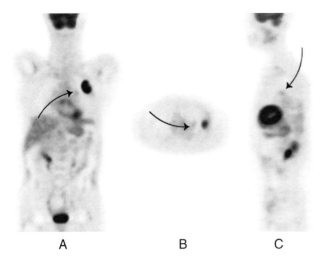

A   B   C

FIGURE 5. PET images in the same planes through the left hilus show faintly increased metabolic activity over background mediastinum, corresponding to borderline lymph node noted on CT (*arrows*). Mediastinoscopy was falsely negative, as shown by the final pathology (6/10 positive lymph nodes). Coronal (**A**), transaxial (**B**), and sagittal (**C**) views are shown.

During the course of these evaluations, the patient developed chest wall pain in the area corresponding to the lesion. Repeat chest CT showed interval growth of the lesion and suggested chest wall involvement. He was treated with left upper lobectomy with in-continuity chest wall resection and mediastinal lymphadenectomy. Pathology showed a 5.5-cm moderately to poorly differentiated squamous cell carcinoma with involvement of chest wall soft tissue, as well as 6 of 10 lymph nodes with metastatic carcinoma. The largest focus of nodal metastasis measured 1 cm (Figure 6; see color plate 5). Post-resection stage was stage IIIA (T3N2M0).

TEACHING POINTS

PET scanning generally is not helpful in evaluating chest wall invasion, or in assessing direct mediastinal or vital organ invasion. Although of high resolution compared with traditional nuclear medicine images, such extension may only be suggested on PET imaging in cases of frank transgression (see Case 24).

Contrast this case with Case 9. Both show very faintly increased nodal uptake, just above background mediastinal activity. In this case, the activity, although markedly disproportionate to the intense primary lesion, corresponded to pathologically proven nodal involvement on histology, despite sampling error at mediastinoscopy. The largest focus of nodal metastatic tumor identified at pathology in this case measures 1 cm, just at the threshold for detectability on PET imaging.

CASE 17 | *Non–small cell lung cancer, with mediastinal involvement*

An asymptomatic 71-year-old woman had a CXR while establishing care with a new physician. This showed an unexpected 6-cm mass in the anterior segment of the RUL, with possible right-sided adenopathy. Chest CT showed the 5 × 6 cm mass in the RUL, with a long margin of anterior pleural abutment. An enlarged right paratracheal lymph node was noted (Figure 1). Bronchoscopic washings yielded a diagnosis of non–small cell carcinoma. PET scan was positive at the site of the RUL mass and at the level of the right paratracheal lymph node seen on CT (Figure 2). She was treated with neoadjuvant chemotherapy and radiation therapy.

TEACHING POINT

The intensity of activity of mediastinal nodes is an important clue in assessing the significance of nodal activity on PET. When the activity of lymph nodes is as intense as that of the primary lesion, such as in this case, the assumption that they are malignant and metastatic can more readily be made. Less intense nodal activity is much less specific. There is overlap between the PET findings of metastases in normal size lymph nodes, and the activity seen in benign postinflammatory or reactive lymph nodes. Mediastinoscopy may be required for differentiation.

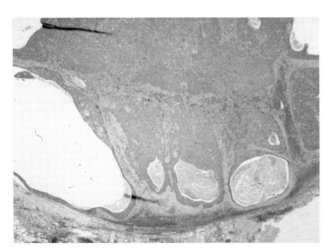

FIGURE 6. Low-power H & E–stained view of the lymph node with the largest focus (1 cm) of metastatic tumor. Cystic degeneration is seen within the tumor. See color plate 5. (Courtesy of Gary Wilcox, MD, Tri City Medical Center, Oceanside, CA.) (See color plate 5.)

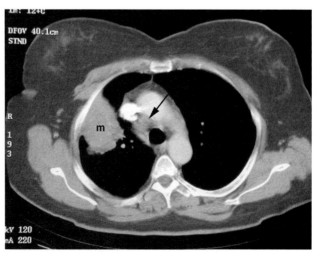

FIGURE 1. Enhanced chest CT section at the aortopulmonary window level shows a 5 × 6-cm pleural-based RUL mass (m) accompanied by an enlarged right paratracheal lymph node (*arrow*).

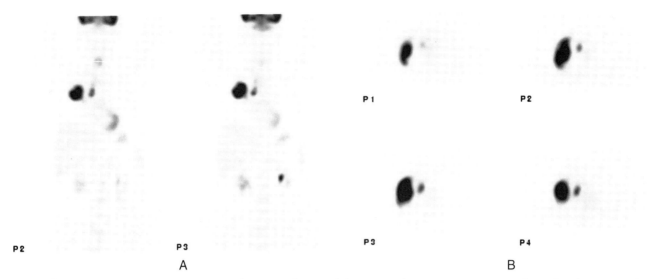

P1   P2

P2   P3   P3   P4

A   B

FIGURE 2. Coronal (**A**) and axial (**B**) PET scan views show intense hypermetabolic activity in the RUL primary tumor, as well as at the right paratracheal nodal level.

CASE 18 | *Lung cancer staging, with mediastinal disease (large cell carcinoma)*

A 75-year-old woman developed a dry cough and right shoulder pain. A CXR showed a large RUL mass. Chest CT showed a low-density, irregularly marginated mass in the posterior segment of the RUL, invaginating into the retrotracheal mediastinum (Figure 1). It was accompanied by a suspicious, enlarged, low-density right paratracheal lymph node. Bronchoscopy showed an RUL endobronchial lesion, but brushings and biopsies were negative. CT-guided biopsy established a diagnosis of large cell lung carcinoma. A PET scan was obtained to confirm the impression of inoperability (Figure 2). It demonstrated the tumor to be necrotic and displayed intense hypermetabolic activity in the metastatic right paratracheal lymph node. The patient

was treated with chemotherapy for quality of life palliation, with second-line therapy begun when she subsequently developed a brain metastasis.

TEACHING POINTS

This patient's lung cancer was inoperable both because of mediastinal invasion and the involvement of mediastinal lymph nodes. In this case, the right paratracheal lymph node was abnormal in morphology (size and density) and displayed metabolic activity comparable to that of the primary lung carcinoma, leaving essentially no doubt of its involvement. Given that increased metabolic activity can be seen in some benign and reactive lymph nodes, less clearly abnormal lymph nodes should be histologically evaluated with mediastinoscopy, so that patients will not be excluded from a potentially curative surgery based only on the suggestion of involvement by PET.

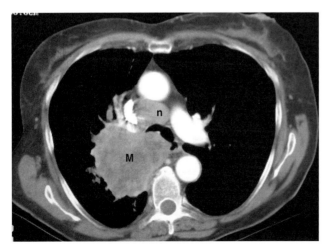

FIGURE 1. Enhanced chest CT image shows a large, low-density, irregularly marginated posterior segment RUL lung carcinoma occluding the right bronchus and invaginating deeply into the retrotracheal mediastinum (M). A pathologically enlarged right paratracheal lymph node is of similar low density to the primary tumor (n).

CASE 19 | Lung cancer staging, with bone metastasis (adenocarcinoma)

A 54-year-old previously healthy man was evaluated with a CXR after a motor vehicle accident and found to have an unsuspected RUL mass. A chest CT confirmed an irregularly marginated RUL mass, accompanied by enlarged prevascular, right paratracheal, right hilar, and subcarinal lymph nodes (Figures 1 and 2). Biopsy of the mass with fluoroscopic guidance proved it to be an adenocarcinoma. PET showed both the lung carcinoma mass and the adenopathy to be metabolically active (Figure 3). A focal site of hypermetabolic activity was also noted in the L4 vertebral body, suggestive of a bone metastasis. This changed the apparent disease stage to stage IV, which was confirmed with bone scan and lumbar spine MRI (Figure 4).

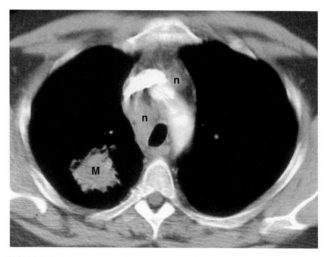

FIGURE 1. Contrast medium–enhanced chest CT, mediastinal window, shows the soft tissue density, irregularly marginated, posterior segment RUL lung carcinoma mass (M). Enlarged lymph nodes are noted in the right paratracheal and prevascular regions (n).

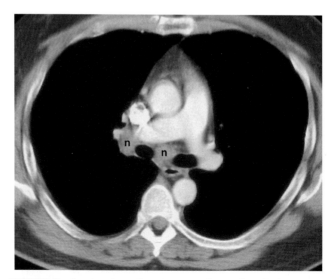

FIGURE 2. A more inferior chest CT section shows enlarged right hilar and subcarinal lymph nodes (n).

FIGURE 2. PET (coronal [**A**] and axial [**B**]) shows the RUL tumor as a ring of hypermetabolism, with central necrosis. The right paratracheal lymph node, enlarged and suspicious on CT, is as metabolically active as the primary tumor and consistent with a nodal metastasis (*arrows*).

P4   P5

P6   P7

A

P4   P5

P6   P7

B

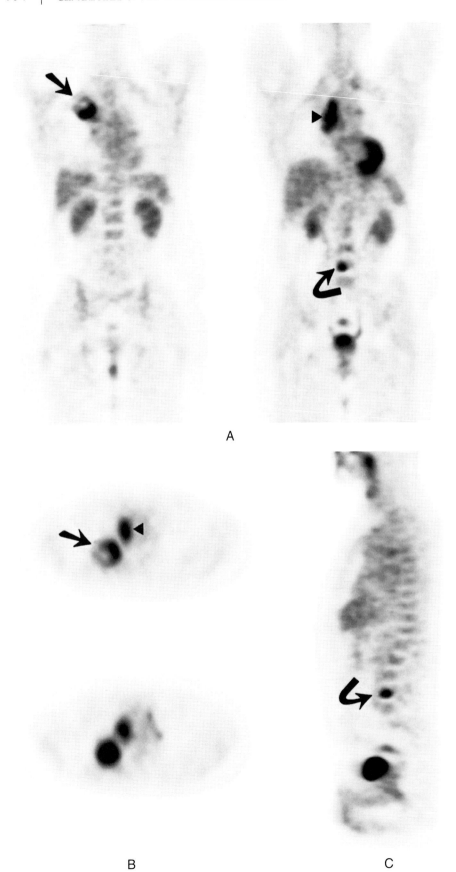

A

B

C

FIGURE 3. On PET (selected coronal [A], axial [B] and sagittal [C] sections), the RUL mass shows central hypometabolism, consistent with necrosis (*arrows*). The right paratracheal nodal mass is as intense in activity as the primary tumor, consistent with nodal metastasis (*arrowheads*). A solitary osseous focus of hypermetabolism, localizing to the L4 vertebral body, is suggestive of a bone metastasis (*curved arrows*).

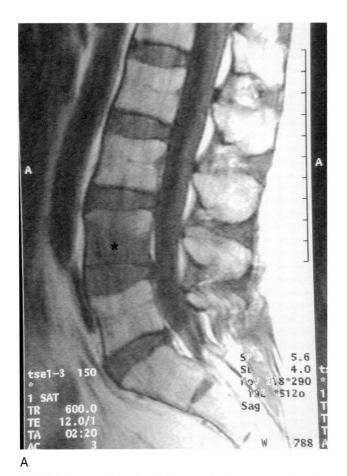

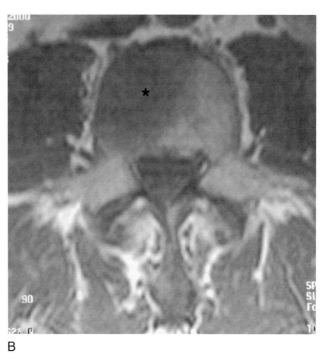

A   B

FIGURE 4. Sagittal (**A**) and axial (**B**) T1-weighted MR images confirm abnormal marrow signal intensity in the right anterior L4 vertebral body, consistent with metastasis (*asterisks*).

TEACHING POINTS

PET scan results frequently will change the apparent stage of a patient's disease. In this case, the chest CT findings suggested stage III disease, with PET suggesting the true diagnosis of stage IV disease. Because nonmalignant processes, such as compression fractures and discogenic disease, can produce spinal findings on PET, it is prudent to confirm suspected solitary osseous metastatic lesions with another modality, preferably MRI.

CASE 20 | Lung cancer staging, with bone metastases (large cell malignancy)

An 83-year-old woman was evaluated with CXR for left shoulder and pleuritic pain and hemoptysis and was found to have a 9-cm pleural-based LUL lung mass (Figure 1). CT showed the mass to abut the posterolateral chest wall without definite rib destruction (Figures 2 and 3). No enlarged lymph nodes were identified. Diagnosis of large cell malignancy with necrosis was made by CT-guided percutaneous biopsy. Further evaluation included bone scintigraphy and PET. The bone scan was abnormal, with increased activity in the right sacroiliac region, thought to be suggestive of metastatic disease (Figure 4). PET imaging showed the LUL primary lesion to be hypometabolic centrally, consistent

with necrosis, with intense FDG accumulation in the periphery of the lesion. In addition, there were multiple sites of abnormal FDG activity localizing to bone, including in the right sacroiliac region noted on bone scan. Abnormally increased hypermetabolic activity was also noted in the left sacroiliac region and in the spine, ribs, sternum, and proximal femora. Osseous metastatic disease was presumed (Figure 5). Pelvic MRI was recommended to confirm this impression. It showed patchy foci of abnormal bone marrow signal in a corresponding distribution, also most consistent with bone metastases (Figures 6 to 8).

TEACHING POINTS

Diffusely increased bone marrow activity can be seen with marrow activation, which is most frequently noted in patients receiving cytokine chemotherapy, such as for lymphoma. See Cases 7 and 8 in Chapter 4. Patchiness of marrow activity and atypical clinical scenario in this case are most consistent with bone metastases.

PET and bone scanning can be complementary in the assessment for bone metastases. It is well documented that lytic metastases, often normal on bone scan, may be visualized as hypermetabolic sites with PET. In this case, PET and MRI show diffuse osseous metastases, much more extensive than suggested by bone scan. However, the converse can occur, and, on occasion, a nonspecific PET scan musculoskeletal finding may be more accurately characterized on bone scan. FDG uptake is noted in benign skeletal processes, such as rib and vertebral compression fractures, analogous to bone scans.

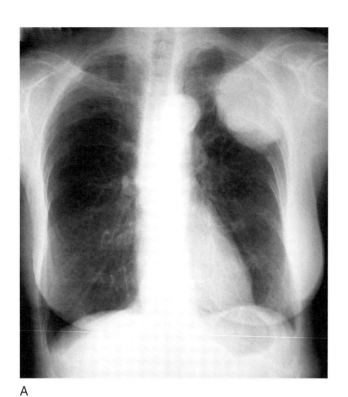
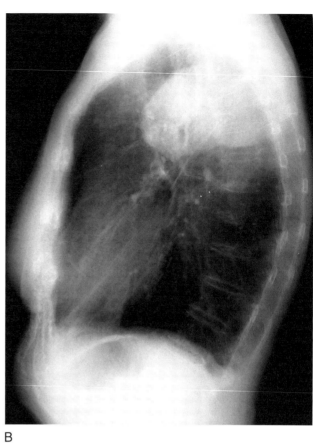

A

B

FIGURE 1. Posteroanterior (**A**) and lateral (**B**) CXR views show a large, smoothly marginated, lobulated, pleural-based mass in the posterior LUL.

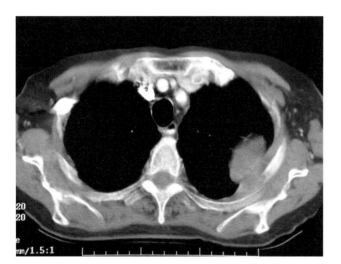
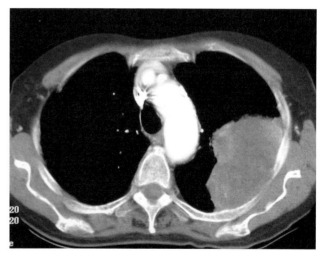

FIGURE 2. Enhanced chest CT section shows the superior aspect of the mass, with thickening of the adjacent pleura.

FIGURE 3. More inferior chest CT section through epicenter of mass shows it to be relatively low density, suggesting necrosis. Broad base of pleural abutment is noted. Tumor extension to intercostal muscle level is suggested without frank rib destruction.

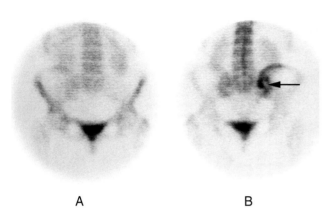

FIGURE 4. Anterior (**A**) and posterior (**B**) pelvis views from a bone scan show focal, inhomogeneous, abnormally increased activity at the right sacroiliac joint level (*arrow*). Pattern is not typical of a joint centered (arthritic or degenerative) process, and metastasis seemed most likely.

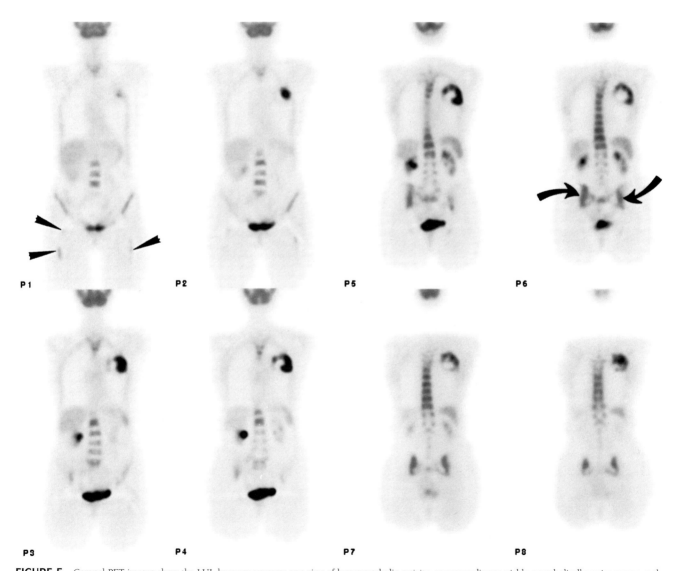

FIGURE 5. Coronal PET images show the LUL lung cancer mass as a ring of hypermetabolic activity, corresponding to viable, metabolically active tumor at the periphery of the lesion, especially laterally. Central necrosis is more easily appreciated on PET than CT. Note asymmetry of activity at sacroiliac joint levels (*arrows*), right greater than left, with both more than normally active, as is the spine. Activity in the spine appears relatively homogeneously increased. Note patchy foci of increased activity in the proximal femora (*arrowheads*). These findings suggested diffuse osseous metastatic disease, much more extensive than was apparent on bone scan.

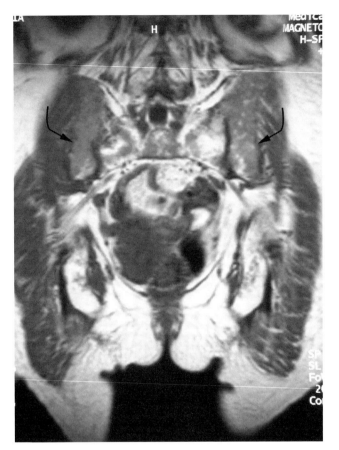

FIGURE 6. T1-weighted coronal MR image through the sacroiliac joints shows abnormally decreased marrow signal intensity of juxtasacroiliac ilia bilaterally (*arrows*). Pictured sacrum and ischia are of more normal fatty marrow signal.

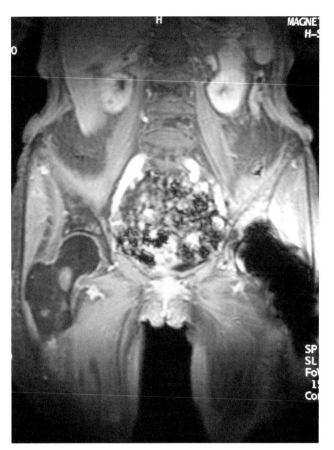

FIGURE 8. Corresponding fat-saturated, enhanced T1-weighted coronal MR image shows right proximal femoral metastases well.

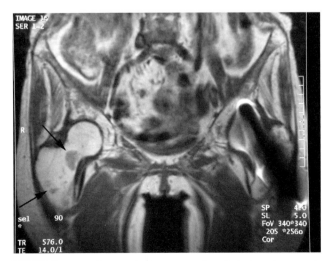

FIGURE 7. Coronal T1-weighted MR image through the hips shows patchy metastatic foci in the right femoral neck and proximal femur (*arrows*) as well as more geographic regions of abnormal marrow signal in the ilia. Left hip pinning susceptibility artifact is noted.

CASE 21 | *Lung cancer staging, stage IV non–small cell lung cancer, with adrenal metastasis*

A 75-year-old woman presented with productive cough and hemoptysis. Past medical history was significant for 60 pack-year smoking history and chronic obstructive pulmonary disease. CXR demonstrated an RLL mass. Chest CT evaluation confirmed a 4 × 4.5-cm RLL mass, with an adjacent 2-cm satellite focus (Figure 1). Liver lesions were noted, thought to be benign, including a probable hemangioma, as well as additional, smaller lesions that were difficult to characterize. Diagnosis of large cell carcinoma was made by CT-guided biopsy of the RLL mass. PET imaging was performed to assess operability. It demonstrated intensely increased metabolic activity in the known lung carcinoma mass, but it also demonstrated hyperintense left adrenal activity, most consistent with an adrenal metastasis and stage IV disease (Figure 2). No abnormal activity was seen in the liver, confirming the CT impression of benign lesions. Concurrently ordered MRI of the liver confirmed hemangiomas and cysts in the liver and demonstrated a small, enhancing left adrenal mass, consistent with a metastasis, which had not been noted prospectively on CT (Figure 3). Because the

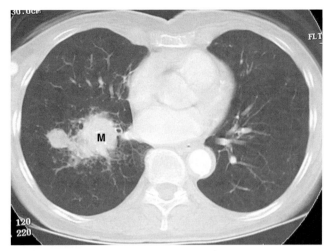

FIGURE 1. Chest CT (lung window) shows 4 × 4.5-cm irregularly marginated RLL mass (M), with surrounding pneumonitis and adjacent, 2-cm satellite-type lesion.

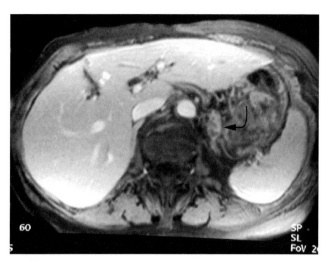

FIGURE 3. Enhanced, fat-saturated axial MR image through the upper abdomen shows small, inhomogeneously enhancing 2 × 1-cm left adrenal metastasis (*arrow*).

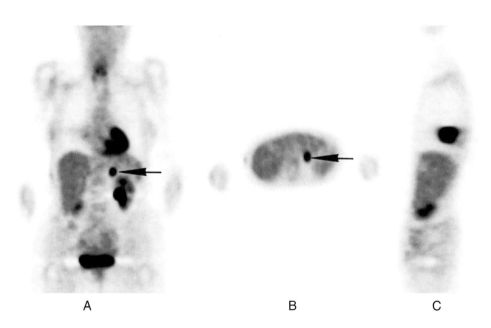

FIGURE 2. Coronal (**A**) and axial (**B**) PET images show hypermetabolic left adrenal activity (*arrows*). Diagnosis of metastatic lung cancer was confirmed by fine-needle aspiration of the adrenal gland. Faint RLL activity on the coronal view is attributable to the pneumonitis associated with the tumor (this section is posterior to the tumor mass). Sagittal (**C**) PET image through the RLL shows marked hyperintensity of the known non–small cell lung cancer.

A   B   C

patient's disease otherwise seemed to be confined to the RLL and she was without other evidence of distant disease, histologic confirmation was obtained of metastatic lung cancer to the adrenal gland by fine-needle aspiration.

TEACHING POINT

PET is an efficient, whole-body method of staging a neoplasm such as the non–small cell lung cancer in this case. The scenario illustrated by this case is a common clinical dilemma. When there is coexisting suspected lung cancer and an indeterminate adrenal mass, this previously required either two percutaneous biopsies (lung and adrenal) or separate MRI adrenal evaluation, with in- and out-of-phase imaging, to differentiate between the two most common causes of adrenal masses: adenomas and metastasis.

CASE 22 | *Lung cancer, restaging post treatment, with adrenal metastasis (large cell carcinoma)*

A 37-year-old man was evaluated for severe back pain with x-rays, that suggested an LUL density. A CXR was obtained for confirmation. It identified a large LUL mass (Figure 1). CT confirmed a 7-cm necrotic mass, extending from the superior hilus to the apex, and abutting the major fissure posteriorly (Figure 2). CT-guided biopsy was positive for large cell carcinoma, with features suggesting adenocarcinoma. During his staging evaluation, the patient was found to have a femoral metastasis, which was treated with radiation, as well as chemotherapy.

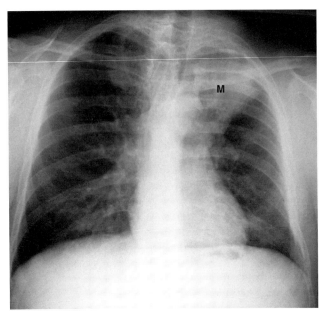

FIGURE 1. Posteroanterior CXR shows a large mass (M), localizing to the LUL.

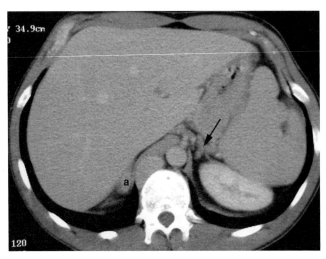

FIGURE 3. Upper abdominal section shows mild enlargement of the right adrenal gland (a), raising the question of adrenal involvement. No abnormality was prospectively suggested of the left adrenal gland (*arrow*).

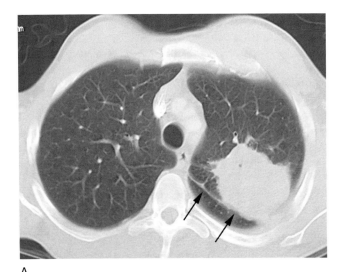

A

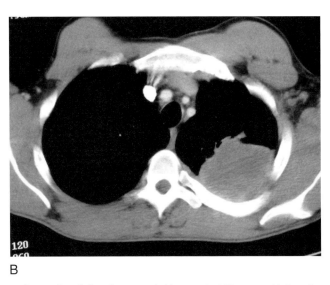

B

FIGURE 2. Lung (**A**) and mediastinal (**B**) windows from an enhanced chest CT confirm a relatively low density, probably necrotic, LUL mass, with irregular, spiculated margins. This typical-appearing lung carcinoma mass abuts the major fissure posteriorly (*arrows*).

He was evaluated with PET scanning approximately a year after diagnosis, while still undergoing chemotherapy. This demonstrated intense persistent activity in the LUL mass, as well as intense hypermetabolism in the left adrenal gland, consistent with metastasis, not previously suspected (Figures 3 and 4). The patient later developed left hand weakness, and brain MRI confirmed intracranial metastatic disease, treated with gamma knife and whole-brain irradiation.

TEACHING POINTS

PET scanning in this case showed persistent activity in the periphery of the in situ, chemotherapeutically treated LUL primary lesion. It also identified unexpected distant metastatic adrenal activity, where no mass was evident morphologically.

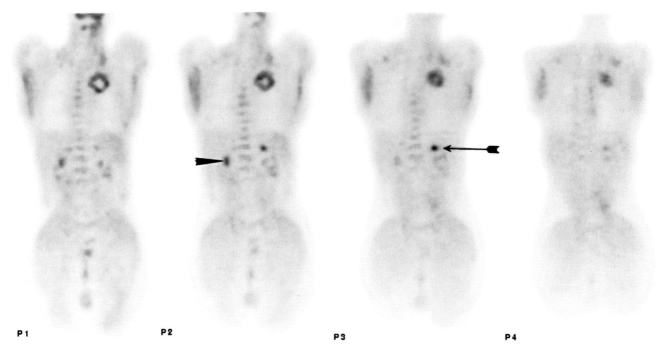

P1   P2   P3   P4

FIGURE 4. PET shows a rind of increased metabolic activity in the centrally hypometabolic and necrotic LUL mass, despite 1 year's treatment with chemotherapy. The small focus of hypermetabolic activity at the left adrenal gland level is consistent with a metastasis (*arrow*). Note activity of similar intensity at the right upper pole renal level, which represents collecting system activity (*arrowhead*). Review of cases on a workstation eases making such distinctions.

CASE 23 | *Squamous cell carcinoma, stage IV, with axillary node involvement*

An 89-year-old previously healthy and active man developed left anterior chest wall pain, radiating into the axilla and arm. CXR showed an anterior LUL mass. Chest CT showed the mass to be 4 cm, pleural based, and extending into the chest wall (Figure 1). The mass was accompanied by an enlarged left axillary lymph node (Figure 2). Histologic sampling of the LUL mass was accomplished with fine-needle aspiration and core biopsy technique, revealing moderately to poorly differentiated squamous cell carcinoma. A bone scan showed uptake in the left second and third anterior ribs, supporting suspected chest wall invasion (Figure 3). PET scan showed intense activity in the LUL mass, as well as activity at the site of the enlarged left axillary lymph node (Figure 4). The patient was referred for irradiation for palliation of symptoms, with initial good response. Eight months later, he again developed increasing left upper anterior chest wall pain, and on reexamination he was found to have new palpable nodules in the left subpectoral and umbilical regions. Palliative chemotherapy for relief of symptoms was then begun.

TEACHING POINT

Chest wall invasion was suggested in this case by symptoms, CT, and localized bone scan activity. PET can only demonstrate chest wall invasion in cases where there is frank extension through the chest wall, when lesional activity actually projects outside the thoracic confines (see Case 24) but generally does not demonstrate lesser chest wall involvement. In this case, activity in the left axillary lymph node helped to confirm the CT and clinical impression of stage IV disease. In a younger patient, in whom more aggressive therapy might have been considered, the patient probably would have undergone an excisional biopsy of the node to confirm involvement.

Caution needs to be exercised in selecting a side for injection if questions of axillary involvement are anticipated. Analogous to nodal activity visualized on bone scans proximal to an injection site, focal axillary activity can be seen on PET scans when the ipsilateral upper extremity is injected. Accordingly, when the involvement of the axilla is of particular interest, the injection should preferentially be made in the contralateral upper extremity.

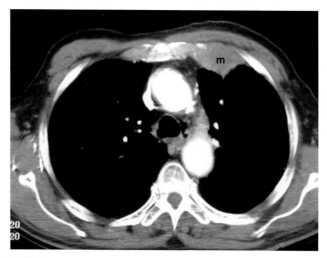

FIGURE 1. Contrast medium–enhanced chest CT at the AP window level shows a triangular pleural-based mass (m) in the anterior LUL, which extends into the intercostal muscle.

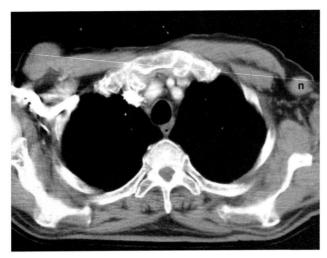

FIGURE 2. A more superior section, through the superior mediastinum, shows an enlarged left axillary lymph node (n), corresponding to the painful, palpable lesion.

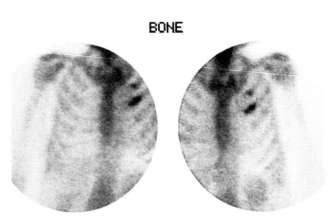

FIGURE 3. Anterior thoracic bone scan images show localized activity in the left anterior second and third ribs, a scintigraphic pattern suggesting chest wall invasion.

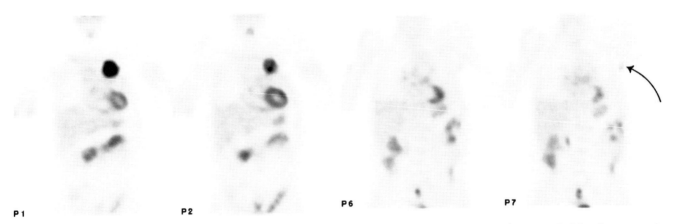

FIGURE 4. Coronal PET images show intense hypermetabolic activity in the LUL squamous cell carcinoma. Activity is also seen in the left axilla, corresponding to the enlarged lymph node, and helping to confirm the impression of stage IV disease (*arrow*).

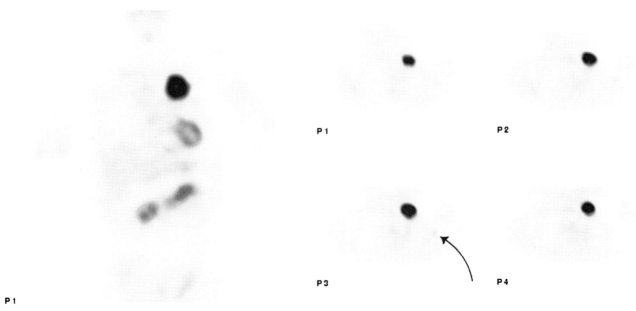

FIGURE 5. Axial PET images through the LUL squamous cell lung cancer do not permit confident prediction of chest wall involvement, better demonstrated in this case on CT and bone scan. Less intense activity in the metastatic left axillary node is also noted (*arrow*).

CASE 24 | Lung cancer (squamous cell carcinoma), with chest wall invasion

A 65-year-old man was evaluated with CXR for complaints of sub-scapular chest wall pain and was found to have an LUL mass. His past medical history was significant for coronary artery disease, status post coronary artery bypass grafting, and chronic obstructive pulmonary disease, with a pack per day smoking habit. Chest CT confirmed the LUL mass to be spiculated and pleural based, with irregularity of the underlying rib suggesting chest wall invasion (Figure 1). No enlarged lymph nodes or distant metastases were seen. Transthoracic needle biopsy yielded a diagnosis of squamous cell carcinoma. PET scan showed pathologic uptake of FDG only at the site of the lesion. The patient underwent induction chemoradiation therapy, with initial remission of pain. Repeat chest CT, 4 months later, showed growth of the mass, with more clear destruction and replacement of the underlying rib (Figure 2). Repeat PET scan, 2 weeks after completion of chemoradiation, showed persistent intense activity at the site of the lesion, which now projected into the chest wall (Figure 3). No new or additional sites of abnormal activity were seen. Surgical resection, with reconstruction of the chest wall, was performed. Final pathology was moderately differentiated squamous cell carcinoma with chest wall involvement. Final margins were negative, and eight hilar lymph nodes were negative for metastatic carcinoma.

TEACHING POINTS

PET scanning is of limited utility in assessing mediastinal, chest wall, or organ invasion. Only fairly florid examples, such as this case of chest wall invasion, will be accurately depicted. This assessment must primarily lie with traditional modalities, namely CT, supplemented with bone scan and MRI in individual cases.

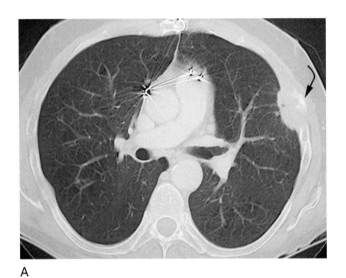

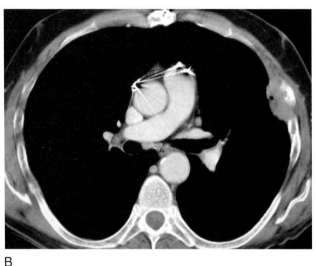

A   B

FIGURE 1. Lung (**A**) and mediastinal (**B**) windows from an enhanced chest CT show an ovoid, peripheral, pleural-based LUL mass, with spiculated margins (*arrow*). Mass appears to extend into the underlying chest wall, with irregularity of the rib. No pathologically enlarged lymph nodes are present.

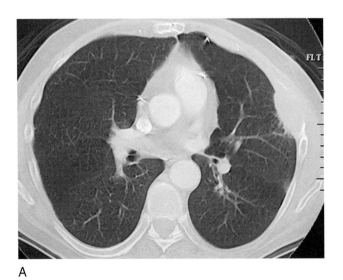

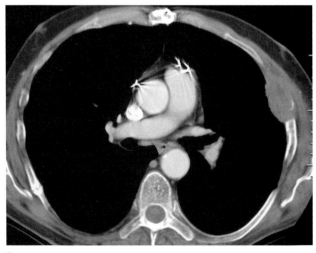

A   B

FIGURE 2. **A** and **B**, Repeat enhanced chest CT, 4 months after chemoradiation, shows interval growth of the mass, increased chest wall penetration, and replacement and destruction of the underlying rib. No other changes were seen.

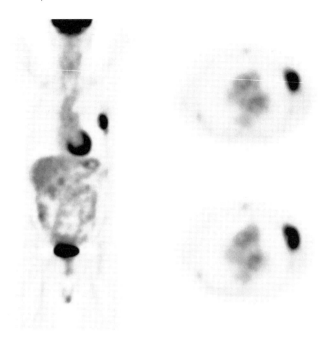

FIGURE 3. PET scan, performed after induction chemoradiation, shows intense activity at the site of the LUL squamous cell carcinoma mass, which projects into the chest wall, best appreciated on the axial images.

In this case, PET was utilized to restage the patient after chemoradiation of his primary lesion, prior to surgery, to confirm that his disease remained confined.

CASE 25 | *Known lung cancer for staging, extensive disease (squamous cell carcinoma)*

A 69-year-old woman presented with a COPD exacerbation. A CXR showed an abnormal right suprahilar density. Chest CT showed this to be bulky, confluent right hilar and mediastinal adenopathy, with a 1.5 cm mass in the posterior segment of the RUL (Figures 1 and 2). A small additional nodule was seen in the lingula (Figure 3). Bronchoscopy showed an extrinsic mass occluding the posterior segment RUL bronchus. Transbronchial biopsy demonstrated moderately differentiated invasive squamous cell carcinoma. PET scan showed intense activity in the confluent right hilar and mediastinal mass, as well as activity in the tiny lingular nodule (Figure 4). Because of the extensive nature of her disease, she was treated with chemotherapy only.

TEACHING POINT

PET scan confirmed inoperable disease in this patient and even identified metabolic activity in the 5-mm lingular nodule. A nodule of this size is problematic for detection on PET scan. However, the demonstration of any activity, however faint, in such a small lesion must be regarded as suspicious.

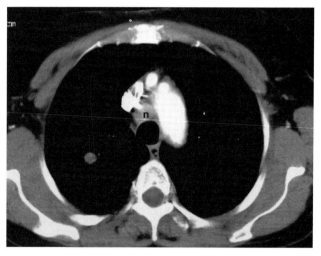

FIGURE 1. Enhanced chest CT shows a lobular soft tissue density nodule in the posterior RUL, accompanied by a suspiciously enlarged right paratracheal lymph node (n).

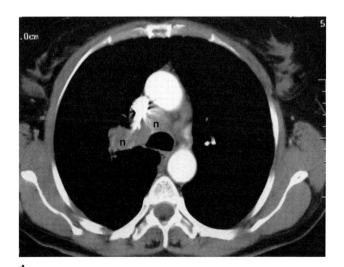

A

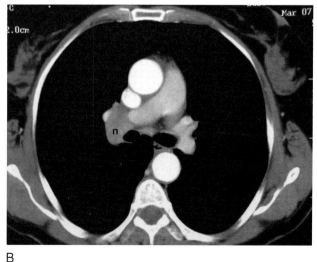

B

FIGURE 2. Contrast medium–enhanced chest CT images (**A** and **B**) through the mediastinum show confluent, bulky adenopathy in the aortopulmonary window, right paratracheal and right hilar levels (n).

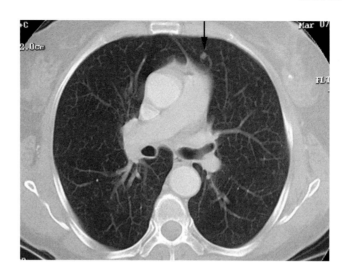

FIGURE 3. In the lingula, chest CT lung windows show a small (5 mm) nodule (*arrow*).

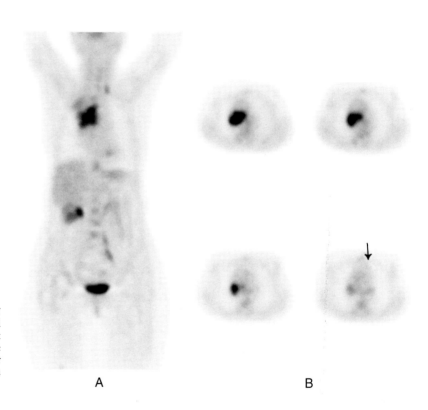

FIGURE 4. Coronal (**A**) and four contiguous axial (**B**) PET images show a hypermetabolic mass at the right paratracheal mediastinal and hilar level, corresponding to the confluent nodal mass noted on CT. The most inferior axial PET image shows metabolic activity at the level of the small lingular nodule (*arrow*). Visualization of any activity on PET in such a small nodule must be considered suspicious.

A   B

CASE 26 | *Lung cancer staging, extensive disease (NSCLC)*

A 62-year-old man with a 50 pack-year smoking history developed a cough. A CXR showed LUL consolidation. When the CXR abnormality persisted after treatment with antibiotics, a chest CT was obtained. This showed dense atelectasis and consolidation of the LUL and a left hilar mass, accompanied by low-density enlarged lymph nodes at prevascular, right paratracheal, aortopulmonary window and left hilar levels (Figures 1 to 3). Bronchoscopic evaluation showed a fungating mass occluding the LUL bronchus. Biopsy identified non–small cell carcinoma. PET scanning confirmed the extensive nature of disease and demonstrated additional disease sites, including the right supraclavicular region (Figure 4). He was referred for chemotherapy for palliation of symptoms and initially demonstrated a response to gemcitabine (Gemzar) and carboplatin, but soon relapsed, with worsening cough, and progressive disease clinically and on CT. He died 4 months after diagnosis.

TEACHING POINTS

Lung carcinoma masses that produce bronchial obstruction and lobar collapse can occasionally be difficult to identify and separate from collapsed lung on CT. This PET scan illustrates intense activity at tumor

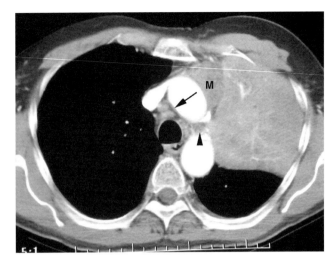

FIGURE 1. Enhanced chest CT at the level of the aortopulmonary window shows dense atelectasis and consolidation of the LUL, with a prevascular nodal mass (M), as well as borderline size right paratracheal lymph nodes (*arrow*). A round, low density lymph node is suspicious as well in the aortopulmonary window, although it is not particularly enlarged (*arrowhead*).

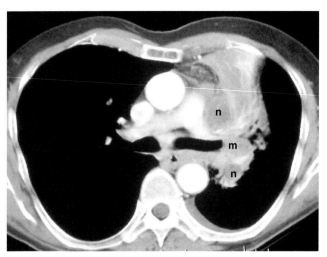

FIGURE 3. A more inferior section, through the right pulmonary artery, again shows atelectasis of the LUL, with occluding left hilar mass (m), with accompanying enlarged, low-density left hilar lymph nodes (n). A small left pleural effusion is also seen.

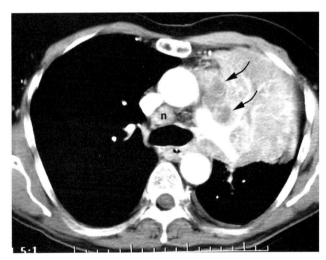

FIGURE 2. More inferior section, through the left pulmonary artery level, shows multiple, low-density masses at the prevascular and left hilar levels (*arrows*), as well as a pathologically enlarged right paratracheal lymph node (n). Densely consolidated LUL is enhanced.

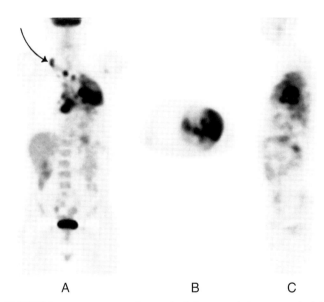

A   B   C

FIGURE 4. PET scan images show markedly hypermetabolic tumor at the left hilar level, as well as activity corresponding to the mediastinal adenopathy depicted on CT. Additional sites of hypermetabolic tumor activity are seen at unexpected sites, including the right supraclavicular region (*arrow*). Less intense activity peripheral to the left hilar tumor activity represents collapsed LUL. Coronal (**A**), transaxial (**B**), and sagittal (**C**) views are shown.

sites, particularly the left hilus, with lesser activity corresponding to the consolidated lung. This examination confirmed extensive, stage IV disease in this patient, even showing unsuspected sites not imaged on CT.

CASE 27 | Lung cancer staging, small cell carcinoma

A 76-year-old woman presented with a cough. She was referred for PET scan evaluation for staging of a small cell lung carcinoma. Chest CT available for correlation showed pathologically enlarged right paratracheal, right hilar, subcarinal, and azygoesophageal recess adenopathy. PET scan showed hypermetabolic disease activity at all of the recognized chest CT abnormalities. It also demonstrated multiple, previously unrecognized foci of disease activity that localized to the abdomen and to bone, consistent with advanced and widely disseminated disease.

TEACHING POINTS

Small cell carcinoma is generally so advanced at diagnosis that patients are not curable by surgery and are treated with chemotherapy and irradiation. Accordingly, the application of PET in lung cancer staging is generally for non–small cell carcinomas. However, small cell lung carcinomas are FDG avid, so if a patient appeared by imaging to have limited-stage disease, PET would be effective in evaluating for distant metastases. In this case, although it appeared by staging CT that this patient's disease was inoperable, PET more fully demonstrated the widely disseminated distribution of disease.

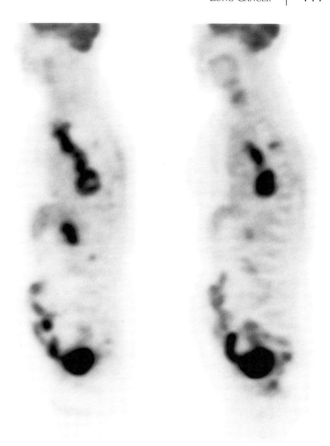

FIGURE 2. Sagittal PET sections show the longitudinal orientation of the right paratracheal and azygoesophageal recess level nodal activity. Foci of pathologic activity in the abdomen and pelvis contrast to normal bowel activity by focality and intensity. A thoracic spine focus of activity is additional evidence of bone involvement.

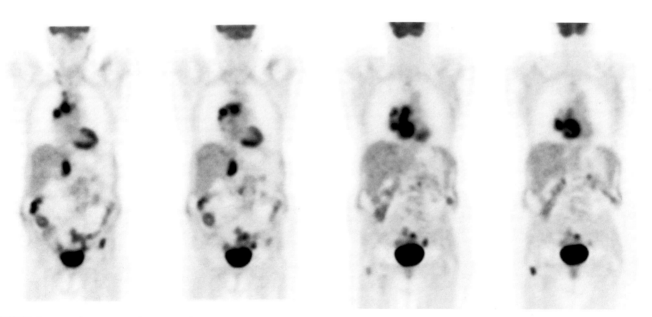

FIGURE 1. Coronal PET images show intense hypermetabolism at multiple levels, including in the chest, abdomen, and bone. Intense thoracic activity is seen where CT showed enlarged mediastinal nodal disease. Marked activity is also noted scattered within the abdomen and pelvis. Bone metastases are suggested by foci in the left acetabulum and the right proximal femur.

CASE 28 | Lung cancer staging, localized pleural involvement (NSCLC and adenocarcinoma)

A 60-year-old woman with a history of left lung fungal infection was followed with CXRs and noted to have a possible LUL nodule. A chest CT showed an irregular LUL infiltrate, with a cavitated, mass-like appearance (Figure 1). Necrotizing pneumonia, tuberculosis, and neoplasm were considered in the differential diagnosis. The patient was initially evaluated with bronchoscopy. Biopsies, brushings, and washings showed no evidence of malignancy. CT-guided biopsy was then performed, yielding a diagnosis of large cell carcinoma. PET scanning was requested for staging (Figure 2). It showed intense LUL activity in the apical-posterior segment, corresponding to the CT lesion. The morphology of the activity, with a peripheral linear component, suggested the possibility of local pleural involvement. The hila and mediastinum and remainder of the PET scan were negative. The patient underwent left upper lobectomy. The specimen showed a focal region of visceral pleural puckering, overlying the 3.2-cm neoplasm. The lung neoplasm showed

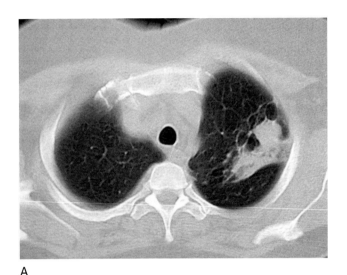
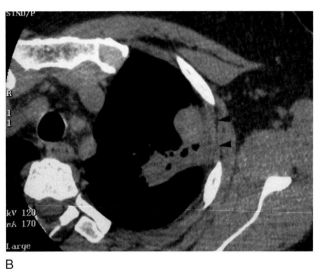

A   B

FIGURE 1. Chest CT images (**A** and **B**) through the LUL abnormality show the process to abut the major fissure posteriorly. There appear to be two components, one more rounded and mass-like anteriorly, the other geographic and infiltrate-like. Note the localized lateral pleural thickening, best seen on the mediastinal window detail view (**B**, *arrowheads*).

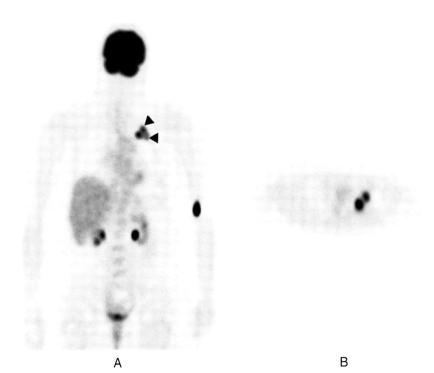

A   B

FIGURE 2. Coronal (**A**) and axial (**B**) PET scan views show corresponding LUL hypermetabolic activity. On the coronal section, the lateral component assumes a linear configuration, suggesting the possibility of localized pleural involvement. This was confirmed histologically and correlated with the CT findings (*arrowheads*). No other disease was seen. Note the left antecubital fossa "injectoma."

a variegated histology, with poorly differentiated solid non–small cell carcinoma and well to moderately differentiated adenocarcinoma. Infiltration through the visceral pleura was noted, as well as lymphatic and vascular invasion. Nine peribronchial lymph nodes were negative for neoplasm, as well as one hilar lymph node. Postoperatively, the patient was treated with radiation and sensitizing chemotherapy.

TEACHING POINT

This case illustrates an unusual manifestation of localized pleural involvement due to direct extension. Hematogenous involvement of the pleural space generally is more nodular and diffuse in distribution (see the next two cases).

 CASE 29 | *Lung cancer staging, pleural adenocarcinoma*

A 41-year-old man presented with a right pleural rub, abdominal distention, shortness of breath with shallow breathing, and occasional stabbing right rib margin pain. A CXR showed a lobular right pleural effusion (Figure 1). Chest CT confirmed a small amount of pleural fluid, with extensive enhancing soft tissue density pleural masses, some focally nodular and others more confluent (Figures 2 to 4). Biopsy confirmed adenocarcinoma. PET scan demonstrates typical findings of pleural neoplasia, with lobular hyperintense activity along pleural surfaces (Figures 5 to 7). No disease was identified elsewhere.

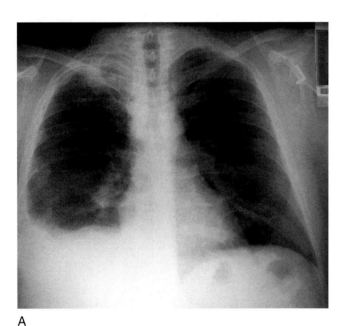

A

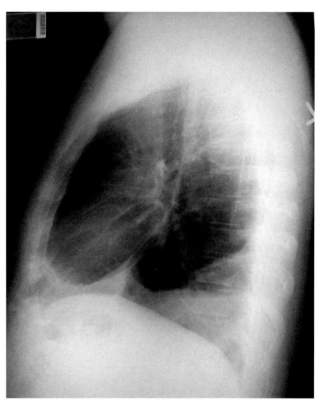

B

FIGURE 1. Posteroanterior (**A**) and lateral (**B**) CXR views show lobular right pleural disease. Differential diagnosis for these findings includes pleural neoplasia (e.g., metastases and mesothelioma) and complicated pleural effusion (empyema with loculations).

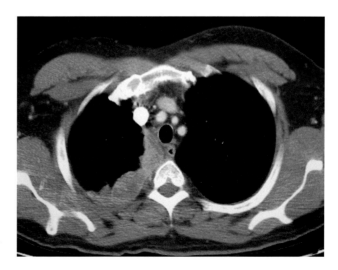

FIGURE 2. Enhanced chest CT image through superior mediastinum shows thick, lobular, enhancing soft tissue neoplasia within the pleural space.

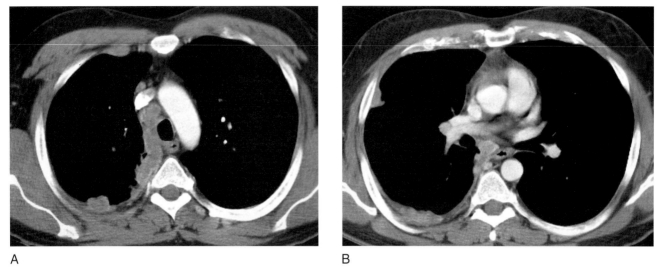

A

B

FIGURE 3. More inferior chest CT sections (**A** and **B**) show similar findings to Figure 2, with focal nodules and more confluent tumor studding pleural surfaces. Both of these sections also show soft tissue nodules at the expected positions of right paratracheal and subcarinal lymph nodes. Without performing a diagnostic pneumothorax, it is not possible to distinguish between mediastinal adenopathy and pleural metastases within invaginations of pleura into the mediastinum.

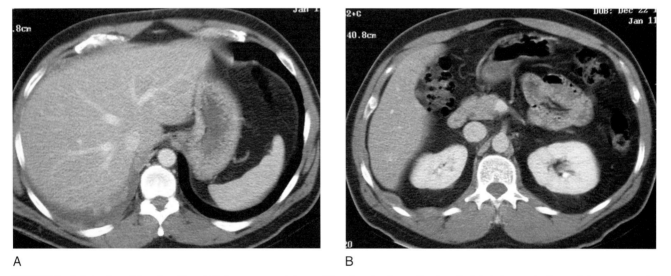

A

B

FIGURE 4. Inferior chest CT sections (**A** and **B**) show tumor nodules studding pleural surfaces. Note how far inferiorly over the liver and down even to the kidney level the posterior costophrenic sulcus and pleural space extend.

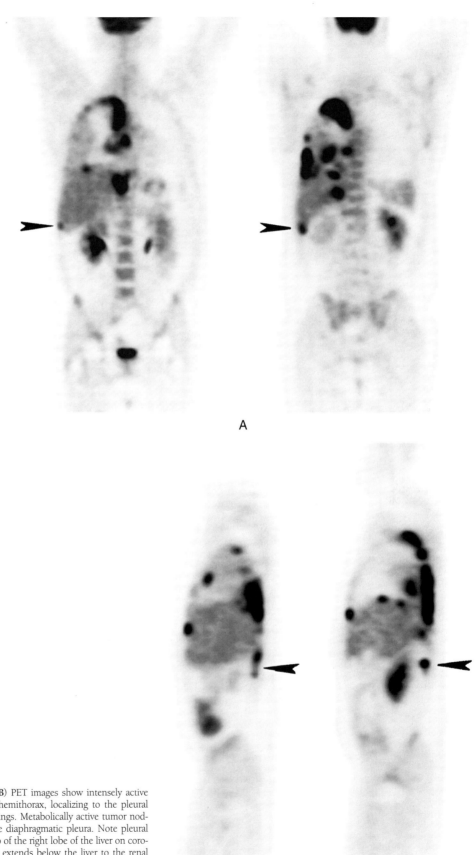

FIGURE 5. Coronal (**A**) and sagittal (**B**) PET images show intensely active tumor along the periphery of the right hemithorax, localizing to the pleural space and correlating with chest CT findings. Metabolically active tumor nodules projecting on the liver dome involve diaphragmatic pleura. Note pleural tumor activity projecting at the inferior tip of the right lobe of the liver on coronal images (*arrowheads*). Similarly, tumor extends below the liver to the renal level in the posterior costophrenic sulcus (*arrowheads*), well seen on sagittal sections.

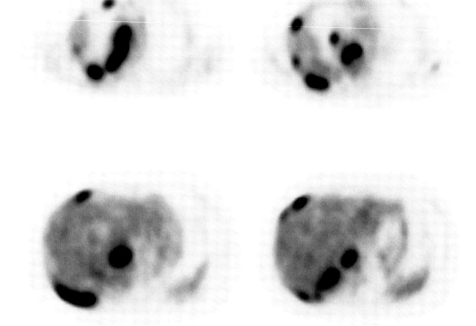

FIGURE 6. Axial PET images correspond in level to CT images in Figure 3.

FIGURE 7. More inferior axial PET images correspond to Figure 4. Note the far medial invagination of costophrenic pleural reflection.

The patient was treated with chemotherapy. After an initial promising response, he later relapsed with widely metastatic disease, including extension to adrenal and bone. He died 9 months after diagnosis.

TEACHING POINTS

PET reminds us, in this case, of important anatomic relationships. A cursory review of this case might initially suggest that this patient has intra-abdominal disease, in addition to extensive right hemithoracic involvement. The tumor nodules projecting in close proximity to the liver, particularly those in far inferior and medial costophrenic pleural reflections, could be mistaken for intra-abdominal metastases. Knowledge of these relationships and imaging correlation ensure accurate anatomic localization and staging of disease. It is also important to have a thorough understanding of the most likely patterns of disease spread for any particular histology, which may help to link findings in individual cases.

CASE 30 | Non–small cell lung carcinoma, metastatic to pleura

A 69-year-old man noted a decrease in energy and shortness of breath in aerobics class and on CXR evaluation was found to have a large right pleural effusion. Contrast-enhanced chest CT showed nodular pleural enhancement in addition to the fluid (Figure 1). A pleural biopsy diagnosed a non–small cell malignancy. PET scan showed a rind of increased metabolic activity surrounding the right lung, consistent with pleural malignancy, but no other sites of disease (Figure 2). He was treated with 6 months of chemotherapy. Repeat PET scan showed

a change in the pattern of the right pleural activity, from a continuous rind, to more discrete pleural nodules, also metabolically active and consistent with progression of pleural malignancy (Figure 3). CT confirmed decreased pleural fluid and replacement with confluent enhancing pleural soft tissue disease (Figure 4). The patient was maintained on a variety of chemotherapy regimens over the next year before dying, 18 months after diagnosis.

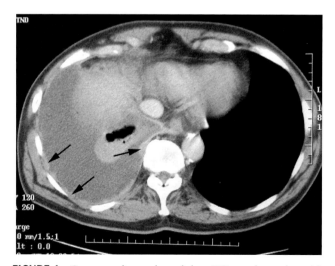

FIGURE 1. Contrast medium–enhanced chest CT image shows a large right pleural effusion. Diffuse nodular enhancement of the pleura is outlined by the fluid (*arrows*). Findings are typical of a malignant pleural effusion, whether from lung primary tumor or metastatic, with mesothelioma in the differential diagnosis as well.

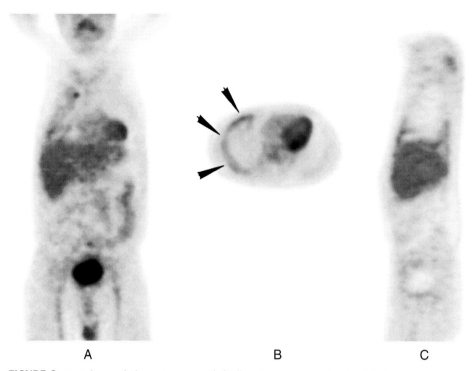

FIGURE 2. PET shows a fairly continuous metabolically active rim surrounding the right lung, consistent with malignant pleural disease (*arrowheads*). Coronal (**A**), transaxial (**B**), and sagittal (**C**) views are shown.

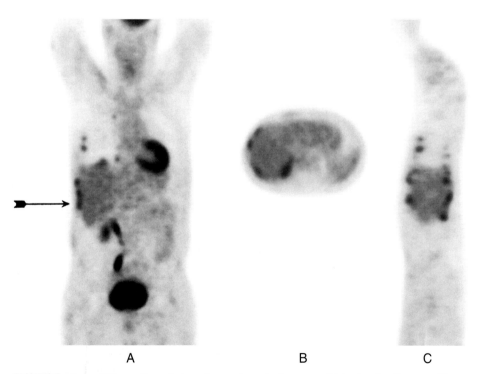

FIGURE 3. Repeat PET scan, 6 months later, shows a change in the pattern of right pleural malignancy, with more discrete linear and nodular foci of intensely increased metabolic activity. Note how far inferiorly the pleural space extends over the liver (*arrow*). Without CT correlation, it could be difficult to localize the activity that projects on the liver surface to the pleural space, rather than the peritoneum. Coronal (**A**), transaxial (**B**), and sagittal (**C**) views are shown.

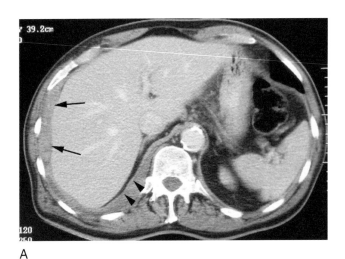
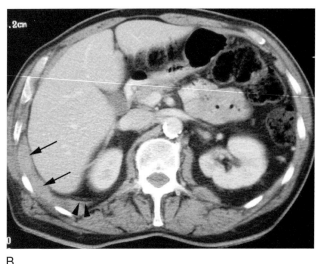

A   B

FIGURE 4. **A** and **B,** CT shows a confluent, enhancing soft tissue density rind of progressive pleural metastases (*arrows*). Correlation of the PET with CT, which shows the disease to be above the diaphragm (*arrowheads*), allows confident localization of the PET findings to the pleural space, and not the peritoneum.

CASE 31 | *Lung cancer restaging, treatment assessment (squamous cell carcinoma)*

A 65-year-old woman was evaluated with a CXR for complaints of progressive low back pain and fatigue. A 2-cm LUL nodule was noted. CT evaluation confirmed a spiculated LUL mass (Figure 1) and noted smooth enlargement of the left adrenal gland as well (Figure 2). CT-guided LUL biopsy was performed, and a diagnosis of small cell, undifferentiated carcinoma was made. She was treated with neoadjuvant chemotherapy for presumed limited-stage small cell lung cancer, prior to small field radiation. CT re-evaluation, after chemotherapy and before irradiation, showed the LUL lesion to have responded minimally and the adrenal gland to be stable. When the mass was noted on follow-up after completion of irradiation to have increased in size, she was re-evaluated for surgery with a negative metastatic work-up. PET scan showed metabolic activity only in the LUL lesion (Figure 3). She underwent a left upper lobectomy with in-continuity hilar and mediastinal lymphadenectomy. Final pathologic diagnosis of the 1.7-cm tumor was poorly differentiated squamous cell carcinoma. Eleven lymph nodes were negative.

TEACHING POINTS

PET scan was utilized in this case to re-stage this patient's disease after chemotherapy and irradiation to confirm the impression of limited-stage disease, prior to surgery. It provided further reassurance that the stable adrenal mass was benign.

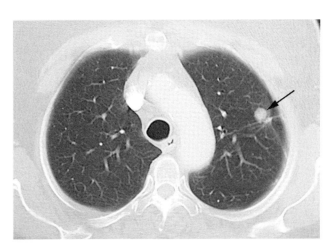

FIGURE 1. Lung window chest CT image shows small, peripheral, relatively well-marginated LUL mass (*arrow*). Lateral pleura is puckered, and there is a tiny pneumothorax.

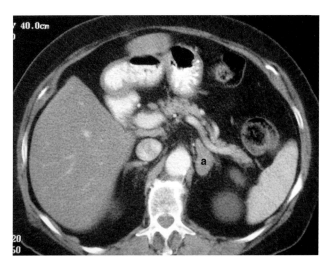

FIGURE 2. Enhanced upper abdominal CT image shows a smoothly marginated left adrenal mass, scintigraphically inactive on PET, consistent with a benign etiology, probably an adenoma (a).

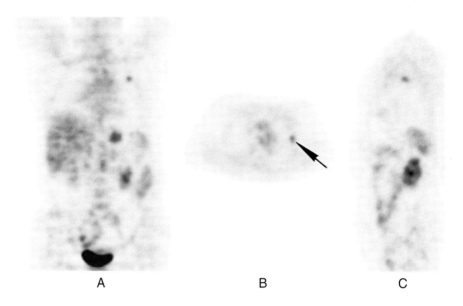

FIGURE 3. Three plane PET images show the hypermetabolic LUL cancer (*arrow*) but no evidence of involvement elsewhere, including in the left adrenal region. Coronal (**A**), transaxial (**B**), and sagittal (**C**) views are shown.

CASE 32 | Lung cancer restaging, radiation therapy effects (squamous cell carcinoma)

A 78-year-old man with LUL squamous cell carcinoma (Figure 1) was treated by irradiation and chemotherapy. He returned for repeat PET scanning 4 months after completion of therapy. PET scan showed complete resolution of the intense LUL tumor activity, replaced by a linear paramediastinal band of less intense activity, consistent with radiation therapy effect (Figure 2). Continued follow-up showed progressive improvement as the radiation-induced inflammation regressed.

TEACHING POINTS

Radiation therapy effects display variable degrees of metabolic activity, depending on the degree of pneumonitis incited and the time course since therapy. Findings due to radiation changes can be relatively intense and at times confused with tumor activity. It is desirable to wait as long as possible after completion of radiation therapy before imaging with PET, optimally a minimum of 2 months. The usually geographic and linear margins of radiation therapy pneumonitis are sufficiently characteristic that recognition of the process is not difficult. What can be disconcerting is the intensity of activity that can be seen in the early postirradiation period and the protracted length of time that it can take to resolve (months to upward of a year).

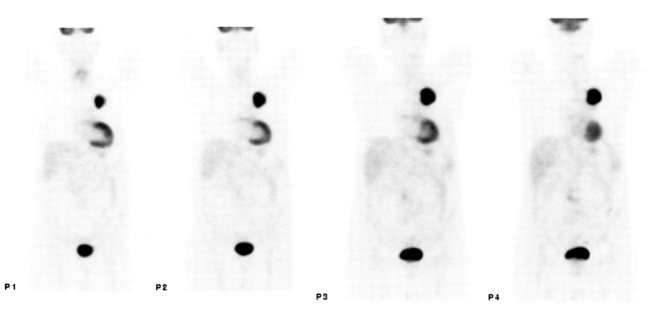

FIGURE 1. Coronal PET scan images at the time of staging work-up show an intensely hypermetabolic LUL focus of tumor activity, corresponding to the known squamous cell carcinoma.

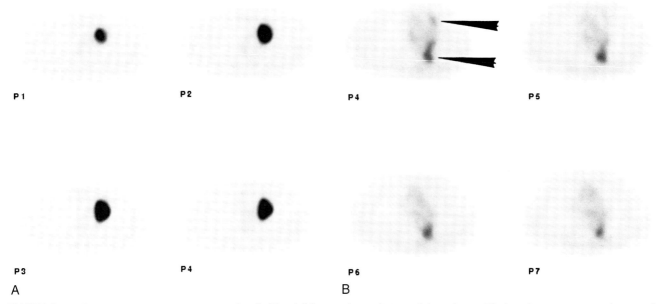

FIGURE 2. Axial PET scan images, juxtaposing original study (**A**) with follow-up after irradiation and chemotherapy (**B**), show the tumor activity to be gone. The follow-up study, 7 months after the first study and 4 months after completion of therapy, shows a less active left paramediastinal band of activity, consistent with radiation therapy effect (*arrowheads*).

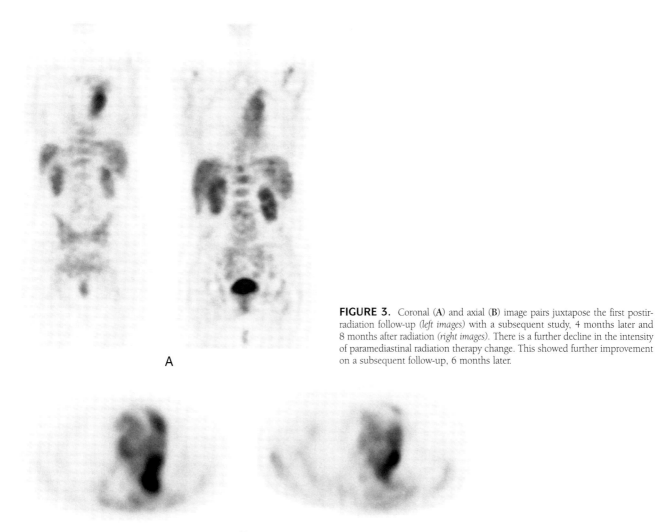

FIGURE 3. Coronal (**A**) and axial (**B**) image pairs juxtapose the first postir-radiation follow-up (*left images*) with a subsequent study, 4 months later and 8 months after radiation (*right images*). There is a further decline in the intensity of paramediastinal radiation therapy change. This showed further improvement on a subsequent follow-up, 6 months later.

CASE 33 | *Bilateral lung cancers*

A 76-year-old woman with emphysema presented with a spontaneous pneumothorax and was found on CXR to have a mass in the posterior RUL. Her past medical history was significant for a 30 pack-year smoking history. CT evaluation showed an irregular 2-cm mass (Figure 1), which was sampled with CT guidance after bronchoscopy revealed only moderate atypia. Pathology showed non–small cell carcinoma. PET evaluation showed two hypermetabolic lesions, one in the posterior RUL corresponding to the known lesion (Figure 2) and another in the superior segment of the LLL (Figure 3), correlating with a smaller, but similar-appearing chest CT lesion (Figure 4). She was considered to have stage IV disease and was treated with chemotherapy with gemcitabine (Gemzar) and carboplatin, with near resolution on follow-up CT. Unfortunately, subsequent brain CT evaluation for headache revealed a presumed brain metastasis.

TEACHING POINTS

The significance of the second lesion in this patient was not fully realized until the PET scan showed it to be hypermetabolic, and therefore

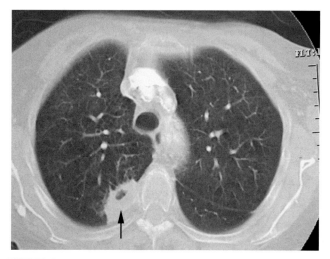

FIGURE 1. Chest CT (lung window) shows a cavitary, pleural-based mass with irregular margins and spiculation, localizing to the posterior segment of the RUL (*arrow*).

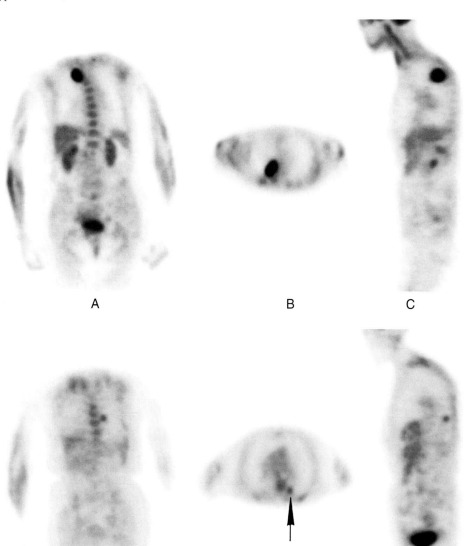

FIGURE 2. PET scan images in coronal (**A**), axial (**B**), and sagittal (**C**) planes show intense hypermetabolic activity at the site of the known posterior RUL non–small cell carcinoma.

A　　　　　　　B　　　　　　　C

FIGURE 3. PET scan images in three planes at another level also show intense activity in a smaller, second lesion in the superior segment of the LLL (*arrow*). Coronal (**A**), transaxial (**B**), and sagittal (**C**) views are shown.

A　　　　　　　B　　　　　　　C

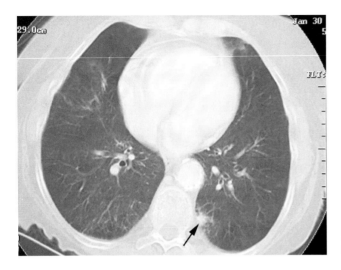

FIGURE 4. Correlation with CT shows the corresponding lesion to be pleural based, small (8 mm), and similar in appearance to the RUL lesion (*arrow*).

almost certainly malignant as well. The course of this patient's management was redirected once it was realized she had multifocal disease. This case also serves to illustrate the ability of PET to demonstrate subcentimeter disease. The threshold for detection of pulmonary nodules depends on lesion size, location, and intrinsic metabolic activity of the tumor. Nodules greater than 1 cm can reliably be seen; and with current instrumentation, nodules of 8 mm can be seen regularly.

CASE 34 | *Breast carcinoma pulmonary metastases mimicking synchronous lung cancers*

An 80-year-old woman with emphysema was found to have an LUL mass on CXR. This was confirmed on chest CT, which also showed a similar-appearing, suspicious RLL lesion (Figure 1). FNA of the LUL lesion was consistent with a non–small cell lung carcinoma.

The patient's past medical history was significant for prior left mastectomy for breast cancer nearly 20 years previous. Lymph nodes were reportedly negative, and she did not undergo additional therapy at that time. She also had a significant past smoking history, on the order of 1.5 packs per day.

The PET scan showed both the LUL and RLL lesions to be hypermetabolic (Figure 2). Based on the information available, this result seemed most consistent with synchronous lung cancers. However, subsequent immunocytochemical stains performed on the material obtained from fine-needle aspiration suggested the cause to be metastatic breast carcinoma.

TEACHING POINT

PET does not discriminate between malignant causes, and although morphology, smoking history, and initial fine-needle aspiration results suggested non–small cell lung cancer, further immunostain study of the aspirated material suggested the final diagnosis of metastases from a breast primary tumor.

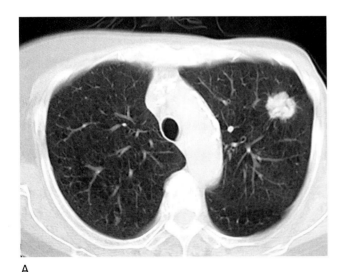

A

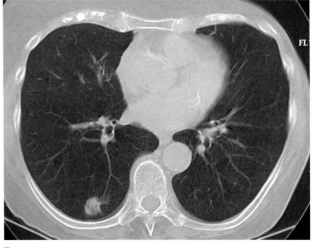

B

FIGURE 1. Two chest CT sections show similar-appearing lung masses, one in the anterior segment of the LUL (**A**) and the other in the superior segment of the RLL (**B**). Both display suspicious morphology, with irregular spiculated margins, suggesting primary bronchogenic cancers in appearance.

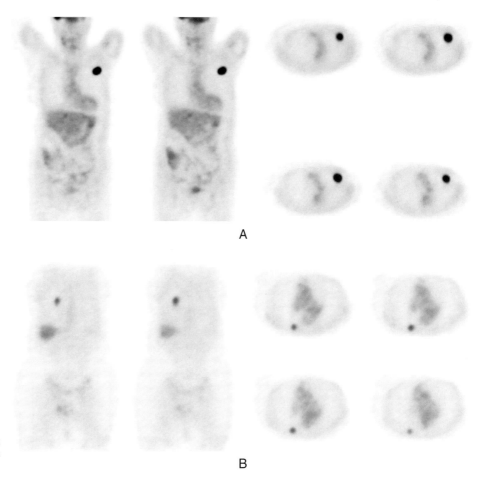

FIGURE 2. **A** and **B**, PET shows both lesions to be hypermetabolic, consistent with malignancy at both sites.

A

B

CASE 35 | *Metastatic endometrial carcinoma to lung and bone*

A 65-year-old woman with a long history of a pack per day tobacco use was found to have a large LLL mass on CXR, obtained to evaluate complaints of chest tightness, hoarseness, and cough. A chest CT confirmed a 6-cm mass in the superior segment of the LLL and left hilus (Figure 1). A bronchoscopy was inconclusive, and so a CT-guided biopsy was performed. Pathology showed adenocarcinoma with foci of squamous metaplasia.

A PET scan was requested to stage the suspected lung cancer. The large LLL mass was intensely hypermetabolic (Figure 2). An additional focus of abnormal activity was noted in the left sacrum, of concern for bone metastasis (Figure 3). A pelvis MRI was then obtained for correlation, which showed an enhancing region of abnormal signal in the left sacrum, consistent with metastasis (Figure 4).

The patient's past medical history included prior hysterectomy 11 years before for endometrial adenocarcinoma with focal squamous differentiation, invasive into the outer third of the uterine myometrium. Her LLL lung mass biopsy specimen was directly compared with her prior uterine carcinoma histology and interpreted as consistent with metastatic endometrial adenocarcinoma.

TEACHING POINTS

This case of metastatic endometrial cancer to lung and bone cannot be distinguished based on imaging from a stage IV bronchogenic carcinoma with bone involvement. The similarity of the patient's lung histology to that of her prior endometrial malignancy was noted by pathology and prompted review of the material from the hysterectomy specimen, enabling the diagnosis to be made. PET imaging first identified the additional sacral disease site, indicating that whatever the histology, the patient had metastatic disease.

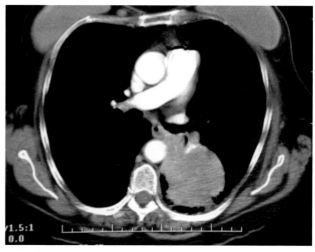

FIGURE 1. Enhanced chest CT image shows a large mass in the superior segment of the LLL, extending into the hilus. Breast implants are present.

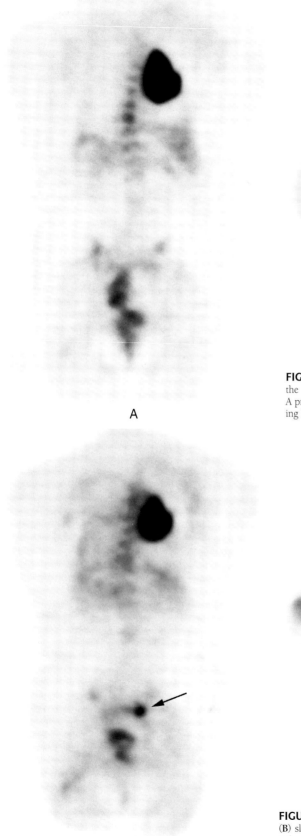

A

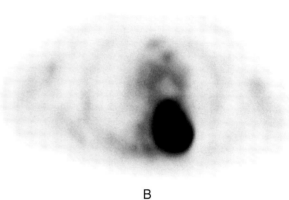

B

FIGURE 2. Coronal (**A**) and axial (**B**) PET images through the LLL show the mass to be intensely hypermetabolic and consistent with a neoplasm. A primary lung carcinoma was suspected based on the patient's heavy smoking history, morphology, and adenocarcinoma histology.

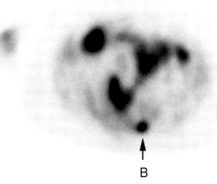

B

FIGURE 3. A more posterior coronal section (**A**) and corresponding axial (**B**) slice show an unexpected left sacral focus of abnormal activity (*arrows*). A bone metastasis was suspected and raised the specter of stage IV lung cancer. Relatively intense bowel activity is seen within the pelvis, particularly on the axial slice.

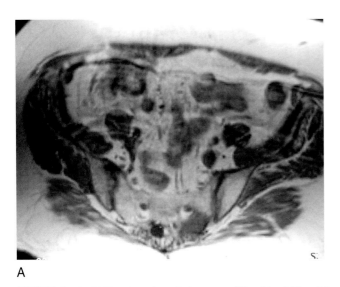

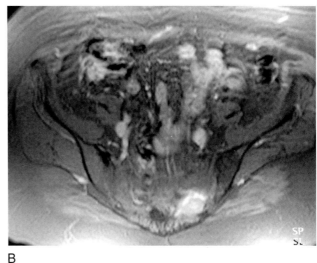

A   B

FIGURE 4. Axial MR sections through the sacrum (T1-weighted [A] and fat-saturated, enhanced T1-weighted [B]) show focal abnormal marrow signal with enhancement in the left sacrum, consistent with a metastasis.

CASE 36 | *Pitfall: Bronchoalveolar cell carcinoma*

A 75-year-old woman with a persistent dry, hacking cough was found on CXR and chest CT to have an LUL infiltrate (Figures 1 to 3). Bronchoscopic evaluation was complicated by severe hemoptysis. No malignancy or infectious etiology was identified. Transthoracic biopsy revealed adenocarcinoma, most likely bronchoalveolar variant. PET scan showed only modest activity at the level of the LUL process (Figures 4 and 5). The patient underwent left upper lobectomy, confirming on pathology a 4-cm well-differentiated non–mucinous-type bronchoalveolar carcinoma (BAC). The tumor was characterized by neoplastic cells growing along alveolar walls. Ten hilar lymph nodes were negative for metastatic tumor.

TEACHING POINTS

BAC is a known potential source of lung cancer false-negative results. This case clearly demonstrates the difficulties affiliated with diagnosis of this disease, which not infrequently is atypical in appearance for lung cancer on CT as well. Tumor growth along alveolar walls can produce opacities that simulate inflammatory processes on CXR and CT. When these infiltrates fail to respond as expected to treatment or if there is interval growth, a neoplastic diagnosis may be suspected. The low level of activity seen with this BAC is more typical of an inflammatory process. If an SUV were measured, it would not meet the most commonly used criterion for malignancy of SUV greater than 2.5.

BAC on PET can produce a spectrum of appearances, from no or little FDG activity to moderate to intense activity more typical of lung cancer. The two additional BAC cases that follow illustrate the spectrum of findings.

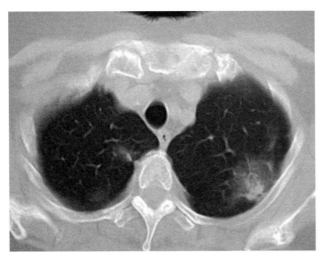

FIGURE 1. Chest CT (lung window) shows an LUL infiltrate. Two smaller, similar-appearing RUL foci are noted as well.

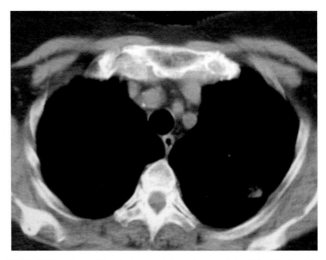

FIGURE 2. Chest CT soft tissue window shows minimal "solidity" of the LUL process.

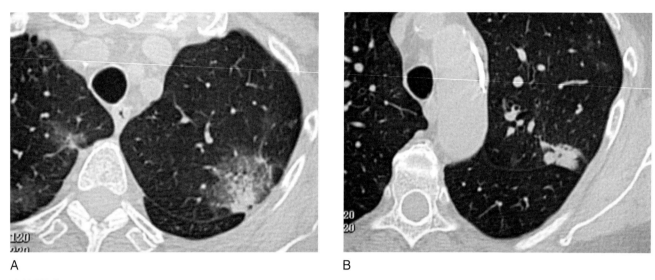

A
B

FIGURE 3. **A** and **B**, High-resolution chest CT sections show the ground-glass appearance of the majority of the process. The more inferior section shows a component that is more mass-like.

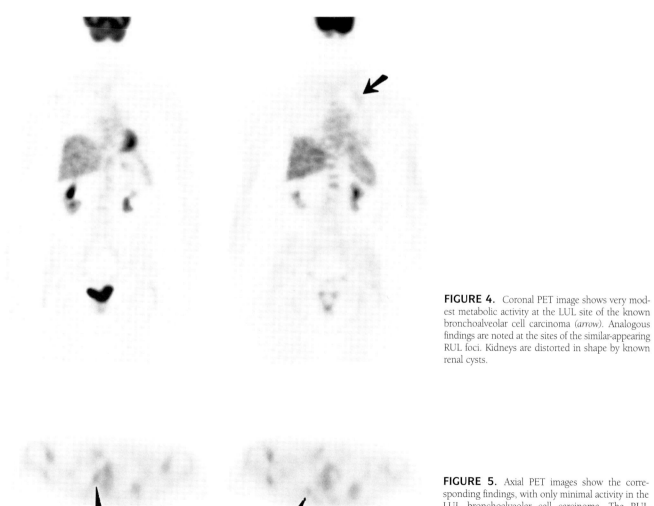

FIGURE 4. Coronal PET image shows very modest metabolic activity at the LUL site of the known bronchoalveolar cell carcinoma (*arrow*). Analogous findings are noted at the sites of the similar-appearing RUL foci. Kidneys are distorted in shape by known renal cysts.

FIGURE 5. Axial PET images show the corresponding findings, with only minimal activity in the LUL bronchoalveolar cell carcinoma. The RUL abnormalities are barely discernible (*arrows*).

CASE 37 | *Pitfall: Bronchoalveolar cell carcinoma*

A CXR was obtained in a 75-year-old female heavy smoker to look for rib fractures after a fall. Instead, an RLL mass was found. The mass was confirmed on CT (Figures 1 and 2), and subsequent biopsy identified well-differentiated adenocarcinoma, suggestive of bronchoalveolar cell carcinoma. On PET imaging, the lesion shows modest metabolic activity, less intense than generally expected with lung cancers (Figure 3).

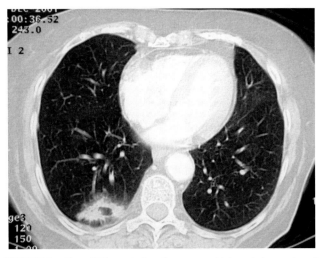

FIGURE 1. Chest CT lung window shows an ovoid, irregularly marginated, cavitary RLL mass. CT appearance is quite suggestive of a lung carcinoma.

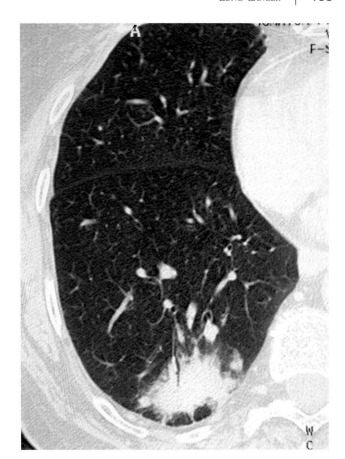

FIGURE 2. High-resolution, thin-section view of a more inferior component of the mass shows the margin spiculation and pleural tags well. An air bronchogram is noted extending into the mass.

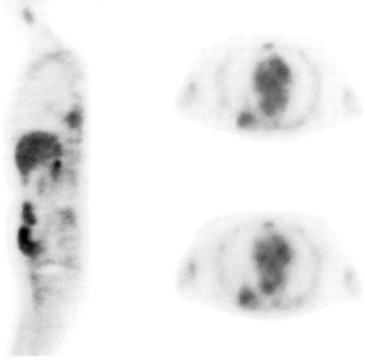

FIGURE 3. Sagittal (**A**) and axial (**B**) views from the PET scan shows modest metabolic activity of the mass. Relatively increased physiologic bowel activity is noted in this patient.

A

B

TEACHING POINTS

Bronchoalveolar cell variety of adenocarcinoma of the lung can be quite variable in PET scan activity level. It can range from negligible to moderate to the intense activity expected with other lung cancers. It is a recognized source of false-negative results. The CT appearance can also be misleading, with some lesions presenting as infiltrates, ranging from ground-glass opacities to focal areas of consolidation. Air bronchograms may be seen, as in this case. The lesions not infrequently suggest inflammatory processes and come to attention when these "pneumonias" fail to resolve as expected after therapy. Caution must be exercised in the PET scan interpretation of these lesions, especially when the activity level on PET is modest and indeterminate. Such lesions require continued imaging surveillance to establish stability over time.

CASE 38 | *Pitfall: Bronchoalveolar cell carcinoma*

A 53-year-old man noted a rattle in his chest when lying down. On CXR, he was noted to have a left lung infiltrate, which did not respond to antibiotics. The infiltrate was initially thought to be a possible aspiration pneumonia, owing to the patient's severe chronic gastroesophageal reflux disease (GERD). Bronchoscopy showed no impacted food or evidence of malignancy. CT showed the process to be mass-like and multinodular (Figures 1 to 3). A CT-guided biopsy demonstrated bronchoalveolar cell adenocarcinoma. PET was requested to help stage this patient's disease (Figures 4 to 6).

TEACHING POINTS

This case provides a further example of the range of possible appearances of bronchoalveolar cell carcinoma (BAC). Case 36 showed a barely visible BAC, which corresponded with a ground-glass opacity on CT. Case 37 showed moderate activity at the site of the air bronchogram containing mass. In this case, two foci with different manifestations of disease show differential activity on PET. Not surprisingly, the largest and most mass-like component shows the most intense activity and is consistent with the expected lung cancer findings on PET.

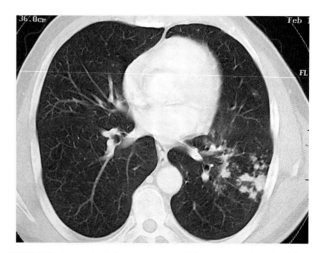

FIGURE 2. A multinodular component of this process is identified below.

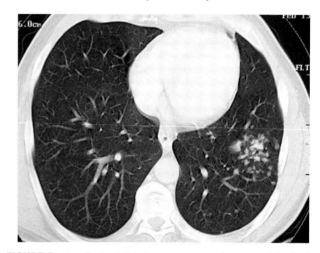

FIGURE 3. Even further inferiorly, there is a triangular region of closely clustered additional nodules.

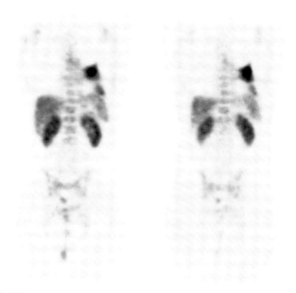

FIGURE 4. Coronal PET image shows two left lower lung hypermetabolic foci. The larger and more active focus in the superior segment of the LLL corresponds with the dominant mass in Figure 1. The left basilar, less active focus correlates with the triangular cluster of nodules in Figure 3.

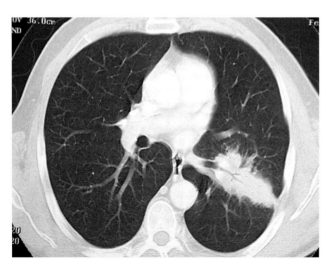

FIGURE 1. An ovoid focus of dense, mass-like consolidation is noted in the superior segment of the LUL. An air bronchogram extends into the mass. Margins are irregular and spiculated.

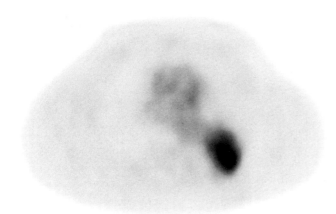

FIGURE 5. Transaxial PET image through the superior segment LLL mass, corresponding to Figure 1.

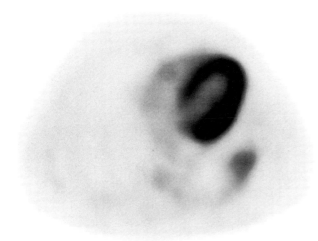

FIGURE 6. Transaxial PET image through the left lung base shows a lower intensity wedge of activity, correlating with the closely grouped nodules in Figure 3. The individual nodules are too small to reliably be visualized on PET, but this closely approximated group is seen as a conglomerate process.

The second component, with closely grouped but small nodules, is visualized as a conglomerate focus of less intense metabolic activity and overlaps in appearance with inflammatory processes. As we have previously noted, BAC has been reported as a potential source of false-negative results on PET and has a highly variable appearance on CT, as well as a range of possible PET findings.

CASE 39 | *Pitfall: Lung cancer false positive, pulmonary infarct*

A 71-year-old man, on warfarin (Coumadin) for pulmonary embolism, had been on treatment for pneumonia for 3 days when he was admitted with progressive dyspnea, hypoxia, and fevers to 102.5° F. CXR showed posterior LUL consolidation, as well as left basilar atelectasis and consolidation and a pleural effusion (Figure 1). Ventilation-perfusion scan showed a new perfusion defect, and Doppler studies of the legs confirmed deep venous thrombosis. CT pulmonary angiography

showed the left lung consolidation to be a wedge-shaped focus, extending from the left hilus to the pleura (Figure 2). A nonocclusive thrombus was visualized in the left pulmonary artery, and a pleural effusion was present. A caval filter was placed for apparently recurrent DVT and pulmonary embolism, despite anticoagulation. This raised the question whether the patient was hypercoagulable and whether the chest CT findings could be secondary to malignancy. PET scan was requested. It showed the peripheral left mid-lung opacity to be quite hypermetabolic (Figure 3). The patient rapidly defervesced while being

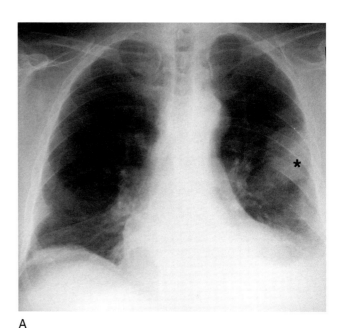

A

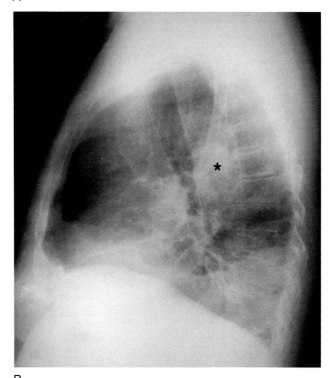

B

FIGURE 1. Posteroanterior (**A**) and lateral (**B**) CXR views show a peripheral, mass-like opacity (*asterisks*) in the left mid-lung zone (posterior LUL), with left basilar atelectasis, consolidation, and pleural fluid.

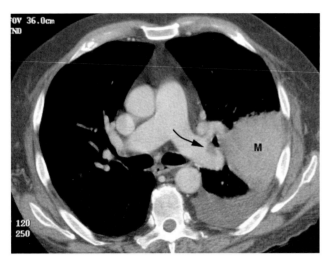

FIGURE 2. Contrast medium–enhanced chest CT through the mass (M) shows it to have a wedge shape, extending from the left hilus to the pleura. A filling defect in the left main pulmonary artery is indicative of pulmonary thrombus (*arrow*). A moderate size left pleural effusion is also noted.

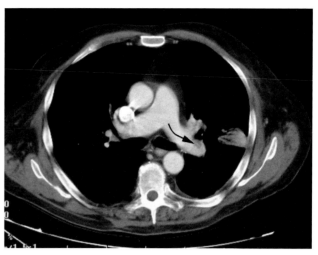

FIGURE 4. Contrast medium–enhanced chest CT, performed 1 month later, at the time of planned CT-guided biopsy, demonstrates persistent thrombus in the left pulmonary artery (*arrow*) but shows the mass-like consolidation to be markedly reduced, consistent with an evolving pulmonary infarct.

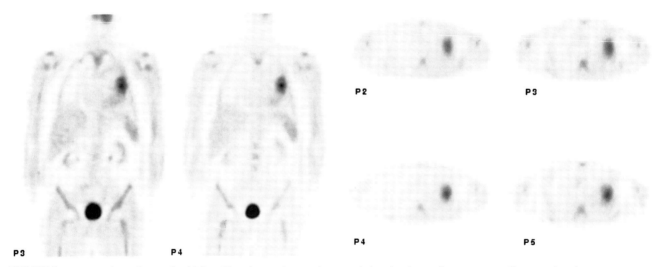

FIGURE 3. PET scan shows the peripheral left mid-lung focus to be quite hypermetabolic. This degree of activity is generally seen with malignant processes, but there is overlap with inflammatory processes. Note also the mild diffuse increase in marrow activity seen in this patient. This was attributed to his known anemia.

treated for pneumonia and pulmonary embolism, and it was elected to follow him in 1 month's time with a repeat chest CT, to be followed by CT-guided biopsy. The follow-up study showed persistent left pulmonary artery thrombus, but the wedge of consolidation present previously had markedly regressed (Figure 4). Accordingly, no biopsy was performed, and a further follow-up CXR showed essentially complete resolution of the opacity.

TEACHING POINTS

There is overlap between hypermetabolism due to malignancy and that seen in active inflammatory processes. This case illustrates this well. The wedge shape of the pulmonary consolidation, coexistence of pulmonary artery thrombus and deep venous thrombosis, symptoms of dyspnea and hypoxia, and resolution of the lesion after treatment for

pulmonary embolism, all suggest this was a pulmonary infarct. Of course, the lesion could have been a wedge-shaped pneumonia, which resolved after treatment as well. Either of these processes may be metabolically active, although not generally to this degree.

CASE 40 | *Pitfall: lung cancer false positive, active tuberculosis*

A 74-year-old male heavy smoker with a chronic cough was found to have an RUL mass on CXR. Calcified bilateral hilar lymph nodes were also seen. He was evaluated with bronchoscopy, which identified acid-fast bacilli, prompting institution of antituberculous therapy. He was then referred for PET scan evaluation. The PET scan showed the RUL

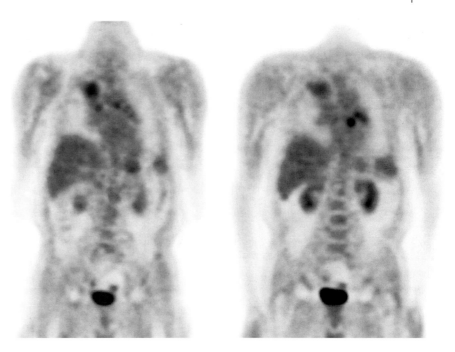

FIGURE 1. Coronal PET images from the initial evaluation show a hypermetabolic RUL mass, accompanied by metabolically active tracheobronchial lymph nodes. Based on the PET scan alone, the findings certainly could represent an RUL lung cancer, with hilar nodal involvement.

mass to be metabolically active and to be accompanied by hypermetabolic nodal foci in the hila (Figure 1). Findings were interpreted as suspicious for lung cancer with nodal involvement, with granulomatous diseases such as tuberculosis in the differential diagnosis. Three months later, with the patient on isoniazid and rifampin, he was re-evaluated with PET imaging. By this time, the patient felt much better. The follow-up PET scan showed marked interval improvement, with near resolution of the RUL mass and partial regression of the nodal activity (Figure 2).

TEACHING POINTS

In the evaluation of suspected lung cancer, active granulomatous diseases, such as tuberculosis and sarcoidosis, are known sources of false-positive PET scan activity. At the time of this patient's first PET scan, he had undergone bronchoscopy, but the results were pending. The PET scan findings are essentially indistinguishable from those of an RUL bronchogenic carcinoma, with hilar nodal involvement. The presence of a large number of calcified hilar lymph nodes on a CXR was the

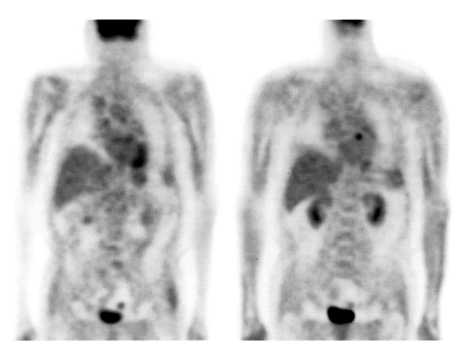

FIGURE 2. Three months later, after therapy with isoniazid and rifampin, the RUL activity has essentially resolved. The tracheobronchial nodal activity is markedly regressed, with the foci fewer, smaller, and decreased in activity.

only initial clue to the ultimate diagnosis in this case. Acid-fast bacilli were demonstrated subsequently, and the patient was treated with an antituberculous regimen before being re-imaged 3 months later. Confirmation of the diagnosis of tuberculosis is provided by the objective improvement demonstrated on follow-up PET imaging after medical therapy only.

CASE 41 | Pitfall: lung cancer false positive, sarcoidosis

A 72-year-old nonsmoking man presented with dyspnea on exertion. His work-up included a low probability ventilation-perfusion scan and a chest CT. CT showed mediastinal lymphadenopathy (Figure 1). Mild to moderately enlarged lymph nodes were identified in the aortopulmonary window, right paratracheal and subcarinal regions, and both hila. No pulmonary parenchymal abnormalities were seen. PET scan evaluation was requested on suspicion of possible metastatic nodal disease or lymphoma. PET imaging confirmed the adenopathy in question to be metabolically active (Figures 2 and 3). No lung parenchymal or other abnormalities were seen. A differential diagnosis of sarcoid, lymphoma, and metastatic disease was entertained. Sarcoid was favored because of the patient's nonsmoking status, and because of the morphology of the nodes, with multiple discrete enlarged, but not confluent or mat-like, lymph nodes. Mediastinoscopy was performed, and pathology showed noncaseating granulomatous lymphadenitis, without acid-fast bacilli or other identifiable organisms. Morphologic features were consistent with the suspected diagnosis of sarcoidosis.

TEACHING POINTS

Active granulomatous processes, such as sarcoidosis, can display significant increased metabolic activity on FDG PET and are potential sources of false-positive results in the evaluation for suspected lung cancer or lymphoma. In typical cases such as this, morphology of the nodal activity may suggest the diagnosis. Sarcoidosis classically presents as bilateral hilar and mediastinal (especially right paratracheal) adenopathy, which may be more remarkable for increased numbers of lymph nodes than for the degree of nodal enlargement, which may be mild.

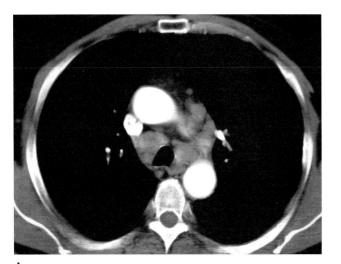

A

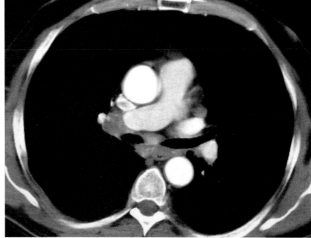

B

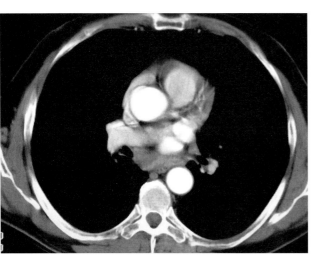

C

FIGURE 1. Enhanced chest CT images (**A** to **C**) show mild to moderately enlarged lymph nodes in right paratracheal, aortopulmonary window, bilateral hilar, and subcarinal regions.

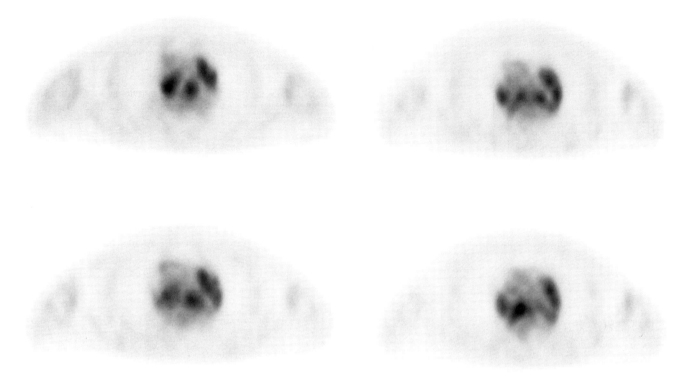

FIGURE 2. Corresponding axial PET scan images show the nodes are metabolically active.

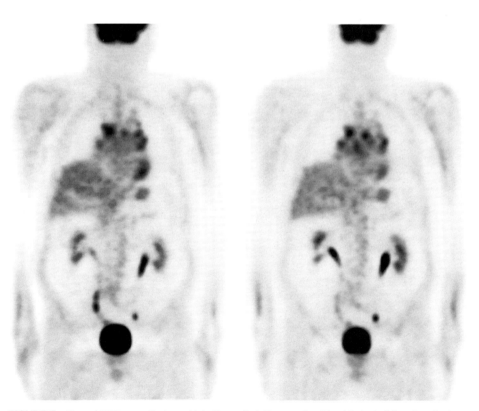

FIGURE 3. Coronal PET images display multiple discrete foci of increased nodal activity in the hila and mediastinum.

Lymphomatous nodal disease tends to be more confluent and mass-like. Of course, other active granulomatous processes, such as tuberculosis, could overlap in appearance with this case (see Case 40).

Although not illustrated here, the PET scan of this patient showed another potentially useful piece of data. In addition to the findings shown here, there was a supraclavicular focus of activity of equal intensity, suggesting another possible site for histologic sampling.

CASE 42 | Pitfall: Lung cancer, size limitation

A 55-year-old woman underwent a surveillance chest CT for follow-up of lung cancer, which showed a new 1-cm cavitary RLL nodule (Figure 1). The patient was 6 months post left upper lobectomy for adenocarcinoma when the new RLL nodule was identified. PET scan was requested for evaluation of the nodule and was negative (Figures 2 and 4). Two months later, after a repeat chest CT showed growth of the nodule to 1.3 cm (Figure 3), the PET scan was repeated. The PET study now identified the metabolically active RLL nodule, at the site of the chest CT abnormality (Figures 2 and 4). The interval change was regarded with suspicion for a growing malignancy, and the patient underwent surgery. Pathology demonstrated an undifferentiated carcinoma, arising in a cyst, confirming the PET finding.

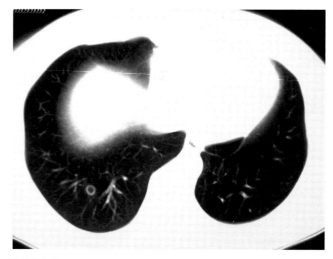

FIGURE 1. Chest CT lung window shows a 1-cm RLL cavitary lung nodule. The wall of the cavity is thin and smooth, characteristics suggesting benignity. However, the lesion was new and the patient had a prior history of lung adenocarcinoma.

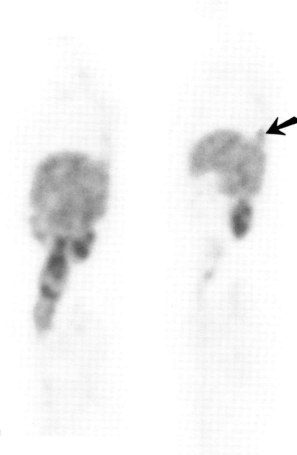

P 1

P 1

FIGURE 2. Two sagittal PET sections, **A** from the first PET scan and **B** from the repeat study 2 months later, showing comparable sections through the RLL. The RLL is clear on the first study, when the nodule in question measured 1 cm on CT. Two months later, when the nodule grew to 1.3 cm on CT, PET now identifies the lesion as a metabolically active nodule (*arrow*).

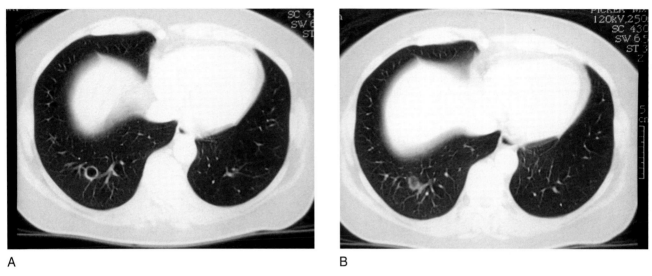

A   B

FIGURE 3. **A** and **B**, Repeat chest CT, 2 months later, shows clear interval growth of the nodule, to 1.3 cm. The lesion is also now visualized on more than one section, with the more inferior section (**B**) suggesting increasing wall thickness of the cavity.

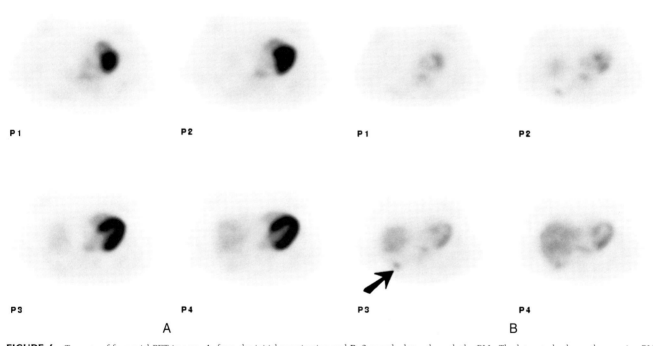

A   B

FIGURE 4. Two sets of four axial PET images, **A**, from the initial examination and **B**, 2 months later, through the RLL. The later study shows the growing RLL nodule to be metabolically active (*arrow*). It is not identifiable on the prior study only 2 months before, even in retrospect. Note marked normal variation in myocardial activity between studies.

TEACHING POINTS

This case illustrates important PET principles regarding size threshold and lesional characteristics in visualization of lung nodules. In addition to absolute size, the metabolic activity of the tumor and growth pattern are important factors in lesion detectability. In general, malignant nodules of 1 cm are reliably demonstrated with PET, with lesions of 8 mm and greater regularly demonstrable with current instrumentation. At the time of initial PET evaluation, this patient's lesion by absolute size was borderline for visualization. However, these size guidelines typically apply to solid nodules. Tumor activity in atypical patterns, such as this small cavitary lesion, will less reliably be detected. Only 2 months later and with interval growth noted on CT to 1.3 cm, this nodule became identifiable on PET.

Lymphoma

Hodgkin's disease (HD) and non-Hodgkin's lymphoma (NHL) account for less than 10% of all malignancies, but their frequency is increasing. Two of the most important prognostic factors are histologic type and extent of disease at initial staging. Imaging plays a critical role in defining the extent of disease and may include CT, MRI, gallium scanning, and, more recently, PET. Important treatment decisions are based on this initial staging. Therapeutic options include radiation therapy (RT), chemotherapy, combination RT/chemotherapy, and bone marrow transplant.

Patients with HD are typically staged I through IV (Table 1), whereas NHL staging divides patients into low-, intermediate-, and high-grade disease. PET appears to be most useful in HD and in intermediate-grade NHL. Management issues, defined by Gambhir and colleagues[1] include staging of disease before treatment, monitoring response to treatment, detecting recurrence, and differential diagnosis.

STAGING BEFORE TREATMENT

In HD, treatment is based primarily on stage, whereas in NHL factors such as natural history of disease assume a more important role. CT is clearly the best modality to provide information about measurable disease and proximity to organs and vascular structures. However, with CT, nodal involvement is generally determined by size alone. As discussed in other sections, lymph nodes larger than 1 cm may be benign and those smaller than 1 cm may be malignant. Additionally, CT may be suboptimal for evaluating the liver, spleen, bone marrow, and sites remote from the area being imaged. Whole-body PET is more sensitive in each of these areas. In summary data from more than 2000 patients, the sensitivity and specificity for PET were significantly better than for CT (PET = 90% sensitive, 93% specific; CT = 81% sensitive and 69% specific). Of note, the positive predictive value of CT was only 48%.[1] These data underscore the important point that many patients will be understaged by CT (perhaps resulting in suboptimal initial treatment) and others will be overstaged (leading to unnecessarily toxic, morbid therapy). Functional imaging with PET does not rely on nodal size for diagnosis. FDG-PET identifies metabolically active malignant tissue. Nearly all lymphomas avidly concentrate FDG, although there does appear to be a relationship between degree of uptake and histologic grade and proliferation rate of the lymphoma cells.[2] Areas where PET has shown added value include liver, spleen, bone marrow (better sensitivity than bone marrow biopsy), and extranodal disease. PET results in a change of stage in approximately 15% of patients.[2] Brief mention should be made of gallium imaging. If it is performed with current protocols (i.e., high dose, delayed views, multiple imaging sessions) and state-of-the-art gamma cameras, gallium imaging can be useful. However, all patients require a baseline study, radiation dosimetry is less favorable than PET, resolution is lower, and physiologic biodistribution can be problematic. Centers with experience with both have replaced gallium imaging with PET.

MONITORING RESPONSE

The use of PET to assess a patient's response to treatment is less well validated an indication than staging or recurrence detection. In theory, a test that could separate responders from nonresponders, early in the course of therapy, should be of great value. Data are accumulating indicating a role for PET in this area. However, much remains to be learned about individual tumor response to chemotherapy and/or irradiation. For example, what is the incidence and duration of the so-called flare phenomenon during chemotherapy (i.e., apparent worsening on scanning in the setting of improvement)? How often will false-negative studies occur during radiation therapy, and how long can false-positive results persist after treatment? In certain anatomical sites (e.g., head and neck), PET may be falsely positive after irradiation for many months. With respect to lymphoma, cumulative data exist on only a few hundred patients. The results are encouraging, showing a 90% sensitivity and 93% specificity.[1]

TABLE 1 ANN ARBOR CLASSIFICATION OF HODGKIN'S DISEASE

STAGE	FINDINGS
I	Involvement of a single lymph node region or lymphoid structure or involvement of a single extralymphatic site (IE)
II	Involvement of two or more lymph node regions on the same side of the diaphragm (II), which may be accompanied by localized, contiguous involvement of an extralymphatic organ or site (IIE)
III	Involvement of lymph node regions on both sides of the diaphragm (III), which may also be accompanied by localized contiguous involvement of an extralymphatic organ or site (IIIE)
IV	Diffuse or disseminated involvement of one or more extralymphatic organs or tissues, with or without associated lymph node involvement.

DETECTING RECURRENCE

Documentation of lymphoma relapse is of more than academic interest. Re-treatment may provide a significant chance of cure or prolonged remission. Post-treatment evaluation addresses two main questions: is there evidence for disease anywhere in the body and what does a residual mass indicate? CT, which relies on the criterion of size, cannot reliably differentiate active tumor from scar/fibrosis. PET can readily make this distinction. With a single test, PET can survey the entire body, including accurate characterization of lymph node–bearing regions, extranodal sites, the spleen, bone marrow, and any residual mass. Data on more than 200 patients show a sensitivity for detection of recurrences of 87%, specificity of 93%, negative predictive value of 90%, and overall accuracy of 88%.[1] The accuracy of CT is below 70%, in large part owing to its inability to distinguish tumorous from fibrotic residual masses.

There are a number of special circumstances where PET is especially valuable in the patient with lymphoma. One important area is the identification of bone marrow involvement. Five to 14% of patients with untreated HD will have bone marrow involvement.[3] In NHL the incidence may be as high as 25% or more.[4,5] In a prospective study comparing FDG-PET with posterior iliac crest bone marrow biopsy, PET identified 10 patients with marrow involvement who were biopsy negative (8 confirmed).[5] This is not unexpected, because the pattern of involvement is typically multifocal rather than diffuse, resulting in sampling error. Bone marrow infiltration places the patient into stage IV, often resulting in significant alterations in treatment approach and prognosis.

Another difficult area to evaluate with conventional imaging studies is the spleen, and to a lesser extent, the liver. Hepatic and splenic involvement figures are 3.2% and 23% for HD and 15.1% and 22% for NHL.[4] A significant number of patients diagnosed as having disease only above the diaphragm by conventional imaging studies prove to be positive in the spleen (and bone marrow) on FDG-PET.

The identification of extranodal disease may also present a problem for conventional imaging modalities.[6] Prospective investigation of 81 patients with HD and NHL showed that 20% to 30% identified as having only supradiaphragmatic involvement by conventional imaging actually demonstrated infradiaphragmatic disease by PET.[4]

In summary, the efficacy and cost-effectiveness of FDG-PET in lymphoma has been established.[7,8] PET can contribute to more accurate staging, characterize a residual mass, and detect recurrence earlier and shows promise for monitoring response to therapy. The relationship between histologic grade and proliferative rate with FDG uptake implies a lowered sensitivity in very low-grade lymphoma (e.g., PET is of no value in mucosa-associated lymphoid tissue [MALT] lymphoma).[9] Finally, conventional imaging modalities (i.e., CT and MRI) are still crucial in the evaluation of patients with lymphoma, owing to their ability to elegantly depict organs, vessels, and other structures and their anatomic relationship to disease sites.

REFERENCES

1. Gambhir SS, Czernin J, Schwimmer J, et al: A tabulated summary of the FDG PET literature. J Nucl Med 2001;42:15S-20S.
2. Delbeke D, Martin WH, Morgan DS, et al: 2-deoxy-2-[F-18] fluoro-D-glucose imaging with positron emission tomography for initial staging of Hodgkin's disease and lymphoma. Mol Imag Biol 2002;4:105-114.
3. Hueltenschmidt B, Sautter-Bihl M-L, Lang O, et al: Whole-body positron emission tomography in the treatment of Hodgkin disease. Cancer 2001;91:302-310.
4. Moog F, Bamgerter M, Diederichs CG, et al: Extranodal malignant lymphoma: Detection with FDG-PET versus CT. Radiology 1998;206:475-481.
5. Moog F, Bamgerter M, Kotzerke J, et al: 18-F-Fluorodeoxyglucose positron emission tomography as a new approach to detect lymphomatous bone marrow. J Clin Oncol 1998;16:603-609.
6. Young CS, Young BL, Smith SM: Staging Hodgkin's disease with 18-FDG PET: Comparison with CT and surgery. Clin Pos Imag 1998;1:161-164.
7. Newman JS, Francis IR, Kaminski MS, et al: Imaging of lymphoma with PET with 2-[F-18]-fluoro-2-deoxy-D-glucose: Correlation with CT. Radiology 1994;190:111-116.
8. Hoh CK, Glaspy J, Rosen P, et al: Whole-body FDG-PET imaging for staging of Hodgkin's disease and lymphoma. J Nucl Med 1997;38:343-348.
9. Hoffman M, Kletter K, Diemling M, et al: Positron emission tomography with fluorine-18-2-deoxy-D-glucose (F18-FDG) does not visualize extranodal B-cell lymphoma of the mucosa-associated lymphoid tissue (MALT) type. Ann Oncol 1999;10:1185-1189.

CASE 1 | *Lymphoma, limited-stage disease, staging*

A 19-year-old man presented with threatened airway compromise. He admitted to several months of difficulty swallowing. Soft tissue neck CT identified a large (4 cm) left mucosal space oropharyngeal mass, accompanied by thickening and mass-like enlargement of the epiglottis and palatine tonsil (Figures 1 and 2). Mildly enlarged internal jugular chain and left posterior triangle lymph nodes were noted. Biopsy of the left tonsil identified B-cell non-Hodgkin's lymphoma.

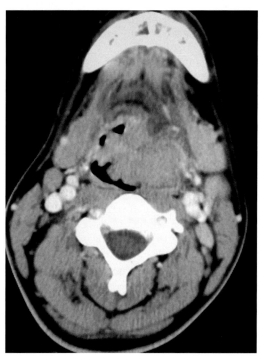

FIGURE 1. Enhanced soft tissue neck CT shows a lobular, exophytic, left mucosal lesion, nearly filling the oropharynx. Mildly prominent lymph nodes are noted in both internal jugular chains and in the left posterior triangle.

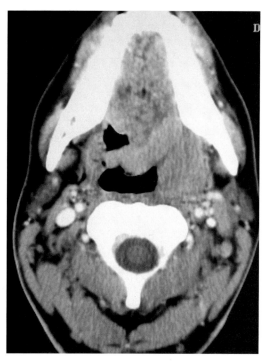

FIGURE 2. A more inferior section shows mass-like enlargement and thickening of the epiglottis and left palatine tonsil. A mildly prominent left internal jugular lymph node is noted.

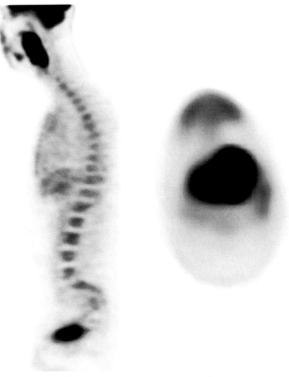

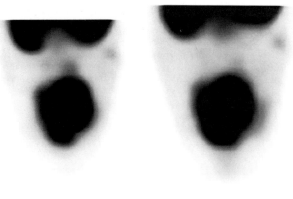

FIGURE 3. Sagittal (**A**), axial (**B**), and two coronal (**C**) PET images show the left oropharyngeal and tonsillar mass to be intensely hypermetabolic. No separate sites of disease activity are identified. Note diffusely increased bone marrow activity, attributable in this case to the patient's anemia.

A   B   C

PET scanning was obtained to aid in initial staging (Figure 3). It showed a large, confluent left oropharyngeal and tonsillar intensely hypermetabolic mass. No other disease site was found. The patient was treated with chemotherapy.

CASE 2 | Lymphoma, staging, isolated neck disease

A 32-year-old healthy man developed a left neck lump that failed to respond to antibiotic therapy. Biopsy showed diffuse large B-cell lymphoma. The patient was otherwise asymptomatic. Staging, with neck, chest, abdomen and pelvis CTs, showed asymmetrical enlargement of the left sternocleidomastoid muscle, but no other disease site was identified (Figure 1). This limited-stage disease was confirmed with PET scan (Figure 2). Follow-up CT after chemotherapy showed reversion to normal.

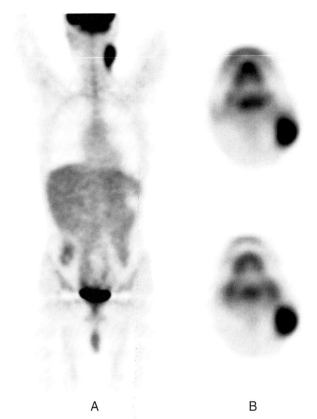

A   **B**

FIGURE 2. Coronal (**A**) and two adjacent axial (**B**) PET images show a left neck ovoid focus of hypermetabolic activity, corresponding to the CT findings and confirming the imaging impression of a solitary locus of disease.

CASE 3 | Lymphoma, staging and treatment assessment, pulmonary parenchymal involvement

An 83-year-old man presented with cough and a 20-pound weight loss. A RLL lung mass proved on percutaneous biopsy to be non-Hodgkin's lymphoma (NHL). PET scan was requested for initial staging and demonstrated intense hypermetabolism of the large RLL mass (Figure 1). He returned for repeat PET scan after four cycles of chemotherapy to assess the efficacy of treatment (Figure 2), feeling well and having regained weight.

TEACHING POINTS

This case illustrates the utility of PET in the evaluation of a less common manifestation of lymphoma, with involvement of lung parenchyma and presentation as a mass. The disease extent was well demonstrated on the staging examination, and an excellent response to chemotherapy is confirmed by repeat scanning after four cycles of chemotherapy.

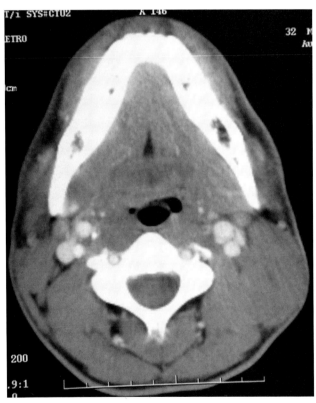

FIGURE 1. Soft tissue neck CT with intravenous contrast shows asymmetrical enlargement of the left sternocleidomastoid muscle, corresponding to the palpable left neck lump. This is secondary either to an isodense nodal mass deep to and indistinguishable from the muscle or to lymphomatous infiltration of the muscle.

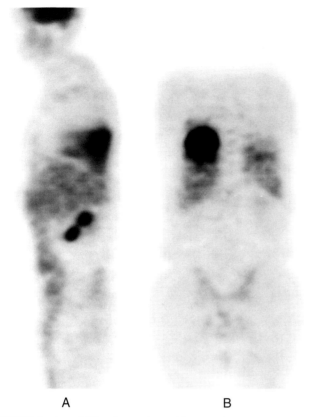

FIGURE 1. Sagittal (**A**) and coronal PET (**B**) images from staging PET scan show a large hypermetabolic region occupying much of the right lower lobe, at the site of the patient's biopsy-confirmed parenchymal non-Hodgkin's lymphoma.

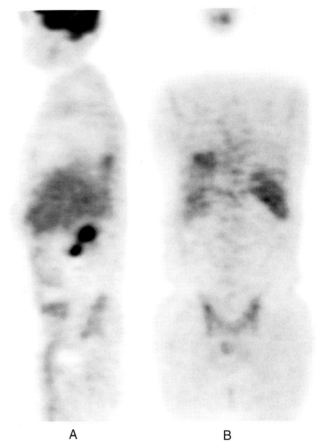

FIGURE 2. Corresponding sagittal (**A**) and coronal (**B**) PET images from the patient's follow-up examination (*right*) show near-complete normalization. Only a small, peripheral rim of residual activity is noted at the site after four cycles of chemotherapy.

CASE 4 | *Unexpected PET identification of limited-stage visceral lymphoma*

A 65-year-old woman was referred for PET imaging for evaluation of a solitary pulmonary nodule. It had been identified on chest CT (Figure 1), obtained because of a question of right hilar enlargement on CXR. The nodule was not evident on PET, suggesting a benign etiology, but its small size (8 mm) was potentially limiting for detection.

However, an additional, unsuspected PET finding was noted, with a hypermetabolic left lobe liver focus (Figure 2). No clear correlate was evident on the images available from the chest CT through this level (Figure 3). MRI was recommended and confirmed an unusual, infiltrating lesion surrounding the left portal vein (Figures 4 to 6). CT-guided biopsy was performed (Figure 7), and pathology identified a diffuse, large B-cell lymphoma.

TEACHING POINTS

This patient's unusual, limited-stage visceral lymphoma was diagnosed almost accidentally and was completely unexpected. This scenario of

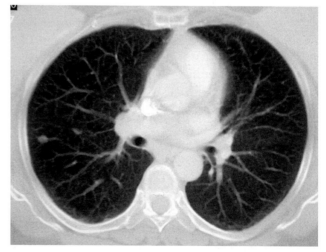

FIGURE 1. Chest CT lung window shows a sub-centimeter RLL peripheral lung nodule.

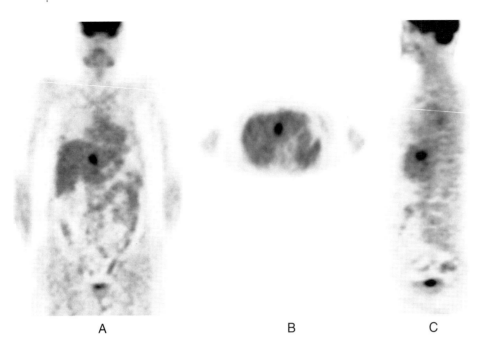

A   B   C

FIGURE 2. PET showed no correlate for the solitary pulmonary nodule, but a focus of pathologic hypermetabolic activity in the left lobe of the liver is apparent. Coronal (**A**), transaxial (**B**), and sagittal (**C**) views are shown.

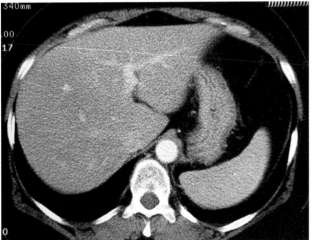

FIGURE 3. Image through the liver from the original chest CT showed no definite correlate for the liver abnormality. MRI was accordingly recommended.

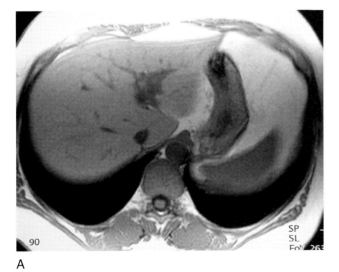

A

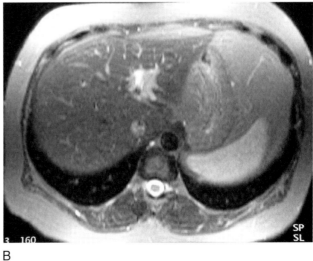

B

FIGURE 4. T1-weighted (**A**) and STIR (**B**) axial MR images at the same left lobe liver level show a corresponding mass, which appears to infiltrate around the left portal vein.

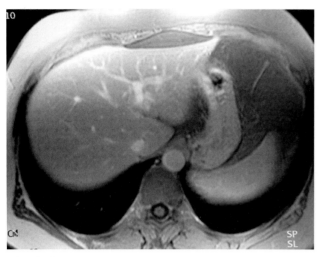

FIGURE 5. Fat-saturated, enhanced T1-weighted axial MR image shows enhancement adjacent to the left portal vein.

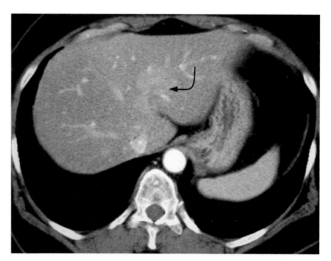

FIGURE 7. Repeat CT, obtained before CT-guided biopsy, shows subtle enhancement at the level of the infiltrating liver mass (*arrow*).

unexpected, significant findings on PET scans obtained for other reasons is a well-recognized phenomenon. Follow-up of 68 unsuspected findings (pathologic activity unrelated to a known or suspected malignant process), drawn from a data base of 1800 scans performed on 1650 patients at Hackensack University Medical Center, yielded a group of 42 patients for which histopathologic correlation was

available (H. Agress Jr., Academy of Molecular Imaging meeting abstract and personal communication, October 2002). Malignant or premalignant findings were diagnosed in 62% of these patients on subsequent work-up (30 significant findings in 26 patients), with the most common abnormalities being colonic, including villous, tubular and tubulovillous adenomas, and adenocarcinomas. In this series, other unsuspected carcinomas identified as a result of unexpected PET findings included two laryngeal, two breast, one gallbladder, one endometrial, one ovarian, one fallopian tube, and one papillary thyroid carcinoma.

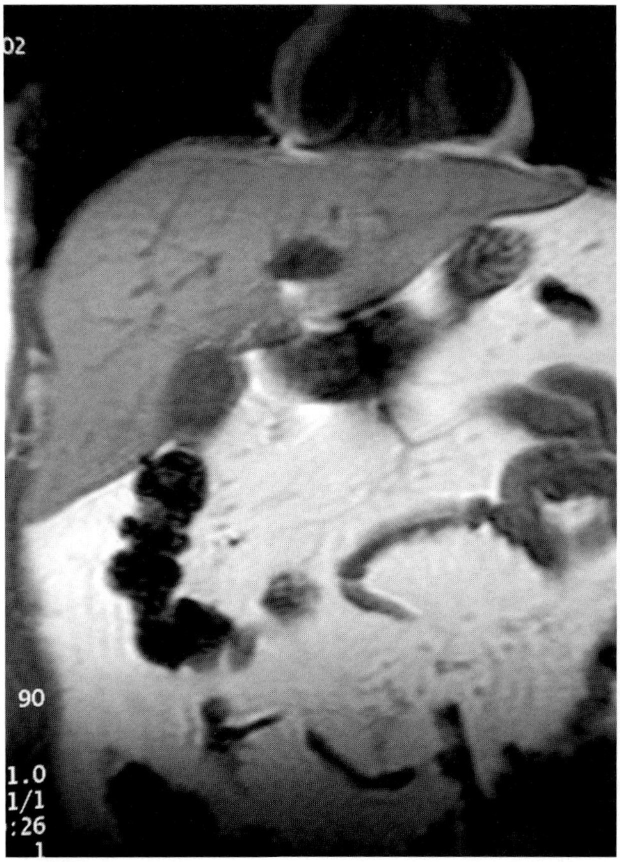

CASE 5 | *Bulky thoracic nodular sclerosing Hodgkin's disease, initial staging and residual mass treatment assessment*

A 38-year-old man presented to the emergency department with chest tightness. A CXR was obtained that showed a huge mediastinal mass (Figure 1). Over the preceding year, he had noted progressive and persistent pruritus and had developed night sweats in recent months. He had not sought medical evaluation until the chest symptoms developed. CT evaluation confirmed a huge mediastinal mass, as well as enlarged axillary lymph nodes (Figure 2). No pathologically enlarged lymph nodes were seen in the abdomen or pelvis (Figure 3). A diagnosis of nodular sclerosing Hodgkin's disease was made by left supraclavicular node biopsy. PET scan confirmed disease to be above the diaphragm, in the mediastinum, axilla, and left neck and supraclavicular regions (Figure 4). A bone marrow biopsy was negative for Hodgkin's disease. The patient was treated with chemotherapy, and the therapeutic response assessed with repeat CT and PET scans. CT showed the mediastinal mass to have shrunk, but a large residual mass remained (Figure 5). The axillary adenopathy had resolved. On PET, all the sites of disease seen previously resolved (Figure 6). The patient then underwent radiation therapy to the large residual mediastinal mass and supraclavicular regions.

TEACHING POINTS

PET served several important functions in the management of this patient's care. During staging, CT showed bulky disease, all above

FIGURE 6. T1-weighted coronal MR image of the left lobe liver lesion.

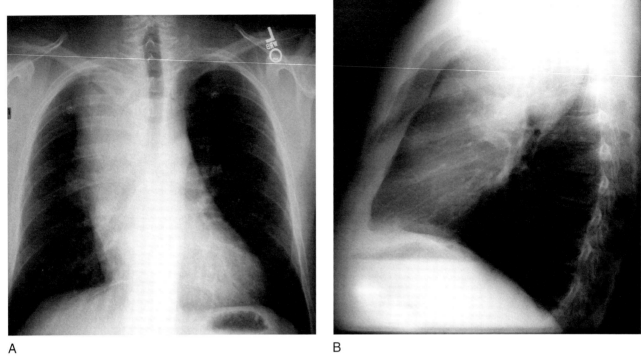

FIGURE 1. Posteroanterior (**A**) and lateral (**B**) CXR films show a large right paratracheal, anterior, and middle mediastinal mass.

the diaphragm. No clear indication by CT of subdiaphragmatic disease was seen, but the negative PET in the abdomen laid the question to rest. It also showed no evidence of bone marrow involvement. Bone marrow biopsy is subject, like all biopsies, to sampling error, potentially leading to understaging in some patients. The negative PET is additional evidence that the bone marrow is negative.

After treatment, although a response was seen, this patient was left with a significant residual mediastinal mass. In the past, the patient may have been subjected to additional chemotherapy and rescanning and /or biopsy in an effort to differentiate between scar/fibrosis and persistent active tumor. The PET scan addresses this residual mass dilemma noninvasively and more definitively than any other available modality.

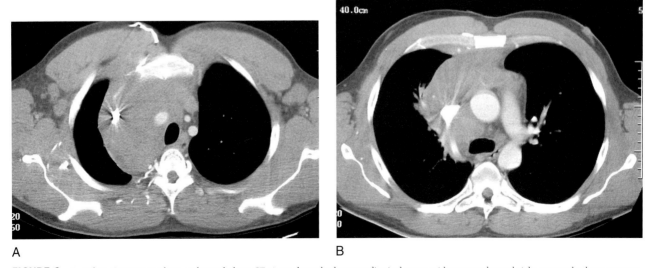

FIGURE 2. **A** and **B**, Contrast medium–enhanced chest CT views show the huge mediastinal mass, with prevascular and right paratracheal components, splaying vessels. The superior vena cava is displaced to the right. Enlarged axillary lymph nodes are noted bilaterally.

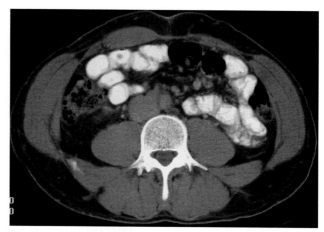

FIGURE 3. In the abdomen, no clear evidence of disease below the diaphragm was seen. Mesenteric vessels and small nodes are seen, not enlarged, but questionably increased in number.

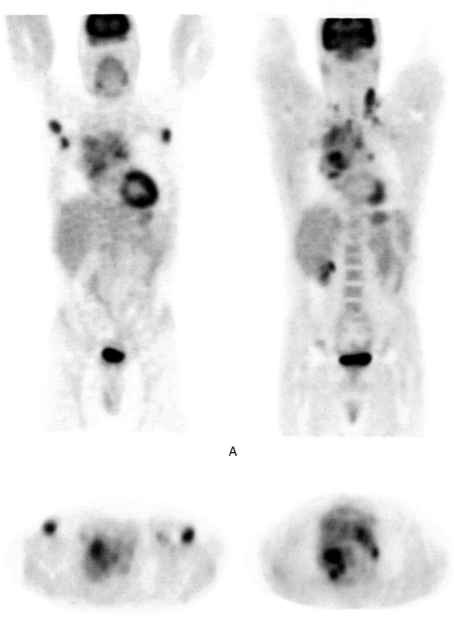

A

B

FIGURE 4. PET images (coronal [A] and axial [B]) confirm lymphoma in the mediastinum, axillae, left neck, and supraclavicular regions. Note the nonuniformity of the activity within the mediastinal mass.

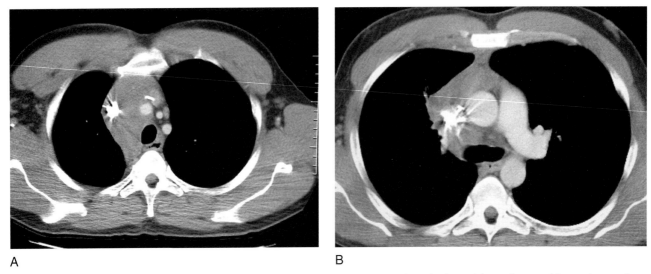

FIGURE 5. Repeat chest CT scans (**A** and **B**), after 4 months and four chemotherapy cycles, show shrinkage of the confluent nodal mass, but significant residual mass remains. The axillary adenopathy has resolved.

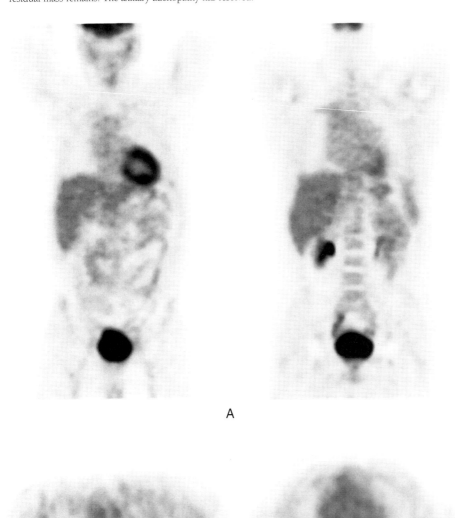

A

B

FIGURE 6. Repeat PET images (comparable coronal [**A**] and axial [**B**] sections to Figure 4) still show a wide mediastinum from the residual mass, but all of the hypermetabolic activity within the mediastinum, axillae, neck, and supraclavicular regions has resolved.

CASE 6 | *Thoracic Hodgkin's disease, initial staging and treatment assessment*

A 37-year-old woman was evaluated with CXR for shortness of breath and found to have mediastinal and hilar adenopathy. Chest CT confirmed moderately bulky mediastinal adenopathy (Figures 1 and 2). A diagnosis of Hodgkin's disease was made by CT-guided biopsy. PET showed extensive pathologic FDG activity in the mediastinum and in the supraclavicular regions, especially the left (Figure 3). The patient was treated with chemotherapy, and reevaluation with repeat CT after six cycles showed improved, but not resolved, adenopathy (Figures 4 and 5). A repeat PET scan showed disappearance of the lymphoma findings noted previously (Figure 6).

TEACHING POINTS

A significant percentage of patients with large lymphomatous masses at the time of diagnosis will have persistent mass(es) after therapy. Even if there is a marked reduction in size on CT, the question remains as to whether there is active tumor, a distinction that cannot be made by anatomic imaging alone. PET, which reflects metabolic activity, more successfully separates benign residual masses from active tumor. However, in up to 10% of PET negative residual masses, active tumor may ultimately be demonstrated, indicating careful follow-up is mandatory.

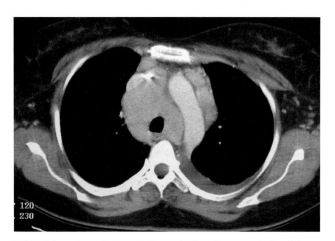

FIGURE 1. Enhanced chest CT shows a bulky right paratracheal nodal mass, as well as prevascular adenopathy and a small left pleural effusion.

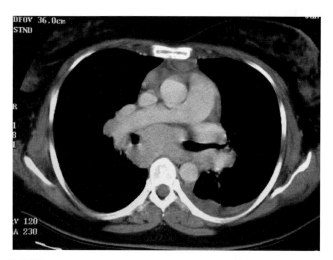

FIGURE 2. A more inferior section shows hilar adenopathy and a subcarinal nodal mass. A small left pleural effusion is again seen.

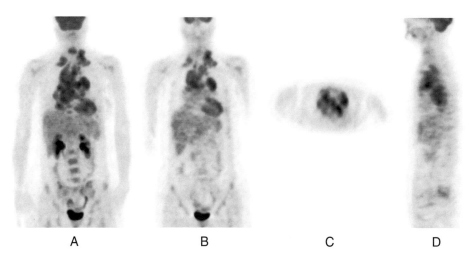

A   B   C   D

FIGURE 3. PET shows inhomogeneous increased FDG activity widening the mediastinum and both hila, with abnormal activity also seen in the supraclavicular regions (left greater than right). Projection (**A**), coronal (**B**), transaxial (**C**), and sagittal (**D**) views are shown.

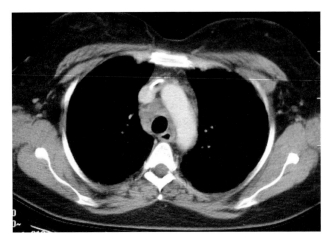

FIGURE 4. Repeat chest CT, after 6 months of chemotherapy, shows improvement compared with the staging examination. The prevascular adenopathy has resolved, but there is still an enlarged right paratracheal lymph node.

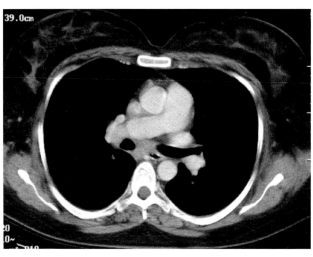

FIGURE 5. The subcarinal nodal mass has also shrunk, but not resolved.

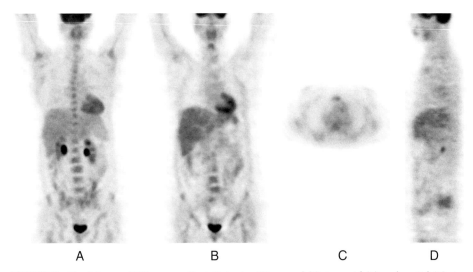

A   B   C   D

FIGURE 6. The follow-up PET has normalized. Projection (**A**), coronal (**B**), transaxial (**C**), and sagittal (**D**) views are shown.

CASE 7 | *Thoracic and abdominal Hodgkin's disease: initial staging, treatment assessment, marrow activation*

A 39-year-old HIV-positive man was diagnosed with Hodgkin's disease from a left posterior cervical lymph node biopsy. PET scan was obtained as part of his staging work-up (Figure 1). It showed extensive nodal involvement, including the mediastinum, left neck, axilla, and retroperitoneum. Hepatosplenomegaly was also noted, without focal visceral disease. After two cycles of chemotherapy, the patient's response was assessed with repeat PET (Figure 2). Marked interval improvement was confirmed, with essentially all of the soft tissue disease resolved. New diffuse increased bone marrow activity was present, consistent with marrow activation due to granulocyte colony-stimulating factor. This appearance of bone marrow resolved on a follow-up, 4 months later, after no additional treatment (Figures 3 and 4).

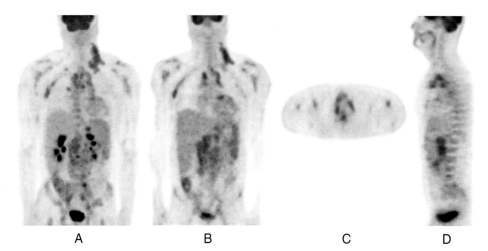

FIGURE 1. Projection (**A**) and coronal (**B**), axial (**C**), and sagittal (**D**) PET images from a staging study, after diagnosis of Hodgkin's disease was made from a left neck node biopsy, show confluent nodal activity in the left neck, mediastinum, right axilla, and retroperitoneum.

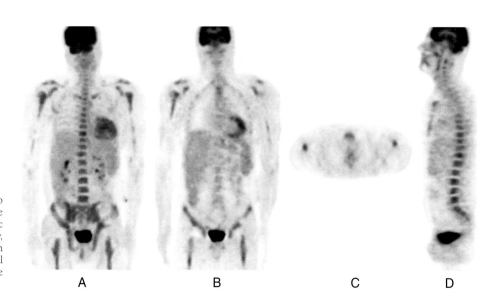

FIGURE 2. Two months later, after two cycles of chemotherapy, all of the disease findings have resolved. There is a dramatic interval change in bone marrow activity, now diffusely increased, consistent with marrow activation. Projection (**A**), coronal (**B**), transaxial (**C**), and sagittal (**D**) views are shown.

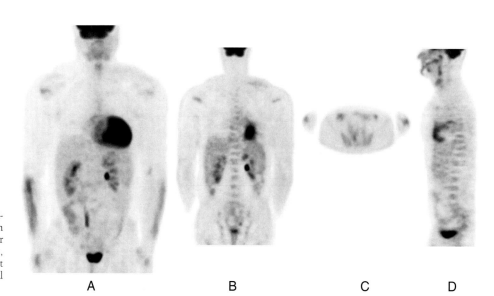

FIGURE 3. The activated marrow findings resolved on a follow-up PET scan 4 months later. Upper extremity muscular activity, seen on the projection image (**A**), may be secondary to the patient's penchant for weight lifting. Coronal (**B**), transaxial (**C**), and sagittal (**D**) views are also shown.

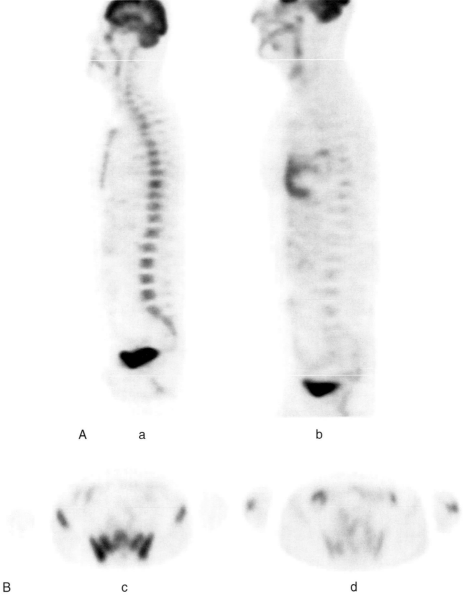

FIGURE 4. Activated marrow: before and after. Paired images, sagittal views (**A**) through spine and axial views (**B**) through pelvis, juxtaposing PET scan obtained during chemotherapy (**a** and **c**) with follow-up 4 months later (**b** and **d**), 3 months after chemotherapy was finished. Bone marrow is normally barely visible, as on the follow-up study on right. Note difficulty of visualizing the sternum. Marrow activation presents as a diffuse and usually fairly uniform increase in marrow activity, seen when chemotherapy includes administration of colony-stimulating factors, and resolves on its own.

CASE 8 | Lymphoma, nodal and visceral involvement, staging and treatment assessment, marrow activation

A 50-year-old woman with follicular, large cell non-Hodgkin's lymphoma, diagnosed from bone marrow biopsy, was staged with CT (Figures 1 to 3) and PET (Figure 4). PET showed foci of increased activity at multiple node group levels, including the axillae, hila, mediastinum, porta hepatis, and retroperitoneum, corresponding to adenopathy on CT. The markedly enlarged spleen was extremely hypermetabolic on PET, indicating visceral disease.

The patient was treated with four cycles of chemotherapy, and returned for follow-up PET scanning, symptomatically much improved.

The repeat PET showed complete resolution of the nodal findings, and the splenic enlargement and hypermetabolism reverted to normal (Figure 5).

TEACHING POINTS

PET has been shown to be highly sensitive in detecting lymphoma in lymph nodes, extranodally (e.g., in viscera), and within bone marrow. In this case, the splenic involvement is the most dramatic manifestation of this patient's disease. The hypermetabolic activity of the enlarged spleen on PET indicated there was visceral involvement, confirmed by the dramatic resolution of these findings after treatment.

This case also illustrates well the typical findings of postchemotherapy marrow activation, thought to be the result of the administration of colony-stimulating factors given with cytotoxic agents.

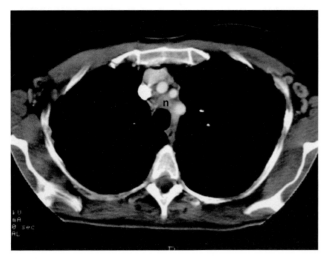

FIGURE 1. Contrast medium–enhanced chest CT shows mildly enlarged right paratracheal (n) and bilateral axillary lymph nodes (left greater than right).

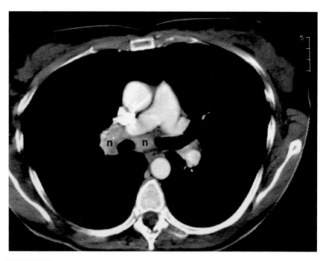

FIGURE 2. A more inferior section shows mildly enlarged hilar and subcarinal lymph nodes (n).

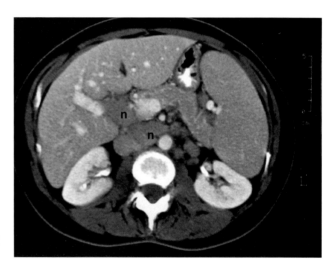

FIGURE 3. An image through the upper abdomen shows splenomegaly and enlarged porta hepatis and aortocaval lymph nodes (n).

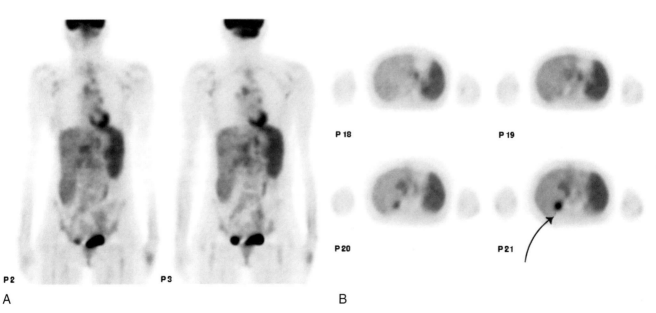

FIGURE 4. Coronal (**A**) and axial (**B**) PET images confirm extensive disease, with foci of increased activity in the axillae, hila, mediastinum, porta hepatis, and retroperitoneum, corresponding to lymphadenopathy seen on CT. The spleen is markedly enlarged and hypermetabolic. Reidel's lobe configuration of the liver is also noted. Intense normal right renal activity is seen on the axial views (*arrow*).

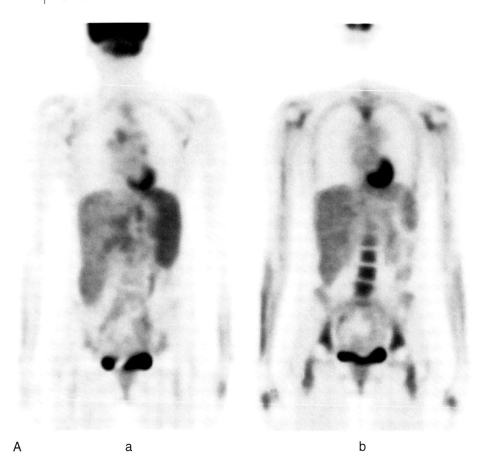

A   a   b

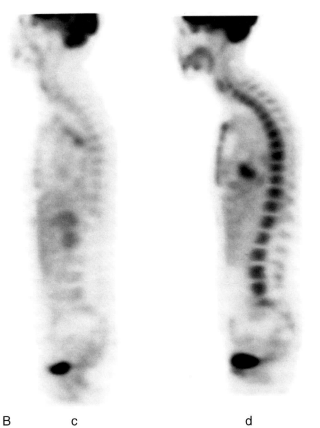

B   c   d

FIGURE 5. Coronal (**A**) and sagittal (**B**) PET images, juxtaposing the initial staging examination (**a** and **c**) with the post-treatment study (**b** and **d**) 3 months later, after four cycles of chemotherapy. The nodal disease in the axillae, mediastinum, hila, porta hepatis, and retroperitoneum (**a** and **c**) has resolved on the follow-up (**b** and **d**). The markedly enlarged and hypermetabolic spleen on the initial study reverted to a normal appearance on the follow-up. The post-chemotherapy examination shows a diffuse, homogeneous increase in bone marrow activity, well seen in the lumbar spine and hips. These PET findings and clinical scenario are typical of marrow activation.

CASE 9 | *Recurrent lymphoma, bone marrow involvement*

A 52-year-old man with a history of non-Hodgkin's lymphoma presented with recurrent bone symptoms, including bone pain, weakness, and malaise. Three years before, the patient was treated with chemotherapy. When his symptoms recurred, he was extensively re-imaged, including with CT, but initial studies showed no evidence of recurrent lymphoma. The patient was evaluated by multiple physicians and offered reassurance and even psychiatric consultation. Only a bone scan was subtly abnormal, with posterior rib inhomogeneity (Figure 1). A PET scan confirmed recurrent lymphoma involving the marrow space extensively (Figure 2). No evidence of nodal or visceral involvement was seen. Subsequent MRI confirmed diffuse abnormal marrow signal intensity abnormality (Figure 3). The patient was treated with two cycles of chemotherapy, and reexamined with PET 2 months later, which showed a dramatic reversion to normal (Figure 4). He finished chemotherapy and underwent stem cell transplantation. His follow-up PET studies have remained normal for 2 years.

TEACHING POINTS

This case is a powerful demonstration of PET's ability to identify disease that may be hard to appreciate by any other means. Discrepancies between PET scan and bone scan findings are not unusual, with bone scans more likely to reflect abnormalities stimulating osteoblastic activity, such as sclerotic metastases. PET can demonstrate lytic or marrow abnormalities that may not be demonstrable on bone scanning.

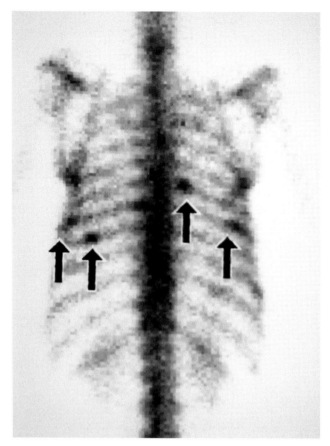

FIGURE 1. Posterior thoracic image from a bone scan shows posterior rib inhomogeneity (*arrows*).

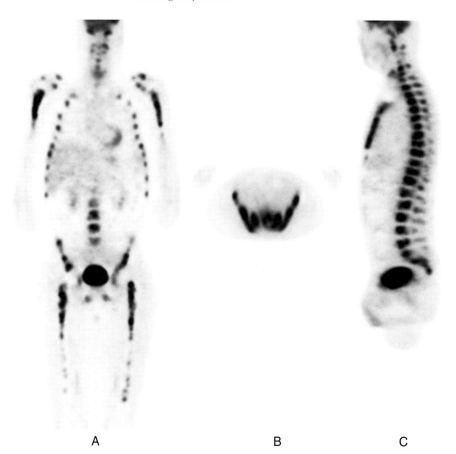

FIGURE 2. PET images (coronal [**A**], axial [**B**], and sagittal [**C**] sections) at the time of diagnosis of recurrent non-Hodgkin's lymphoma, show diffuse, hyperintense, heterogeneous marrow activity, consistent with extensive marrow involvement. Activity is so extensive it is nearly confluent in areas. Patchiness is best appreciated in the femurs. No visceral or nodal disease is suggested.

A   B   C

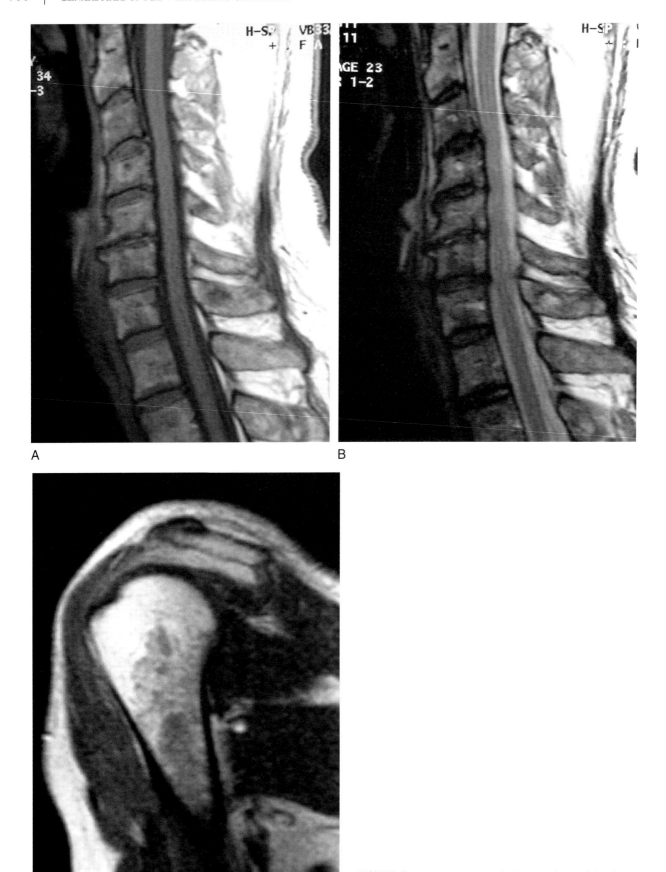

FIGURE 3. MR imaging obtained subsequently (T1- [A] and T2-weighted [B] fast spin-echo sagittal views of the cervical spine and T1-weighted sagittal [C] of the humerus) confirms diffusely abnormal, mottled marrow signal intensity.

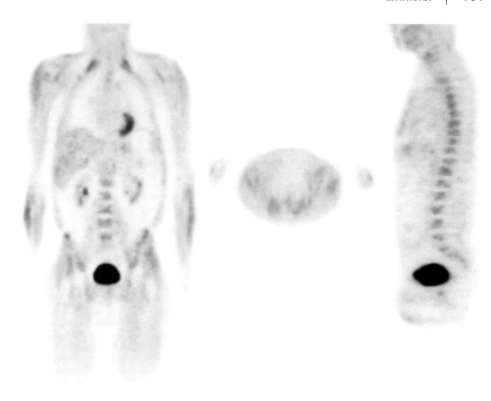

FIGURE 4. Repeat PET image, 2 months later (after two cycles of chemotherapy), shows reversion to normal. Multiple follow-up studies over the next 2 years remain normal. Coronal (**A**), transaxial (**B**), and sagittal (**C**) views are shown.

A   B   C

CASE 10 | *Recurrent pelvic non-Hodgkin's lymphoma, radiation therapy follow-up*

A 50-year-old man, 2 years post diagnosis of non-Hodgkin's lymphoma, was evaluated with PET imaging for a growing pelvic abnormality seen on CT. He was initially diagnosed with NHL when he presented with lower extremity swelling and was found to have retroperitoneal and pelvic lymphadenopathy. He was successfully treated with chemotherapy and rituximab (Rituxan), as confirmed by a negative PET scan. His right kidney was noted to be atrophic (Figure 1) apparently secondary to lymphomatous nodal encasement of the ureter. On an ensuing follow-up CT, a growing pelvic abnormality was noted (Figure 2). Suspected lymphoma recurrence was evaluated with PET scanning, which showed a new corresponding right hemipelvic focus of activity (Figure 3). This recurrence was treated with radiation therapy, which concluded 7 months before he was reexamined with PET. This follow-up PET was normal, indicating an effective radiation therapy response. Concurrent CT follow-up showed little change in the visible residual mass.

TEACHING POINTS

PET scanning provided valuable ancillary information at several important junctures in this patient's care. Although the patient was not evaluated at initial staging, PET scanning was performed after completion of chemotherapy and was negative. When a recurrence was suspected based on a CT change, it was confirmed with PET, which showed this to be new and the only site of active disease. The localized recurrence could be treated with radiation instead of systemic therapy. The CT findings after radiation were little changed. The residual mass was inactive on repeat PET, indicating a successful response to radiation.

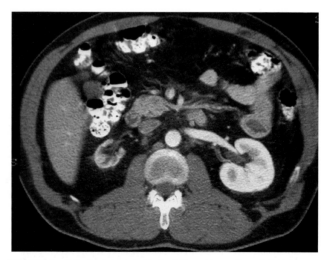

FIGURE 1. Enhanced CT through the kidneys shows the right kidney to be tiny and atrophic.

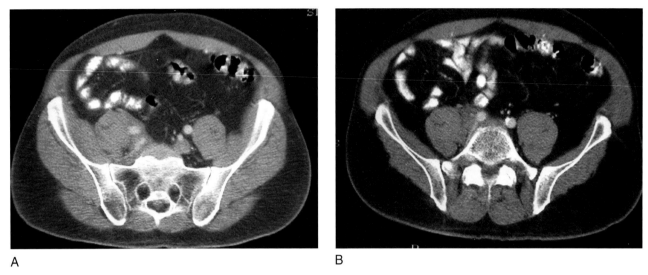

A   B

FIGURE 2. In the pelvis (two levels, **A** and **B**), a confluent nodal mass encases the right iliac vessels and presumably the ureter (not separately visualized).

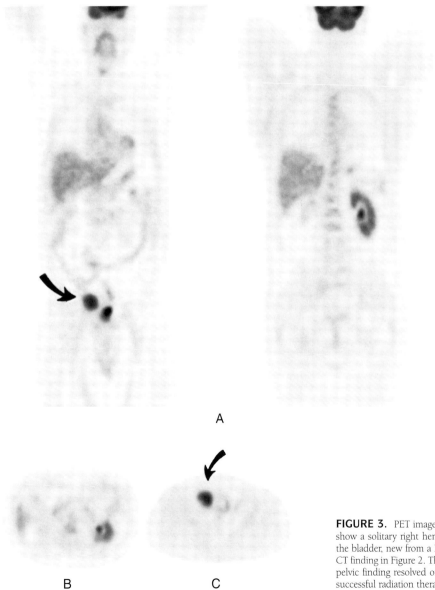

A

B   C

FIGURE 3. PET images (coronal [**A**] and axial [**B**, abdomen; and **C**, pelvis]) show a solitary right hemipelvic focus of activity *(arrow)*, above and lateral to the bladder, new from a PET scan 11 months before and corresponding to the CT finding in Figure 2. The tiny, atrophic right kidney is barely visible. The right pelvic finding resolved on a subsequent PET scan 10 months later, indicating successful radiation therapy, although CT findings were little changed.

CASE 11 | *Mantle cell lymphoma, radiation response*

A 56-year-old man with a history of mantle cell, non-Hodgkin's lymphoma was evaluated with PET imaging when an intra-abdominal recurrence was detected. His tumor had initially been identified 2 years before in the left neck and was irradiated. About 1.5 years later, he developed painless jaundice and was found on ultrasonography and CT to have a mass at the level of the pancreatic head (Figure 1). Biopsy confirmed recurrent mantle cell lymphoma, and he was referred for PET imaging for restaging. PET scanning confirmed the RUQ mass to be intensely hypermetabolic (Figure 2). No other sites of involvement were found. He was treated with radiation therapy and stented to relieve the obstructive jaundice and reevaluated with PET imaging 4.5 months later. The previously identified mass was no longer visualized, indicating a favorable response to radiation (Figure 3).

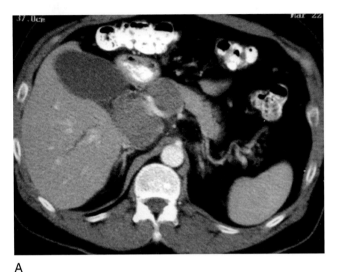

A

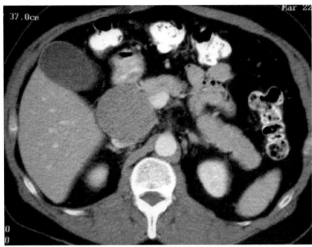

B

C

FIGURE 1. Enhanced abdominal CT images (**A** to **C**), from superior to inferior, show a homogeneous retropancreatic mass, which displaces anteriorly the uncinate process of the pancreas and compresses posteriorly the inferior vena cava. Mild resulting biliary ductal dilatation is seen on the most superior slice.

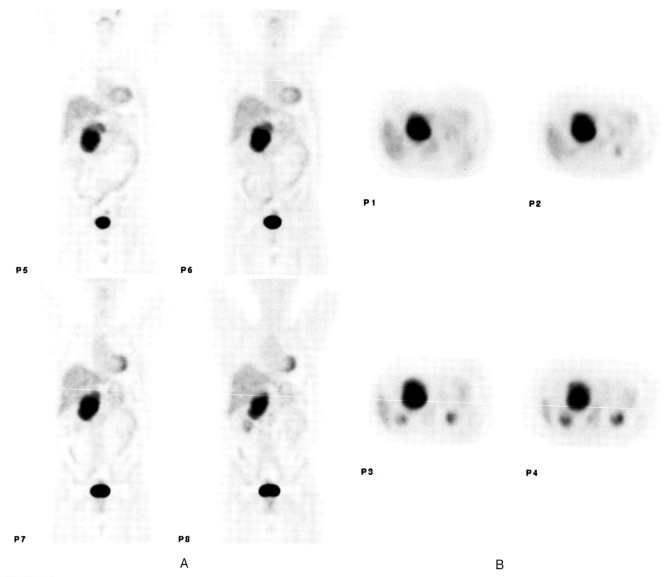

FIGURE 2. Coronal (**A**) and axial (**B**) PET slices show a large, ovoid, hypermetabolic RUQ mass, at the level of the pancreatic head and corresponding to the biopsy-confirmed mantle cell lymphoma recurrence.

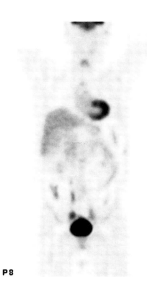

FIGURE 3. Repeat PET scan, 4.5 months later, after radiation to the peripancreatic recurrence, shows no residual at the site.

CASE 12 | *Mediastinal recurrent lymphoma, response to chemotherapy*

A 60-year-old man with a history of mesenteric non-Hodgkin's lymphoma developed new disease in the chest. He had been diagnosed about a year before when he presented with lower abdominal pain. The diagnosis was established at laparoscopic surgery after fine-needle aspiration showed small lymphocytes, nondiagnostic for lymphoma, and he was treated postoperatively with chemotherapy.

When CT showed a marked increase in mediastinal disease (Figure 1), he was referred for PET scanning for restaging (Figure 2). Bulky hypermetabolic disease was confirmed in the chest. Chemotherapy was resumed, and after 12 cycles, he was reevaluated with CT and PET scanning. Although CT showed clear improvement, there continued to be a sizeable low-density lymph node in the aortopulmonary window (Figure 3). His PET scan had completely normalized, including at the site of the residual nodal mass (Figure 4).

TEACHING POINTS

This patient's recurrent lymphoma became evident on CT follow-up. The initial restaging PET scan demonstrates the disease distribution and confirms that this patient's lymphoma is well depicted with FDG-PET. When his measurable disease failed to resolve on anatomic imaging after completion of chemotherapy, the demonstration on PET of normalization is reassuring that the residual mass is scar/fibrosis. This patient has been stable on CT and PET follow-up for 1.5 years.

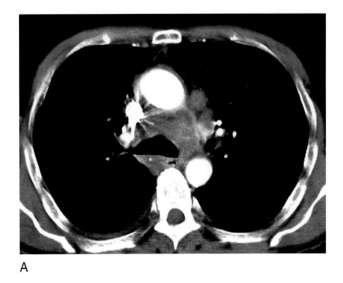

A

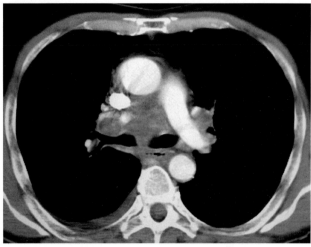

B

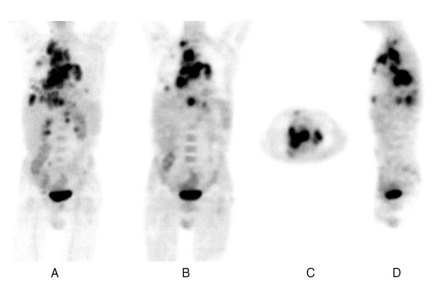

C

FIGURE 1. A to C, Bulky, low-density lymph nodes are seen in the aortopulmonary window, bilateral hila, and subcarinal regions and had progressed from a prior study 1 year before.

FIGURE 2. PET projection and volume images confirm the intense hypermetabolism and extensive distribution of the recurrent lymphoma. Projection image (A) and coronal (B), transaxial (C), and sagittal (D) views are shown.

A B C D

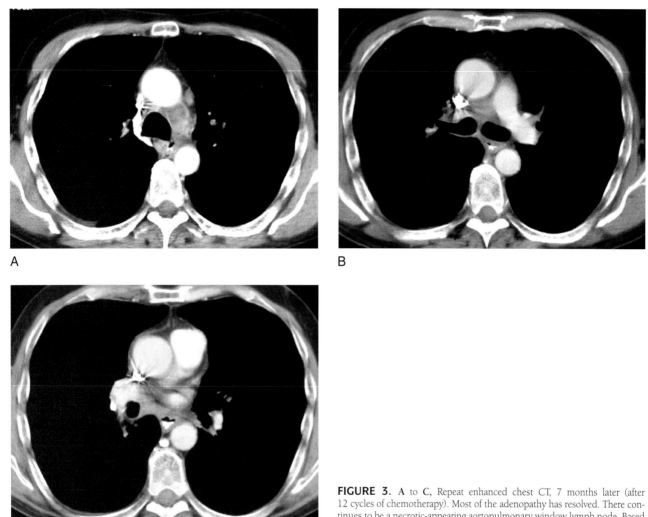

A

B

C

FIGURE 3. A to C, Repeat enhanced chest CT, 7 months later (after 12 cycles of chemotherapy). Most of the adenopathy has resolved. There continues to be a necrotic-appearing aortopulmonary window lymph node. Based on CT alone, active lymphoma cannot be differentiated from an inactive residual fibrotic mass.

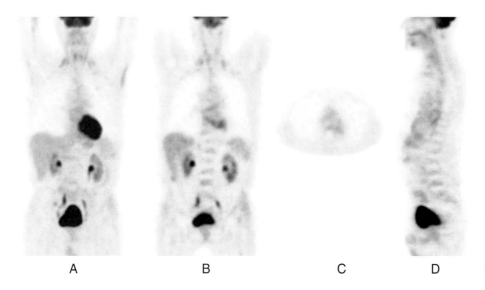

A   B   C   D

FIGURE 4. All pathologic findings have resolved on the corresponding, follow-up PET scan, 7 months after the first PET scan. Projection image (A) and coronal (B), transaxial (C), and sagittal (D) views are shown.

CASE 13 | *Mesenteric non-Hodgkin's lymphoma, residual mass assessment*

A 68-year-old man presented with abdominal pain, with intractable nausea and vomiting. Physical examination showed a large palpable abdominal mass. CT localized the mass to the mesentery (Figure 1). Biopsy proved diffuse large B-cell lymphoma. The non-Hodgkin's lymphoma was treated with chemotherapy, with incomplete radiographic regression . The residual mass was further treated with radiation, with no further shrinkage on CT (Figure 2).

Two months after completion of radiation therapy, PET was requested to assess the significance of the residual mass (Figure 3). It showed a small focus of intense localized metabolic activity in the LLQ, corresponding to the residual mass on CT. The case was discussed at tumor board. If the activity represented persistent tumor, surgical excision of the remaining mass would be considered. The possibility that the activity represented a persistent radiation therapy effect

was considered, given that the scan took place only 2 months after completion of therapy. PET was repeated 1 month later, which showed the abnormal focus to be smaller and decreased in activity, an encouraging trend. The patient did undergo surgical excision of the mass, with fat necrosis and fibrosis identified, but no evidence of lymphoma.

TEACHING POINTS

No staging PET scan was performed in this patient. Fortunately, the background level of bowel activity in this patient was low, allowing the focal abnormal activity of the mesenteric process to be readily visualized on PET. Without a prior PET study, the significance of the activity in the residual mass was uncertain, and at that one data point could have represented persistent lymphoma activity or radiation treatment effect. The first PET scan was performed 2 months after completion of radiation therapy. The regressing activity on the repeat PET study, 1 month later, suggests a resolving radiation therapy effect, which might have been confirmable noninvasively with further improvement on subsequent PET scans and/or continued residual mass stability on CT.

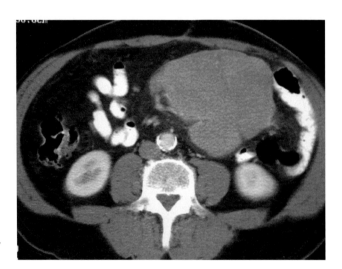

FIGURE 1. Enhanced CT through the mid abdomen shows a lobular, homogeneous soft tissue density mesenteric mass.

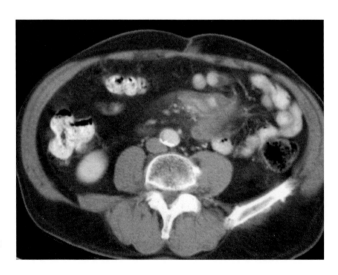

FIGURE 2. CT scan, 8 months later (after six cycles of CHOP chemotherapy, seven cycles of rituximab [Rituxan], and radiation therapy) shows an unchanging residual mass.

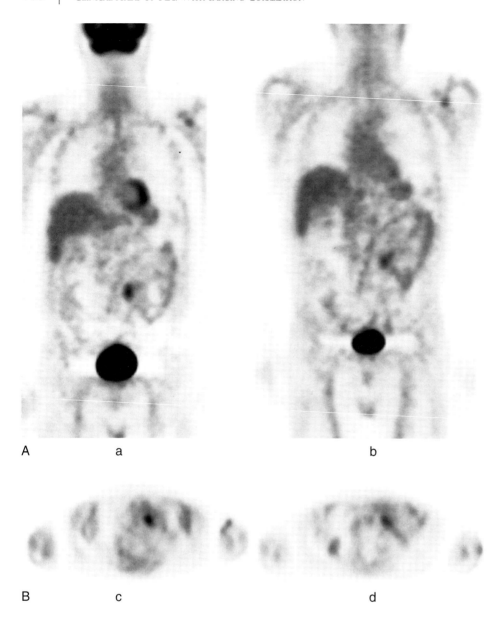

A   a   b

B   c   d

FIGURE 3. Coronal (**A**) and axial (**B**) PET scans (**a** and **c** 2 months after completion of radiation, **b** and **d** 1 month later) show a small focus of locally intense activity in the LLQ on the initial PET study, which is smaller and diminished in activity 1 month later. The trend suggested regressing radiation therapy effect.

Radiation therapy provokes hyperemia and inflammation, and metabolic activity at the site of treated lesions can persist for months to upward of a year. The optimal timing of PET scans after radiation to mitigate these effects is variable, but we try to wait as long as possible and prefer a minimum of 2 months.

CASE 14 | Lymphoma, staging and treatment assessment, head and neck presentation

A 78-year-old man presented with a 6-month history of hoarseness and progressive dysphagia to the point of choking. Imaging evaluation with barium swallow and soft tissue neck MRI identified a left base of tongue mass, on the order of 5 cm. MRI also showed associated left neck adenopathy. He was evaluated endoscopically and biopsied for a suspected head and neck carcinoma. Pathology instead identified a diffuse large, B-cell non-Hodgkin's lymphoma. PET was requested to complete the patient's staging. It confirmed intense hypermetabolic activity at the base of tongue, extending more to the left, with additional nodules of activity in left neck lymph nodes (Figure 1). He was treated with chemotherapy, with an immediate, excellent clinical response. When he was reevaluated with PET after completion of six chemotherapy cycles, he felt well, had regained lost weight, and had no difficulty eating. However, the repeat PET scan showed a smaller, but persistent base of tongue focus of activity, equal in intensity to the original PET scan (Figure 2). The nodal left neck foci of activity noted before had resolved. The PET scan findings clearly displayed evidence of persistent and active disease, despite a clinical examination suggesting the patient had had a definitive response to chemotherapy.

TEACHING POINTS

This patient's initial imaging evaluations all suggested a head and neck carcinoma, the most common cause of a mass in this region. The staging PET findings confirm the disease distribution but are nonspecific as to histology, as are most imaging modalities. The findings displayed here of base of tongue lymphoma could easily have been produced by a squamous cell carcinoma, the diagnosis expected before biopsy.

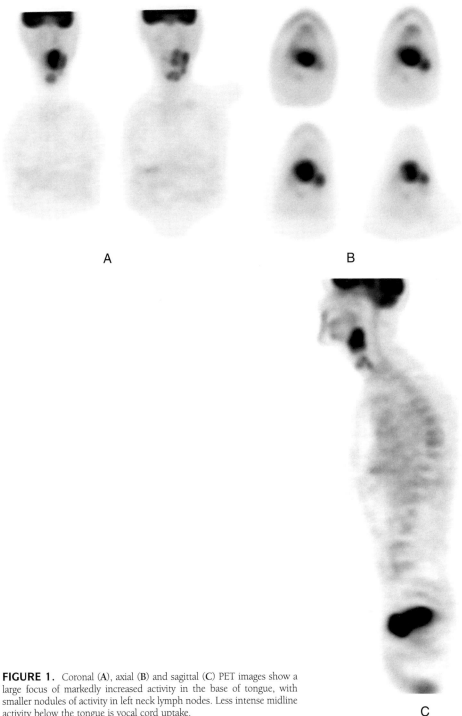

FIGURE 1. Coronal (**A**), axial (**B**) and sagittal (**C**) PET images show a large focus of markedly increased activity in the base of tongue, with smaller nodules of activity in left neck lymph nodes. Less intense midline activity below the tongue is vocal cord uptake.

The most important function PET served in this patient's care was in assessing the response to chemotherapy. The patient was thought clinically to have had an excellent result, with much improved physical examination findings and symptoms. Typically, with nonulcerated, predominantly submucosal lesions like this, underestimation of disease by direct inspection is common. PET serves an important function here by indicating the clear need for additional therapy.

The question may arise as to the timing of PET with regard to chemotherapy. Although there is no clear consensus on optimal timing, most would agree that waiting 6 weeks after chemotherapy is desirable, if possible. However, studies are very often successfully performed earlier.

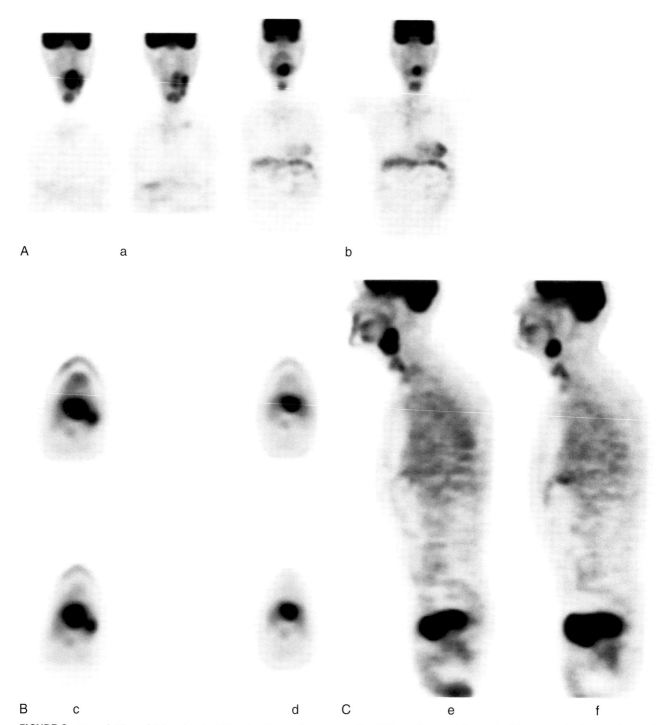

A   a   b

B   c   d   C   e   f

FIGURE 2. Coronal (**A**), axial (**B**), and sagittal (**C**) pairs of images juxtapose the first PET scan (**a, c,** and **e**) with the follow-up study after completion of chemotherapy (**b, d,** and **f**). Improvement is seen, but the persistent activity in the smaller base of tongue focus has not diminished in intensity. The smaller left neck nodal foci of activity have resolved. Less intense vocal cord activity, due to talking during the uptake period, is well demonstrated on the coronal images and is seen also on the sagittal images.

CASE 15 | *Recurrent lymphoma, pediatric patient*

A 10-year-old boy, previously treated for Hodgkin's disease, was referred for PET imaging when a biopsy-proven retroperitoneal recurrence was identified. He had been diagnosed 1.5 years before and treated with chemotherapy, irradiation, and splenectomy. A recurrence was identified a year later in liver, lung, and retroperitoneum. This was treated with a second course of chemotherapy and stem cell transplantation, which concluded 3 months before. Development of fever and back pain led to identification of retroperitoneal disease, which was confirmed with biopsy. PET imaging was requested to assess the disease burden and showed extensive paraspinal chains of activity, corresponding to retrocrural and retroperitoneal nodal disease (Figure 1).

TEACHING POINTS

There are approximately 10,000 new cases of cancer per year in the United States in children younger than the age of 16. For most of these patients, standard imaging studies (CT, MRI, ultrasound, nuclear examinations) suffice for diagnosis and monitoring. However, in certain malignancies, PET has proven beneficial. As this case illustrates, lymphoma is one example.

In selected patients, FDG-PET may be helpful in imaging musculoskeletal tumors and neuroblastoma. The use of PET to identify a seizure focus is well established.

An important issue with any imaging study is radiation dosimetry. For FDG-PET, the bladder wall receives the highest exposure and the absorbed dose is higher than in adults in the brain, heart, liver, pancreas, and bladder wall. Fortunately, the total absorbed dose from a PET scan is typically less than that from standard nuclear studies. Specific issues in children include alleviation of anxiety about the study, immobilization, sedation (must administer >30 minutes before FDG injection), and dose (adjust for body weight or body surface area; minimum 1 to 1.5 mCi).

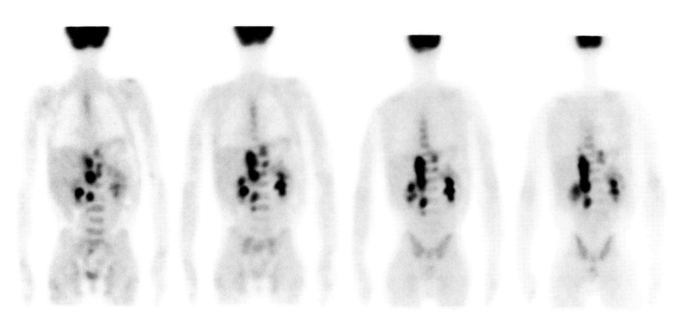

FIGURE 1. Coronal PET images show paraspinal chains of abnormal activity (right greater than left), corresponding with retrocrural and retroperitoneal nodal disease.

CASE 16 | *Lymphoma follow-up, thymic rebound*

A 20-year-old man was referred for PET imaging after decompressive spinal surgery and chemotherapy for intraspinal high-grade B-cell diffuse malignant lymphoma. He had presented with back pain and paraparesis, and MRI evaluation found an intraspinal epidural mass spanning T12-L3. At the time of referral for PET imaging, the patient was 6 months postoperative and had concluded chemotherapy 1 month before. His MRI findings had improved considerably, but he was left with residual signal abnormalities in lumbar spine vertebrae. PET was requested to help assess their significance. It showed no abnormalities.

Because the patient was considered to be high risk, he was closely followed, with repeat MRI and PET scanning 2 months later.

There continued to be stable persistent marrow signal abnormalities in the lumbar spine on MRI, which were not active on PET. New prevascular mediastinal activity was now noted, consistent with thymic rebound (Figure 1). This was corroborated with CT (Figure 2).

TEACHING POINTS

Thymic activity can be seen as a normal variant in young patients, even into their 30s. Normal thymic activity may be suppressed as a consequence of chemotherapy. The subsequent follow-up of these patients with CT and PET may show the development of new tissue or activity representing the rebounding thymus. When its characteristic appearance and location are recognized, there is no diagnostic dilemma. However, failure to remember the thymus as a possible cause of mediastinal activity in a young patient could lead to misdiagnoses.

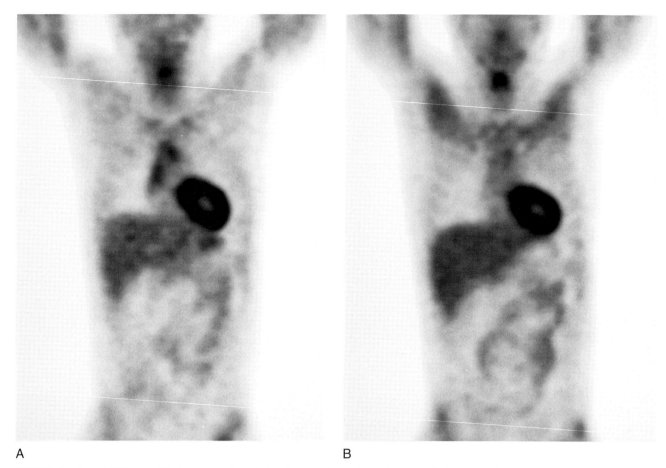

A   B

FIGURE 1. Coronal PET image (**A**) shows triangular, sail-shaped prevascular mediastinal activity, which was new from the PET scan obtained 2 months before (**B**). At this time, the patient was 3 months out from the conclusion of his chemotherapy.

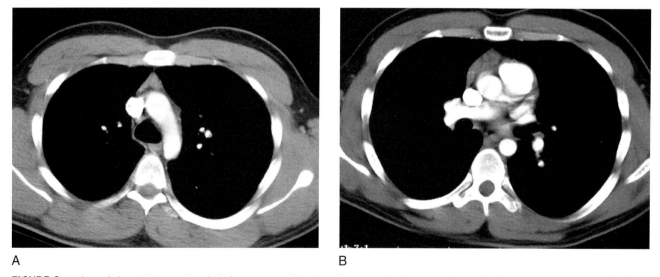

A   B

FIGURE 2. Enhanced chest CT images (**A** and **B**) show corresponding triangular prevascular tissue, consistent with thymus in a young patient. The lower section shows the right limb of the thymus to extend farther inferiorly than the left in this patient, as on the PET scan.

CHAPTER

5

Melanoma

Cutaneous melanoma is a malignancy of increasing incidence. Current estimates are that 1 in 75 Americans will develop melanoma in their lifetime.[1] Risk factors include multiple atypical nevi, freckles, lighter hair color, inability to tan, excess sun exposure, familial history, and perhaps disorders of DNA repair.[1,2] Spread may occur via lymphatics or hematogenously. Once distant metastases are identified, the median survival is 4 to 6 months.[3] However, approximately 20% of patients presenting with only local nodal metastases may be cured by surgery. It has also been shown that isolated distant metastases may be amenable to surgical cure. Accurate staging and surveillance, therefore, are crucial to optimal patient care. PET has proven to be an important addition to conventional methods of evaluation (e.g., clinical examination, plain radiography, CT, MRI, ultrasonography, bone scan, sentinel node biopsy).

STAGING

A number of staging classifications exist (Tables 1 to 3).[1]

Combined data on more than 1600 patients for staging revealed a 91% accuracy for PET.[2] With the exception of small

TABLE 1 CLINICAL STAGING OF MALIGNANT MELANOMA

Stage	Findings
I	No metastases detectable
II	Metastases within 3 cm of primary lesion (primary tumor with "satellitosis")
a	Metastases > 3 cm from primary
b	Metastases at lymph nodes
c	Both
III	Regional metastases
IV	Distant metastases

From Ak L, Stokkel MOM, Bergman W, et al: Cutaneous malignant melanoma: Clinical aspects, imaging modalities and treatment. Eur J Nucl Med 2000;27:447-458.

TABLE 2 BRESLOW CLASSIFICATION SYSTEM

Stage	Depth of Invasion	Category
I	< 0.75 mm	Thin melanoma
II	0.76 to 3.99 mm	Intermediate melanoma
III	> 4 mm	Thick melanoma

From Ak L, Stokkel MOM, Bergman W, et al: Cutaneous malignant melanoma: Clinical aspects, imaging modalities and treatment. Eur J Nucl Med 2000;27:447-458.

lung metastases, PET was more sensitive than CT in detecting metastases.[4] There are a number of locations where PET has proven to be superior to CT, including the mediastinum and hilar regions (note that PET will often be positive in normal-sized lymph nodes), abdomen, and peripheral lymph nodes (often not imaged by conventional CT examinations). A word of caution about the investigation of regional nodal activity with PET is in order. Although a prospective study of this application showed an 88% sensitivity for PET, false-negative results may be expected in micrometastatic disease.[5]

Another advantage of PET is the identification of unsuspected distant metastases. Two important reasons this is of

TABLE 3 CLARK'S CLASSIFICATION SCHEME

Level	Finding
I	In situ melanoma
II	Infiltrates papillary dermis without filling it completely
III	Tumor invades the papillary-reticular dermal interface
IV	Tumoral invasion of the reticular dermis
V	Tumoral invasion of the subcutaneous tissue

From Ak L, Stokkel MOM, Bergman W, et al: Cutaneous malignant melanoma: Clinical aspects, imaging modalities and treatment. Eur J Nucl Med 2000;27:447-458.

value are (1) patients may be spared noncurative, potentially disfiguring surgery and (2) earlier referral can be made for some of the newer, innovative forms of systemic therapy. Based on our current understanding of the strengths and weaknesses of PET in melanoma, consideration should be given to PET for staging and the investigation of suspected recurrence.[6-8] Brain involvement remains the purview of MRI, CT is more sensitive in the lungs, and sentinel node biopsy is the preferred study to identify the first node draining the primary tumor site.[9]

REFERENCES

1. Ak L, Stokkel MPM, Bergman W, et al: Cutaneous malignant melanoma: Clinical aspects, imaging modalities and treatment. Eur J Nucl Med 2000;27:447-458.
2. Gambhir SS, Czernin J, Schwimmer J, et al: A tabulated summary of the FDG PET literature. J Nucl Med 2001;42:13S-15S.
3. Macfarlane DJ, Sondak V, Johnson T, et al: Prospective evaluation of 2-[18F]-2-deoxy-D-glucose positron emission tomography in staging of regional lymph nodes in patients with cutaneous malignant melanoma. J Clin Oncol 1998;16:1770-1776.
4. Rinne D, Baum RP, Hor G, et al: Primary staging and follow-up of high risk melanoma patients with whole-body ^{18}F-flurodeoxyglucose positron emission tomography. Cancer 1998;82:1664-1671.
5. Crippar F, Leutner M, Belli F, et al: Which kinds of lymph node metastases can FDG PET detect? A clinical study in melanoma. J Nucl Med 2000;41:1491-1494.
6. Eigtved A, Anderson AP, Dahlstrom K, et al: Use of fluorine-18 fluorodeoxyglucose positron emission tomography in the detection of silent metastases from malignant melanoma. Eur J Nucl Med 2000; 27:70-75.
7. Holden WD, White RL, Zuger JH, et al: Effectiveness of positron emission tomography for the detection of melanoma metastases. Ann Surg 1998;227:764-771.
8. Acland KM, O'Doherty MJ, Russell-Jones R, et al: The value of positron emission tomography scanning in the detection of subclinical metastatic melanoma. J Clin Acad Dermatol 2000;42:606-611.
9. Nguyen AT, Akhurst T, Larsen SM, et al: PET scanning with ^{18}F-2-fluoro-2-deoxy-D-glucose (FDG) in patients with melanoma: Benefits and limitations. Clin Pos Imag 1999;2:93-98.

CASE 1 | *Staging, persistent disease at operative site*

A 41-year-old woman with metastatic melanoma presented with left axillary adenopathy (Figure 1). Work-up, including mammography, was negative, and ultimately the histologic diagnosis of metastatic melanoma was made by excisional biopsy. Two lymph nodes were removed, both positive. Two weeks later, she underwent left axillary dissection, with 10 of 12 additional lymph nodes positive. Total-body skin examination, including benign biopsies of lesions of the left anterior thigh, left medial ankle, and right posterior shoulder region, failed to identify a primary site. PET scanning was requested to aid in staging. This was performed 2 weeks after surgery, at which time the patient noted swelling in the operative bed.

The PET scan showed clear evidence of persistent disease in the left axilla, as well as findings of a postoperative seroma (Figure 2). A skin primary site was not found. The only other finding of note was moderate intensity focal activity in the left hemipelvis (Figure 3). Comparison with pelvis CT showed a correlate of a cystic left ovary, suggesting a corpus luteum cyst (Figure 4).

TEACHING POINTS

PET scanning was requested for staging and to search for a primary lesion in this patient with axillary metastatic melanoma presenting without an antecedent skin lesion. The results confirmed the negative whole-body skin examination. The persistent disease in the left axilla was unexpected. Fortunately, although performed only 2 weeks postoperatively, the PET findings of residual axillary melanoma and postoperative seroma were quite distinct.

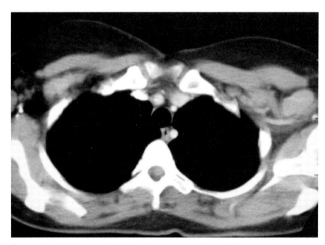

A

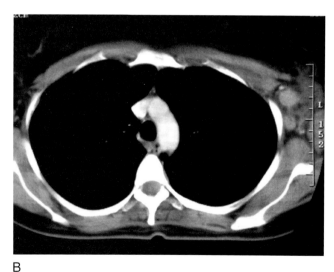

B

FIGURE 1. Enhanced chest CT images (**A** and **B**), after diagnosis made by excisional biopsy and before axillary dissection, show multiple enlarged, enhancing left axillary lymph nodes.

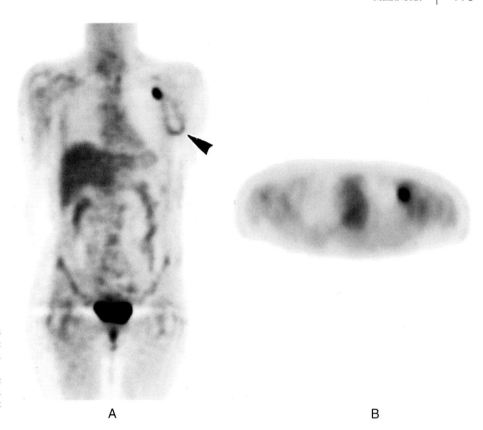

FIGURE 2. Postoperative PET scan images (**A** and **B**) show a ring of modest metabolic activity in the left axilla, consistent with an organizing post-surgical seroma *(arrowhead)*. However, this clearly differs from the intense hypermetabolic nodular activity in the high left anterior axilla, indicative of persistent melanoma.

A

B

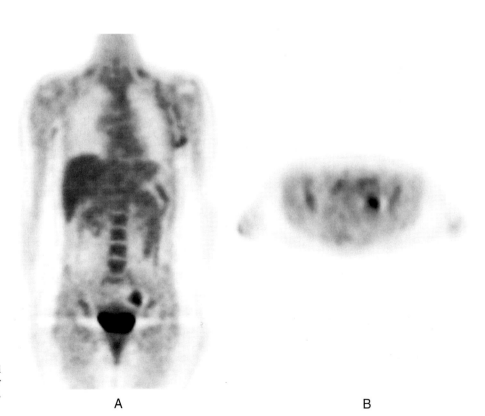

FIGURE 3. Additional coronal (**A**) and axial (**B**) PET scan images through the pelvis show a moderately active left hemipelvic focus, more localized and intense than bowel.

A

B

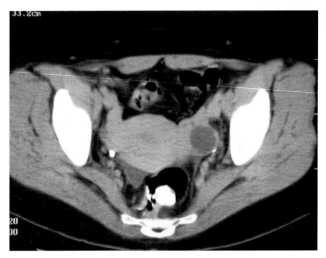

FIGURE 4. Enhanced pelvis CT image for correlation shows a cystic left ovary at the level in question. Corpus luteum cysts can be a benign source of activity on FDG-PET.

CASE 2 | Initial staging and restaging, disease progression despite chemotherapy

A 43-year-old woman was diagnosed with a left great toe melanoma at the time of surgery for an ulcerated lesion. One month later, she underwent wider excision of the toe and left inguinal dissection after lymphoscintigraphy. Two lymph nodes were positive. PET scan evaluation was performed 2 weeks after surgery, at which time there was relatively intense and somewhat lumpy left inguinal activity noted, thought suggestive of residual melanoma (Figures 1 and 2). The patient was treated with chemotherapy for 4 months and rescanned with PET. The repeat study showed a clear, marked progression of metastatic disease at the left groin level.

TEACHING POINTS

Assessing a surgical scar site for residual neoplastic disease can be difficult with any modality. As with anatomic techniques, the ease of evaluating such sites increases the longer one can wait before imaging. Most surgical scars display fairly characteristic, linear, relatively modest and readily recognizable activity, especially when the evaluation takes

FIGURE 1. Coronal PET images (**A** is from initial PET scan; **B** is 4.5 months later) show progression of left inguinal metastatic disease, despite interval chemotherapy. The initial study was obtained only 2 weeks after surgery, which identified two positive lymph nodes. Although the activity is linear in overall configuration and the surgery is relatively recent, the activity seemed both more intense and thicker and somewhat more nodular than usually seen in the postoperative setting. Based on these observations, residual melanoma was questioned at this level, and the patient was treated with chemotherapy. The follow-up 4.5 months later shows progressive disease at this level, with a large, lobular focus of intense activity, with adjacent smaller satellites of presumably nodal disease noted in addition.

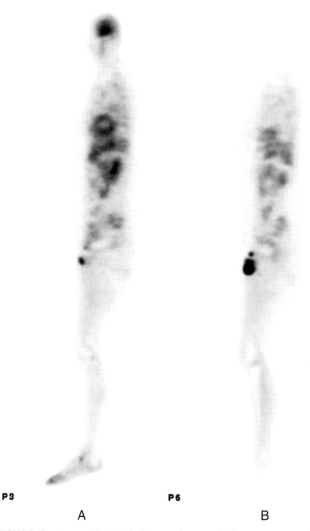

FIGURE 2. Comparable PET findings in the sagittal plane. Again, original study is shown in **A** and follow-up study is shown in **B**, showing progression.

place a month or more later. The evaluation of this scar site was complicated by the recent time course. Even allowing for this, careful scrutiny of it showed concerning features. The activity, linear in overall configuration, is very thick and intense, with subtle nodularity suggested. The suspicions raised were borne out by the clear, subsequent disease progression later demonstrated, despite interval chemotherapy.

CASE 3 | *Staging, unexpected additional disease site*

A 40-year-old woman was recently diagnosed with a 2.5-mm thick right thigh melanoma. The mole in question had been present for years and was sampled when the patient noted gradual growth and intermittent bleeding. The margins of the excision were clean. Shortly after the biopsy and diagnosis of melanoma, the patient noted a small right groin lump. She underwent an inguinal lymph node biopsy, as well as wider excision of the thigh lesion site. The wider thigh excision did not show any residual melanoma, but the groin lymph node was positive for metastatic melanoma. The patient was referred for PET scan for staging, before planned more extensive right inguinal dissection.

PET scan showed linear foci of mild activity at the thigh and inguinal surgical sites, consistent with uptake at the scars but not suggestive of persistent melanoma (Figures 1 and 2). However, an unexpected round, intense focus of hypermetabolism was seen within the right pelvis, thought likely nodal and metastatic (Figures 3 and 4). MRI was recommended to further evaluate this, and a corresponding, enhancing conglomerate right obturator nodal mass was identified (Figure 5).

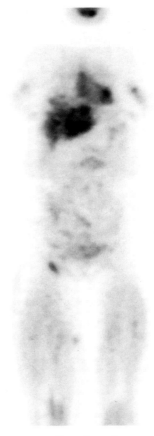

FIGURE 2. Just posterior to Figure 1, another coronal PET section shows an oblique linear focus of activity at the right groin level, consistent with post-surgical change. No foci of melanoma are suggested by PET at this level.

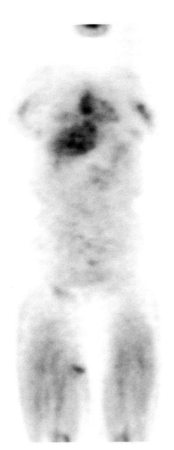

FIGURE 1. Far anterior coronal PET image shows a transverse, linear focus of activity at the right medial mid-thigh level, at the site of the excised melanoma. The low-level activity is consistent with surgical scar uptake.

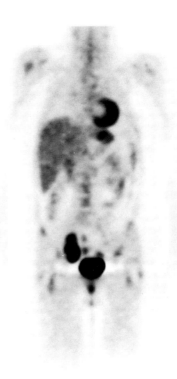

FIGURE 3. A coronal PET image through the urinary bladder shows a lobular, ovoid markedly hypermetabolic focus in the right hemipelvis, just supero-lateral to the bladder.

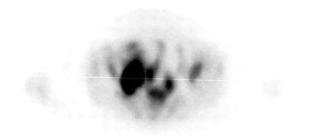

FIGURE 4. Axial PET section through the right hemipelvic abnormality, corresponding to Figure 3. A nodal site of metastatic melanoma within the pelvis was suggested based on PET, and MRI confirmation was recommended.

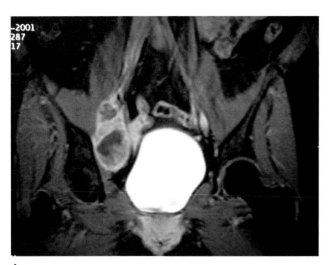

A

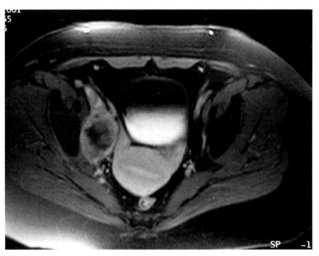

B

FIGURE 5. Coronal (**A**) and axial (**B**) fat-saturated, enhanced T1-weighted MR images through the pelvis show a heterogeneously enhancing ovoid right obturator nodal mass, corresponding precisely with the PET finding.

TEACHING POINTS

PET was used as the first imaging test in the staging of this patient and demonstrated unexpected disease within the pelvis, which was subsequently confirmed on MRI. The traditional approach of anatomic imaging (usually with chest, abdomen, and pelvis CT) first, and then PET, was reversed in this case. In clinical practice, this is occurring with

increasing frequency, with PET directing which portion of the body is subsequently imaged. The risk of this strategy is that certain forms of neoplasia, (e.g., small pulmonary metastases and peritoneal carcinomatosis [see Case 16 in Chapter 6 and Case 7 in Chapter 7]), which may be readily recognized on CT, might not be apparent on PET due to size limitations.

CASE 4 | *Staging, multiple unexpected additional disease sites*

A 59-year-old man was diagnosed with metastatic malignant melanoma in a right inguinal node, which he first noted 2 years before excision with little growth over time. The patient did not have a lower extremity skin lesion. He was treated with adjuvant interferon. PET scanning became available 7 months into a planned year course of interferon and showed metabolically active foci at a number of unsuspected sites in the left thigh, which were not detectable on physical examination (Figure 1). The patient was reevaluated with PET 6 months later, after completion of a year of interferon therapy, with complete normalization of his study (Figure 2). He has remained free of evidence of disease, on maintenance interferon and granulocyte-macrophage colony-stimulating factor, 17 months later.

TEACHING POINTS

In this patient, the initial PET scan identified a number of unsuspected disease sites, and PET proved efficacious in treatment assessment and follow-up. PET scanning is highly sensitive for identification of malignant melanoma, even in skin sites without a physical examination correlate, and is useful in staging, restaging, and treatment monitoring.

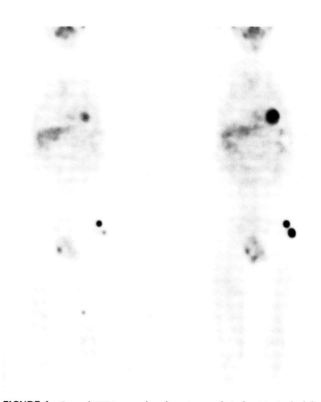

FIGURE 1. Coronal PET images show hyperintense foci of activity in the left proximal lateral thigh, with an additional focus in the left distal medial thigh, which were unsuspected and did not correlate with identifiable skin lesions, consistent with metastatic melanoma.

CASE 5 | *Melanoma, restaging, solitary recurrent disease site (axilla)*

A 47-year-old woman with a past history of right cheek and arm melanomas presented with a right axillary lump. Biopsy confirmed melanoma. The patient's history of right cheek melanoma was remote and estimated by the patient to have been 17 years before. Her right lower arm melanoma lesion had been excised 9 years before. She was referred for PET scanning for staging. PET showed a large right axillary hypermetabolic mass but no additional disease site (Figure 1).

TEACHING POINT

The importance of this PET scan is in what is not identified, namely, that there are no other disease sites, other than the known right axillary recurrence. This reassuring piece of data influences treatment decisions. A solitary site of recurrent disease favors surgical management over systemic therapy alone.

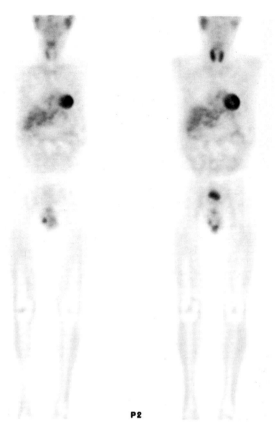

P1   P2

FIGURE 2. Six months later, repeat PET scan shows complete normalization with resolution of the abnormal findings. Note thyroid gland activity, which can be seen as a normal variant.

FIGURE 1. Coronal (**A**) and axial (**B**) PET images show a large hypermetabolic mass in the right axilla, at the site of the known melanoma recurrence, but no additional disease sites.

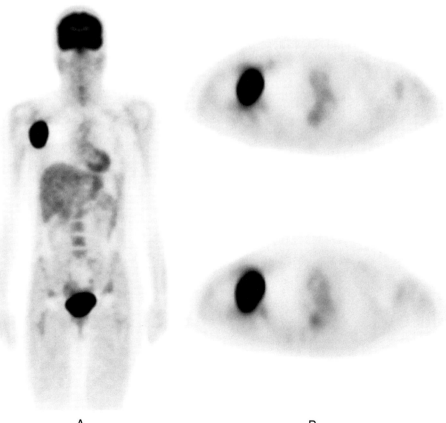

A   B

CASE 6 | *Restaging, recurrent facial disease*

An 86-year-old man with a history of recurrent facial malignant melanoma was evaluated with PET when he presented with a clinically evident subcutaneous recurrence in the right infraorbital cheek and right nasolabial fold.

His past history of melanoma dated back 8 years when he first presented with a forehead lesion. A recurrence occurred approximately 4 years later when he developed a right cheek (lower eyelid) lesion, confirmed surgically to be metastatic melanoma. Subsequent development

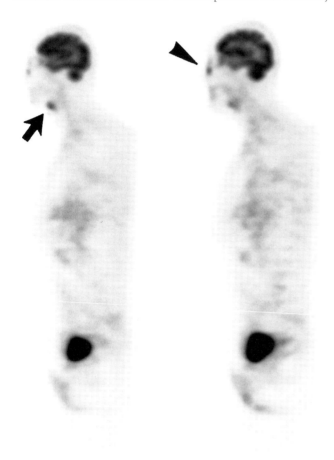

FIGURE 1. Sagittal PET images show two discrete sites of pathologically increased activity. One is at the right submandibular level (*arrow*), and the other is at the site of the clinically apparent right infraorbital recurrence (*arrowhead*).

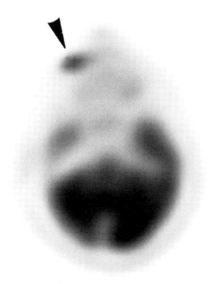

FIGURE 2. Axial PET image through the right infraorbital region shows an asymmetrical focus of increased activity at the paranasal level (*arrowhead*).

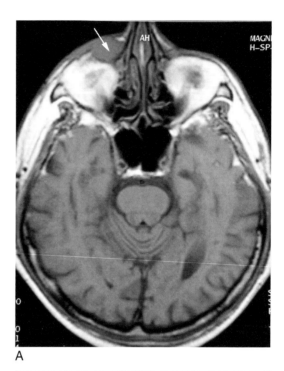

A

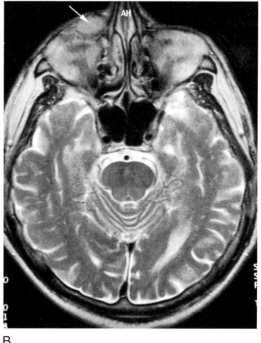

B

FIGURE 3. T1- (**A**) and T2-weighted (**B**) axial MR images through the same level confirm a corresponding superficial discrete tumor nodule (*arrows*).

of a larger recurrence in this region, a 1.5-cm lower eyelid nodule, was excised 8 months before. When he again developed clinical evidence of infraorbital recurrence, as well as subcutaneous nasolabial nodularity, he was referred for PET imaging to restage him.

PET identified two discrete abnormalities (Figures 1, 2, and 4). One was at the right paranasal, infraorbital level of the prior recurrences. A previously unsuspected site of disease was also found at the

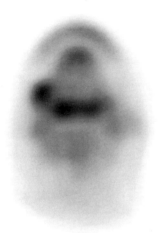

FIGURE 4. Axial PET image at the submandibular level shows an asymmetrical right submandibular focus of activity, thought suggestive of nodal disease.

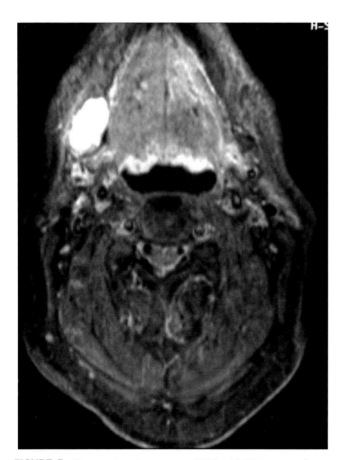

FIGURE 5. Short tau inversion recovery (STIR) axial MR image confirms a mass lesion at this level, most consistent with a pathologically enlarged lymph node.

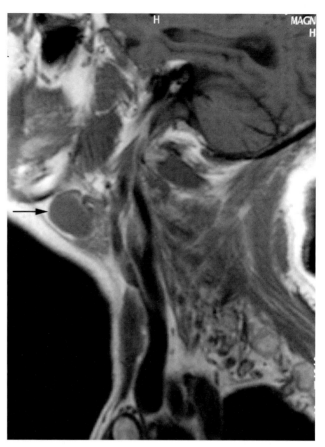

FIGURE 6. Sagittal T1-weighted MR image shows the lymph node in relation to the adjacent submandibular gland *(arrow)*.

right submandibular level. MRI was subsequently obtained and confirmed mass lesions at both sites (Figures 3, 5, and 6). At surgery, the patient underwent debulking of the right lower lid recurrence, with biopsy of three 0.5-cm diameter nasolabial fold nodules. An enlarged submandibular lymph node that appeared to be involved with melanoma was also resected. Pathology confirmed metastatic melanoma to the dermis at all facial sites, with positive margins. The submandibular lymph node proved to be almost totally effaced by metastatic melanoma. Because of the positive margins, the patient underwent radiation therapy. Radiation therapy was foreshortened when chest CT toward the end of the planned course identified lung metastases.

TEACHING POINTS

In this case, PET confirmed a clinically suspected recurrence in the infraorbital cheek and identified an unsuspected submandibular nodal metastasis, which was subsequently confirmed on MRI and pathologically. Small (0.5 cm) nasolabial subcutaneous metastases were not identified on PET, presumably secondary to their size.

CASE 7 | Restaging, progressive facial recurrences

A 71-year-old woman, status post extensive right sinonasal surgery for melanoma involving the right naris and filling the nasal cavity, was evaluated with PET when a recurrence was identified 7 months later in the right infraorbital cheek. At the original surgery, the lesion measured 2.8 cm and was treated with right medial maxillectomy, right near-total

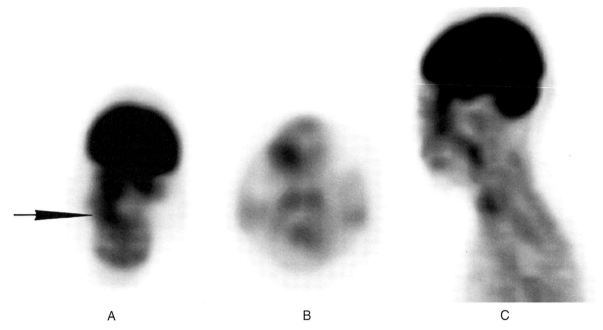

A   B   C

FIGURE 1. Coronal (**A**), axial (**B**), and sagittal (**C**) PET sections through the right infraorbital region show an asymmetrical hypermetabolic focus, corresponding to the fine-needle aspiration–confirmed malignant melanoma recurrence (*arrow*). This was excised and treated by postoperative irradiation.

septectomy, and right upper palatectomy. A right upper neck dissection was also performed with excision of a sentinel node.

When the right infraorbital cheek lump developed, it was evaluated with fine-needle aspiration, which confirmed malignant melanoma. PET scan identified hypermetabolic activity at this level, without additional sites of disease (Figure 1). The recurrence was excised and treated with postoperative radiation. Three months after finishing

radiation therapy, the patient developed nose bleeding and right-sided headache and pressure sensation. CT and MRI showed recurrent disease, filling the right maxillary sinus, with bony erosion and extension into the inferior orbit and pterygopalatine fossa. Aggressive local surgery was being considered when the patient was referred for PET scanning. In addition to confirming extensive locally recurrent tumor, bone metastases were identified on PET imaging (Figure 2).

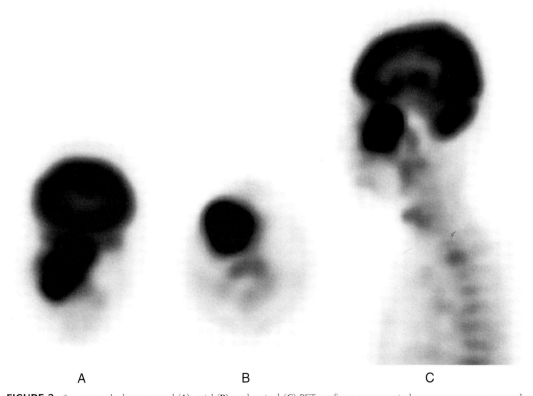

A   B   C

FIGURE 2. Seven months later: coronal (**A**), axial (**B**), and sagittal (**C**) PET confirms an aggressively recurrent tumor, centered at the right maxillary sinus and extending into the inferior orbit and pterygopalatine fossa, corresponding to imaging findings. In addition, there is new evidence of bone metastases, demonstrated here on the sagittal section in the upper thoracic spine.

TEACHING POINTS

The high metabolic rate of melanomas and PET's whole-body imaging capability make FDG PET particularly useful in the evaluation of melanoma. At any one time, PET can survey a whole body to accurately stage malignant melanoma. Of course, as in this case, PET can make no predictions as to the aggressiveness of a particular tumor or the rate at which recurrences may occur. Although the initial PET scan in this patient showed only local disease at the time of her first recurrence, the follow-up PET showed more extensive disease than expected, including bone metastases, at a time when aggressive surgery was being considered for this patient.

CASE 8 | Melanoma, restaging, lung and brain metastases

An 81-year-old man, 3 years post excision of a superficial left shoulder melanoma, presented with speech slurring. He was found to have a right temporal lobe mass (Figures 1 to 3). A metastasis was suspected.

He was also evaluated with chest and abdominal CT, which identified two right lung nodules, both 1.1 cm in size and also suspected to be metastases (Figure 4). PET imaging was requested to assess these findings. All three lesions were metabolically active (Figures 5 to 7). A percutaneous lung biopsy was subsequently performed that confirmed non–small cell malignancy, consistent with metastatic melanoma. The presumed intracranial metastasis was treated with gamma knife therapy.

TEACHING POINTS

PET imaging was utilized in this patient to assess the significance of the lung nodules and to aid in determining the best site from which to pursue a histologic diagnosis. If the lung lesions had been negative, a brain biopsy might have been pursued for diagnosis. The demonstration of hypermetabolism of all identified lesions strengthened the working supposition of metastatic disease and directed initial histologic sampling efforts at the lung, a less morbid avenue than brain biopsy.

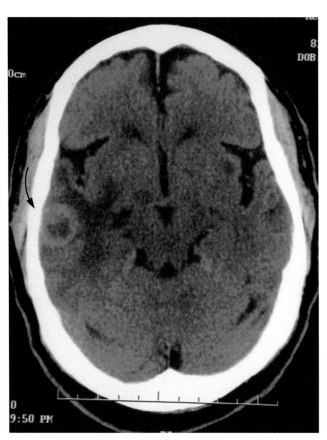

FIGURE 1. Unenhanced head CT shows a round right temporal lobe lesion (*arrow*), with associated edema.

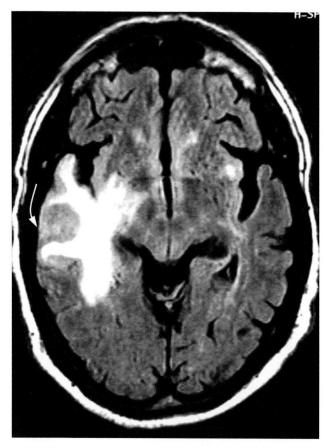

FIGURE 2. FLAIR axial MR image shows the lesion (*arrow*) to be nearly isointense to brain parenchyma. It is outlined by the extensive vasogenic edema.

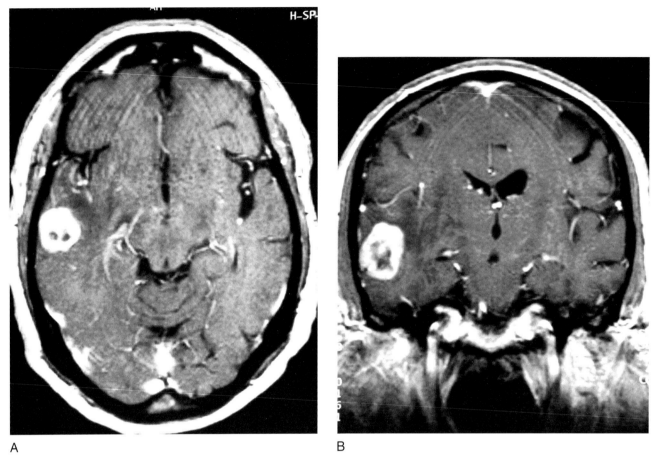

FIGURE 3. Enhanced T1-weighted axial (**A**) and coronal (**B**) MR images show the lesion to ring enhance. No other lesions were identified. Based on this patient's known history of melanoma, a brain metastasis was suspected.

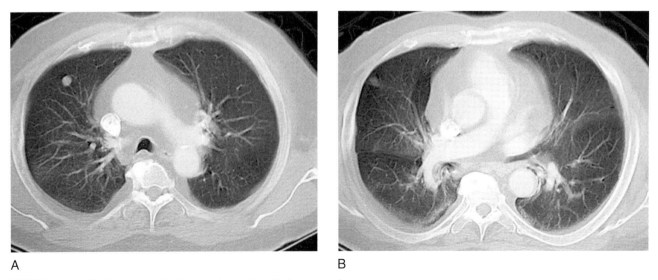

FIGURE 4. A and B, Two 1.1-cm right lung nodules on chest CT also suggested metastases.

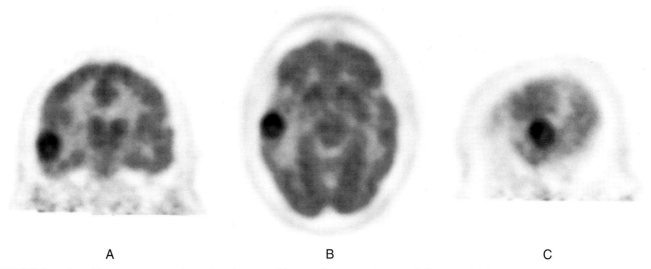

A   B   C

FIGURE 5. Dedicated brain PET imaging shows the right temporal lesion to be intensely hypermetabolic. Coronal (**A**), transaxial (**B**), and sagittal (**C**) views are shown.

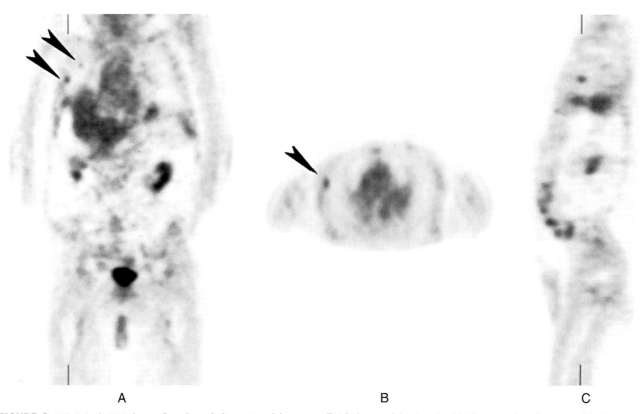

A   B   C

FIGURE 6. Whole-body PET also confirmed metabolic activity of the two small right lung nodules (*arrowheads*). The unusual configuration of the liver seen on the coronal image is secondary to large, stable and unchanged liver cysts. Coronal (**A**), transaxial (**B**), and sagittal (**C**) views are depicted.

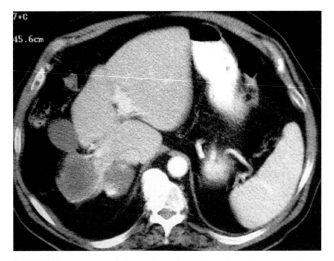

FIGURE 7. Enhanced abdominal CT through the liver shows it to have a bizarre appearance, with three adjacent right lobe presumed cysts. Two are complex in appearance, whereas the third is characteristic. These near water density lesions had not changed from prior studies and, other than producing an unusual contour of the liver on PET, were scintigraphically inapparent, helping confirm their presumed benign nature.

CASE 9 | Restaging; lung, hilar, liver, and osseous metastases

A 40-year-old woman was diagnosed with a mid-back melanoma 1 year before a CXR suggested the possibility of metastatic disease. She had been treated surgically with wide excision and left axillary node dissection. PET scan showed much more extensive abnormalities than had been suspected. In addition to right lower lobe pulmonary parenchymal foci, hypermetabolic disease sites were found in the right hilus, liver, and bone (Figure 1).

TEACHING POINTS

Metastatic melanoma can present in myriad ways, making imaging surveillance by anatomic modalities difficult. CT and bone scan may well have demonstrated these abnormalities, but PET provides a very sensitive, full-body alternative. PET upstaged this patient's apparent disease status considerably, a scenario observed all too frequently in melanoma patients.

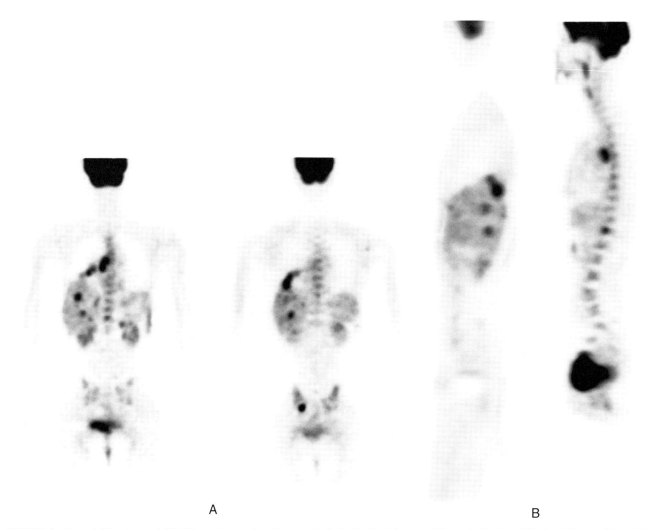

A

B

FIGURE 1. Coronal (**A**) and sagittal (**B**) PET scan images show hypermetabolic foci in the right chest (hilus and right lower lobe lung), liver, and bone (right sacroiliac joint region and T12).

CASE 10 | *Restaging, extensive disease, treatment assessment*

A 43-year-old man with metastatic melanoma was followed with PET imaging as he underwent treatment for liver metastases. He was first diagnosed with melanoma from the right trapezius level 4 years before and was treated with wide excision and lymphadenectomy. A subsequent subcutaneous recurrence 15 months later was excised and a radical neck dissection was performed. Lymph nodes reportedly were negative. He was then treated with vaccine therapy for 1 year before a recurrence was noted in the same region, and he was treated with biochemotherapy. Six months before his first PET evaluation, another subcutaneous recurrence was identified, as well as liver metastases. This was treated with right intrahepatic infusions of cisplatin and vinblastine, as well as left hepatic lobe embolization, performed 2 months before PET scanning. PET scan showed extensive disease, with the largest single focus in the left liver (Figure 1). Additional hepatic metastases were also noted, as well as foci in the mediastinum and other soft tissues.

He was reevaluated 1 month later to assess the progress of his right lobe intrahepatic chemotherapeutic infusions (Figure 2). There did appear to be improvement within the right liver. However, extensive scattered extrahepatic metastases appeared progressive. Systemic chemotherapy was administered, and the patient was rescanned with PET 2 months later (Figure 3). Clear progression was demonstrated on PET, with the left lobe of the liver being essentially replaced, with new right lobe liver disease. An increase in number and intensity of extrahepatic disease foci was noted.

TEACHING POINTS

PET imaging's whole-body capability and the high metabolic rate of malignant melanoma make it uniquely suitable to the imaging follow-up of the melanoma patient. In a complex case such as this, where a patient may receive both systemic and local therapies, it lends itself particularly well to assessing the disease response.

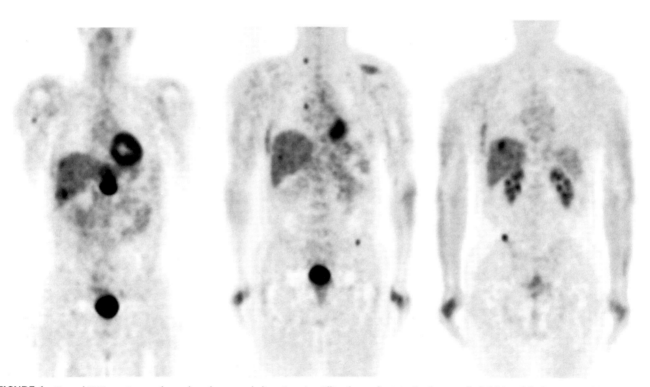

FIGURE 1. Coronal PET scan images show a large hypermetabolic epigastric midline focus of activity, localizing to the left lobe of the liver. Four additional small foci of right lobe liver involvement can be seen on these sections. Scattered additional disease sites are depicted, including at the right hilar level and at the right thoracic inlet, right upper arm, left buttock, and right ileal regions.

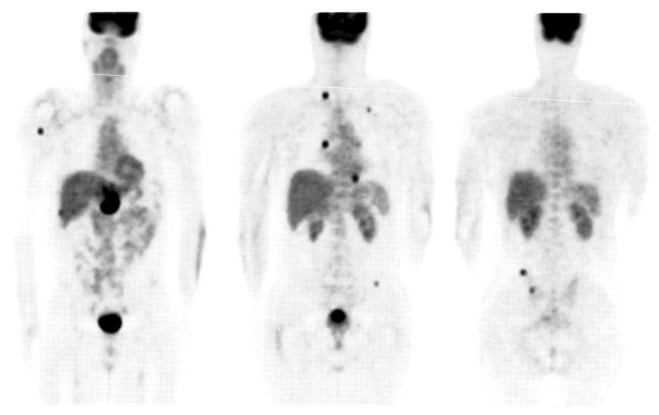

FIGURE 2. Repeat PET scan, 1 month later, to assess right hepatic intra-arterial chemotherapy: The same three coronal levels are shown to allow comparison. Although the treated right lobe liver lesions are clearly improved, progression is evident elsewhere. The left lobe lesion appears larger, and the scattered smaller disease sites are larger and more intense in activity, with a few new sites now noted.

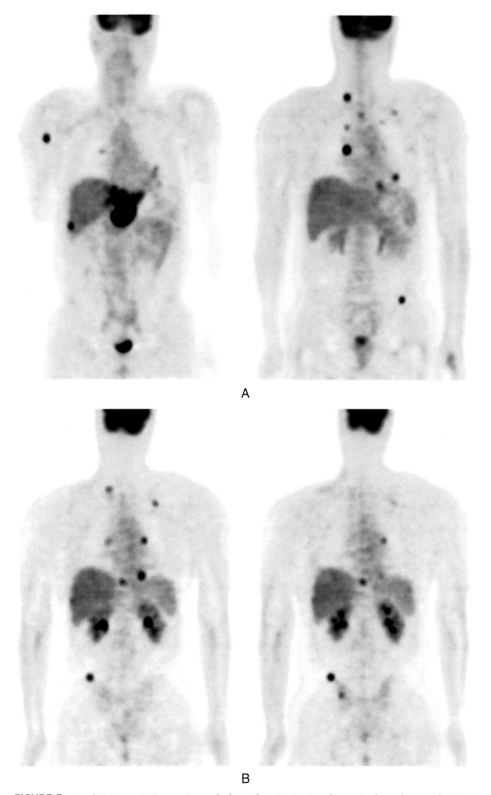

FIGURE 3. **A** and **B,** Repeat PET scans, 2 months later, after reinstitution of systemic chemotherapy. Clear interval progression is seen. The left liver lesion now appears to occupy the entire lobe, and multiple new soft tissue and osseous disease sites are evident.

CASE 11 | Restaging, advanced disease (carcinomatosis)

A 75-year-old woman was diagnosed with vaginal melanoma after presenting with spotting. She underwent vaginectomy and two courses of chemotherapy. At the time of referral for PET imaging, the patient had biopsy-proven disease of the perineum, and cystectomy and rectal resection were being contemplated. Abdominal distention was noted, and ascites was suspected. The patient's disease status was assessed with CT (Figures 1 to 4) and PET imaging (Figures 5 to 8).

TEACHING POINTS

At the time of this patient's imaging restaging, she was known to have locally persistent or recurrent disease by perineal biopsy and a more aggressive surgery was being contemplated. The extent of her advanced disease was not fully appreciated until these studies were obtained and correlated. Clearly, this patient would not have benefited from additional surgery.

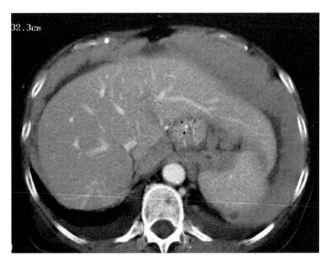

FIGURE 1. Enhanced abdominal CT shows a thick enhancing collar of soft tissue encircling the liver and spleen, consistent with massive peritoneal carcinomatosis. There are small bilateral pleural effusions as well.

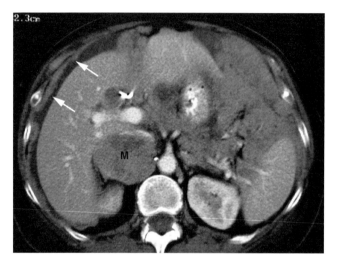

FIGURE 2. A more inferior abdominal CT section shows a large, inhomogeneously enhancing adrenal mass (M), anteriorly displacing the inferior vena cava. Enhancement, thickening, and nodularity of the peritoneal lining is well seen against the perihepatic ascites (*arrows*). Confluent soft tissue tumor infiltration is seen in the perisplenic region.

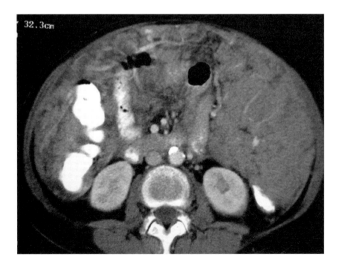

FIGURE 3. A thick mantle of peritoneal tumor and omental cake is seen at a more inferior section.

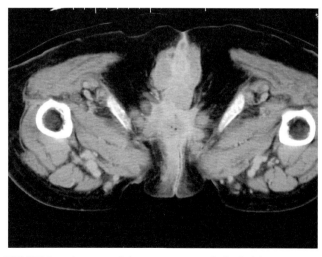

FIGURE 4. Enhancing nodular tumor is seen at the level of the perineum.

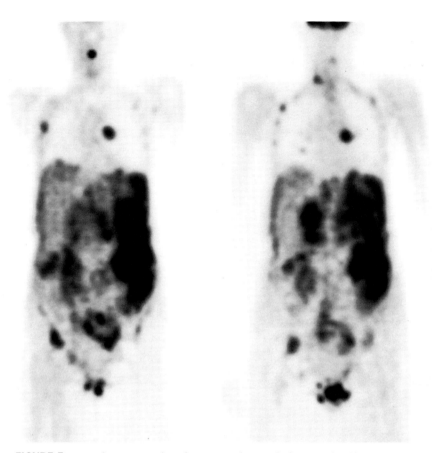

FIGURE 5. Coronal PET images show the extensive disease. The liver is outlined by a peritoneal sheet of tumor activity, and the bulky left upper quadrant tumor activity is confluent. Lobular tumor activity is seen at the level of the perineum. In addition to these findings, which correlate well with the abdominal and pelvis CT abnormalities, scattered tumor foci are identified in the chest and neck, including in bone.

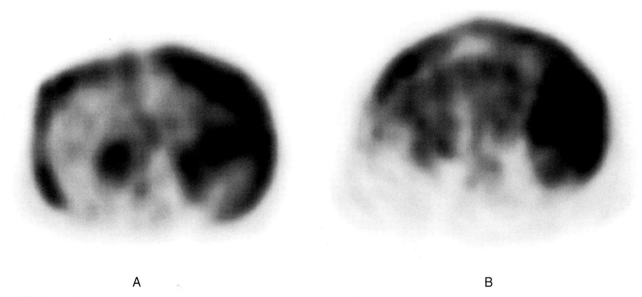

A   B

FIGURE 6. Axial PET sections, corresponding to the CT slices. The higher section (**A**) shows the modest metabolic activity of the liver and spleen as negative defects against the intensely metabolically active surrounding peritoneal carcinomatosis. The more inferior section (**B**) corresponds in level to Figure 3 and again shows the peritoneal tumor and omental cake to be highly metabolically active.

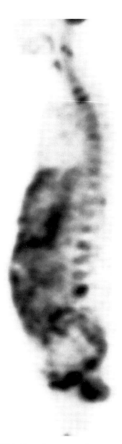

FIGURE 7. Axial PET section through the perineum, corresponding to Figure 4, shows bulky, multinodular metabolically active tumor.

FIGURE 8. Sagittal PET slice shows another perspective on the extensive disease and its distribution and better demonstrates the osseous involvement of the spine.

Colorectal Cancer

In the United States approximately 150,000 new cases of colorectal cancer are diagnosed each year.[1] The recurrence rate is 30% to 40%, with a significant number of patients presenting with an isolated liver metastasis. Accurate staging of patients with colorectal cancer may improve survival statistics as well as reduce the number of unsuccessful curative-intent surgeries for recurrent disease. PET imaging has shown efficacy in staging, in evaluating suspected recurrence, and in assessing response to treatment. Table 1 outlines the current colorectal staging system, whereas Table 2 compares staging and survival.

Currently used imaging modalities include CT, MRI, transrectal ultrasonography, scintigraphy with monoclonal antibodies, and PET. Most often, the first study ordered is CT; however, sensitivity, negative predictive value, and overall accuracy are significantly better with PET.[2] Additionally, CT may miss up to 7% of patients with hepatic metastases and underestimate the number of lobes involved in up to 33%.[3] The addition of PET to the diagnostic algorithm for colorectal cancer has resulted in an improvement in accuracy, provided a unique problem-solving tool, and demonstrated cost-effectiveness.

In a report on 134 patient studies for diagnosis/staging, PET showed an accuracy of 94% versus 81% for CT.[2,4]

The data on recurrence are substantial; evaluation of patient studies (2244) showed a 94% accuracy for PET versus 80% for CT. The sensitivity and specificity for PET versus CT were 94% versus 79% and 87% versus 73%, respectively.[2] Additional series suggest PET is valuable to maximize information.[5-8] Anatomical definition and structural relationships clearly are the purview of anatomic studies such as CT and MRI.

One of the more common scenarios in the management of patients with colorectal carcinoma is the postoperative/posttherapy patient who presents with a rising carcinoembryonic antigen (CEA) level. This serum tumor marker has become one of the mainstays of longitudinal follow-up. A significant number of patients with an elevated CEA level will have negative conventional studies.[9] PET is extremely valuable in this group. In one study, 63 of 72 (87%) patients with a rising CEA level and negative CT/MRI were found to have lesions with PET.[10]

PROBLEM SOLVING

Arguably, one of PET's major contributions to the evaluation of patients with cancer is its use as a problem-solving modality. This is applicable to many types of cancer, including colorectal. The differentiation of scar/post-surgical change/postirradiation change from active tumor is problematic for anatomic-based imaging modalities. PET is uniquely able to make this distinction. In the vast majority of cases, a region of abnormality on CT or MRI that demonstrates hypermetabolism (i.e., increased FDG accumulation) is active tumor until proven otherwise. A negative PET in the area of question denotes benignity. Caveats include postirradiation inflammatory changes (which may last weeks to months) and coexisting areas of inflammation/infection, which often will show increased FDG accumulation. Small perivesicular sites may be problematic but may often be resolved with sagittal or transaxial views. Some investigators recommend bladder catheterization (with or without instillation of saline), diuretic administration before pelvic imaging, or even repeat pelvic imaging after the initial scan (post void).

Surgery for recurrent colorectal cancer is another area where PET can play a vital role. The liver is the sole site of metastasis in 20% to 40% of colorectal cancer cases, and approximately 14,000 patients present each year with an isolated liver metastasis as their first recurrence. Because early detection and prompt surgical resection may be curative, an accurate method to identify these patients, and differentiate them from those with multicentric disease, is desirable. PET is ideally suited. Virtually all studies report a sensitivity for detection of hepatic metastases of more than 90%.[2] More importantly, the ability of PET in a single examination to identify additional metastatic sites elsewhere in the body can save a patient a noncurative hepatic resection, with its attendant morbidity and even mortality. This can result in major cost savings. For these reasons, the identification of a presumed liver metastasis on surveillance CT should prompt whole-body PET to better assess the patient for operability. A large cooperative study reviewed the relationship between follow-up tests (not including PET) and salvage

TABLE 1 CURRENT COLORECTAL STAGING SYSTEM

PRIMARY TUMOR (T)

Tx	Primary tumor cannot be assessed
T0	No evidence of primary tumor
Tis	Carcinoma in situ
T1	Tumor invades submucosa
T2	Tumor invades muscularis propria
T3	Tumor invades through muscularis propria into the subserosa or into nonperitonealized pericolic or perirectal tissues
T4	Tumor perforates the visceral peritoneum or cavity or invades other organs or structures

REGIONAL LYMPH NODES (N)

Nx	Regional lymph nodes cannot be assessed
N0	No regional lymph node metastasis
N1	Metastasis in four or more pericolic or perirectal lymph nodes
N2	Metastasis in any lymph node along the course of a name vascular trunk

DISTANT METASTASIS (M)

Mx	Presence of distant metastasis cannot be assessed
M1	No distant metastasis
M1	Distant metastasis

STAGE	TNM SUBSETS		
O	Tis	N0	M0
I	T1	N0	M0
	T2	N0	M0
II	T3	N0	M0
	T4	N0	M0
III	Any T	N1	M0
	Any T	N2	M0
IV	Any T	Any N	M1

TABLE 2 STAGING AND FIVE-YEAR SURVIVAL FOR COLORECTAL CANCER

CLASSIFICATION	DESCRIPTION			5-YEAR SURVIVAL (%)
DUKES				
A	Tumor limited to bowel			85
B	Extension of the tumor into perirectal adipose tissue			64
C	Nodal metastasis regardless of tumor presentation			33
D	Distant metastases			5
TNM				
0	Tis	N0	M0	100
1	T1	N0	M0	100
	T2	N0	M0	85
2	T3	N0	M0	70
	T4	N0	M0	30
3	Any T	N1	M0	60
	Any T	N2,3		30
4	Any T	N	M1	3

surgery, assessing outcomes and documenting surgical mortality. This retrospective cohort study looked at 548 patients with colon cancer recurrence. Curative-intent surgery was performed in 109 patients (20%), with a 5-year disease-free survival rate of 23%. Whereas the authors conclude that second operations can result in long-term disease-free intervals, it is suspected that a significant percentage of the 77% who did not achieve long-term survival may have been spared a second, curative-intent surgery by more accurate restaging.[11]

COST-EFFECTIVENESS

Data exist attesting to the economic impact of PET in the evaluation of colorectal cancer.[12,13] The average savings per patient may be more than $4000 and is primarily related to procedures avoided based on information provided by PET.

To summarize, FDG-PET should be considered an integral part of the diagnostic armamentarium for colorectal carcinoma. It is extremely valuable for staging, detecting recurrence, and monitoring response to therapy. It plays a pivotal role in selecting patients for curative-intent second surgery, can differentiate tumor recurrence from post-treatment changes, is highly accurate for staging, and has been demonstrated to be cost-effective.

REFERENCES

1. Meta J, Seltzer M, Schiepers C, et al: Impact of ^{18}F-FDG PET on managing patients with colorectal cancer: The referring physician's perspective. J Nucl Med 2001;42:586-590.
2. Gambhir SS, Czernin J, Schwimmer J, et al: A tabulated summary of the FDG PET literature. J Nucl Med 2001;42:95-125.
3. Steele G Jr, Bleday R, Mayer R, et al: A prospective evaluation of hepatic resection for colorectal carcinoma metastases to the liver: Gastrointestinal tumor study group protocol 6584. J Clin Oncol 1991;9:1105-1112.
4. Abdel-Nabi H, Doerr RJ, Lamonica DM, et al: Staging of primary colorectal carcinomas with fluorine-18 fluorodeoxyglucose whole-body PET: Correlation with histopathologic and CT findings. Radiology 1998;206: 755-760.
5. Jarnagin WR, Fong Y, Ky A, et al: Liver resection for metastatic colorectal cancer: Assessing the risk of occult irresectable disease. J Am Coll Surg 1999;188:33-42.
6. Whiteford MH, Whiteford HM, Ye LF, et al: Usefulness of FDG-PET scan in the assessment of suspected metastatic or recurrent adenocarcinoma of the colon and rectum. Dis Colon Rectum 2000;43:759-770.
7. Lai DT, Fulham M, Stephen MS, et al: The role of whole-body positron emission tomography with [^{18}F] fluorodeoxyglucose in identifying operable colorectal cancer metastases to the liver. Arch Surg 1996;131:703-707.
8. Delbeke D: Oncological applications of FDG-PET imaging: Brain tumors, colorectal cancer, lymphoma and melanoma. J Nucl Med 1999;40: 591-603.
9. Flanagan FL, Dehdashti F, Ogunbiyi OA, et al: Utility of FDG-PET for investigating unexplained plasma CEA elevation in patients with colorectal cancer. Ann Surg 1998;227:319-323.
10. Maldonado A, Sancho F, Cerdan J, et al: FDG-PET in the detection of recurrence in colorectal cancer based on rising CEA level: Experience in 72 patients. Clin Pos Imag 2000;3:170.
11. Goldberg RM, Fleming TR, Tangen CM, et al: Surgery for recurrent colon cancer: Strategies for identifying resectable recurrence and success rates after resection. Ann Intern Med 1998;129:27-35.
12. Gambhir SS, Valk P, Shepherd J, et al: Cost effective analysis modeling of the role of FDG PET in management of patients with recurrent colorectal cancer [abstract]. J Nucl Med 1997;38:90P.
13. Hustinx R, Benard F, Alavi A: Whole-body FDG-PET imaging in the management of patients with cancer. Semin Nucl Med 2002;32:35-46.

CASE 1 | Initial staging, no additional disease site (rectal cancer)

A 43-year-old man with blood in his stool was found to have a rectal carcinoma. CT staging raised the question of liver metastases. PET scan was requested preoperatively to address this issue. It showed no evidence of liver metastases. Localized rectal activity was identified at the primary site (Figure 1).

TEACHING POINTS

PET scanning is used in the evaluation of colorectal carcinoma most often when a recurrence is suspected. It is also useful to assess the efficacy of treatment, such as of liver metastases. Less commonly, PET is utilized at the time of initial diagnosis. Identification of an in situ primary lesion is somewhat dependent on luck, because recognition of a lesion depends on it being hypermetabolic compared with the rest of the bowel. In the majority of patients in whom overall bowel activity is low, this is not difficult. However, even normal patients may have relatively intense diffuse bowel activity as a variant; and in these patients, recognition of a primary lesion could be hampered.

PET also is of limited utility in the local staging of a primary tumor. Local nodal involvement most commonly would present as activity confluent with the primary tumor and so would not be recognized separately. This is analogous to the difficulty PET has in identifying para-esophageal lymph node involvement in staging esophageal carcinomas. PET does excel at identification of distant metastases and should be able to resolve preoperative imaging dilemmas.

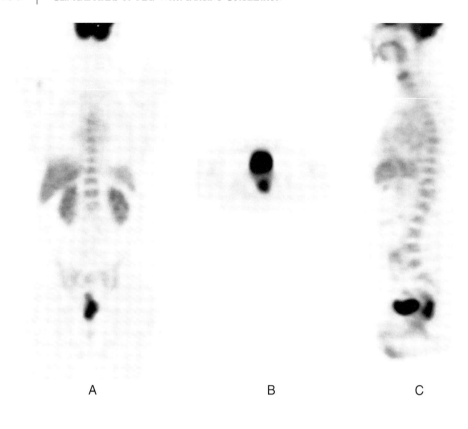

A   B   C

FIGURE 1. Localized hypermetabolic activity is identified at the rectal level, in a patient with little other bowel activity, and corresponds with the patient's in situ primary lesion. Coronal (**A**), axial (**B**), and sagittal (**C**) views are shown.

CASE 2 | *Initial staging, involved adjacent lymph node*

An 80-year-old woman presented with intermittent rectal bleeding. Colonoscopic evaluation identified a large annular rectal mass. Superficial biopsy identified adenocarcinoma in situ arising within a villous adenoma. CT evaluation showed a large enhancing rectal mass, with a 2-cm adjacent tumor nodule or lymph node (Figures 1 and 2). The patient's CEA value was elevated at 108 units.

Advanced disease was suspected after the CT evaluation, based on the large size of the rectal mass and a suspected perirectal lymph node. The CT also showed a small focus of liver hypodensity, with a differential diagnosis of focal fat deposition versus metastasis.

PET scan was requested to aid in staging (Figures 3 and 4). It showed intense hypermetabolic activity of the rectal carcinoma, as well as the adjacent suspected perirectal lymph node at the right upper margin of the mass. No evidence of liver metastases was seen. There was a marked diffuse increase in bone marrow activity, which was regarded with suspicion for bone metastases. However, a spine survey

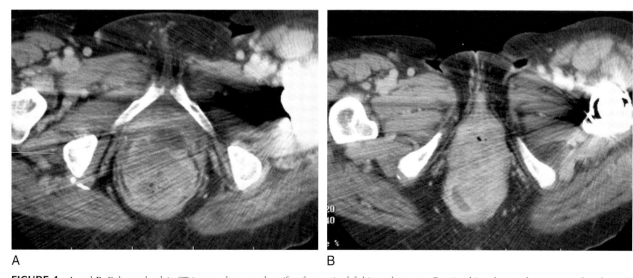

A   B

FIGURE 1. A and **B,** Enhanced pelvis CT images show streak artifact from prior left hip replacement. Despite this, a large, inhomogeneously enhancing rectal mass is recognized.

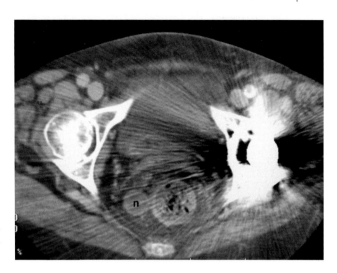

FIGURE 2. At the upper margin of the rectal mass, an adjacent low density 2-cm presumed perirectal lymph node (n) is seen. The patient has previously undergone a hysterectomy.

MRI showed normal bone marrow, with no evidence of osseous metastases. Presumably, the patient's anemia, secondary to the recurrent gastrointestinal bleeding, accounts for the abnormal marrow activity.

TEACHING POINTS

This large in situ rectal carcinoma mass displayed marked hypermetabolism, which contrasted strongly to the low background level of bowel activity elsewhere in this patient. In this case, this activity corresponded well with the morphologic abnormalities on CT, and there is no real diagnostic dilemma as to the significance of this activity. However, the very real variability of normal bowel activity can produce perplexing interpretive quandaries in less florid cases. This case also is exceptional in that it is not usually possible to assess the activity of pericolonic lymph nodes on PET, separate from the primary lesion activity.

Increased marrow activity raises a differential diagnosis of bone metastases, or marrow activation, secondary either to red marrow recruitment in anemia or to stimulating factors administered in the course of chemotherapy. The uniformity of the marrow activity is an important clue, as well as the clinical history. Activated marrow, whether due to anemia or chemotherapy, is usually homogeneous, whereas bone metastatic activity more often is inhomogeneous. In this case, despite the homogeneity of the increased activity, concern remained as to possible diffuse bone metastases. This possibility was investigated with MRI and excluded. The patient was anemic, owing to ongoing gastrointestinal bleeding, presumably accounting for the marrow activity.

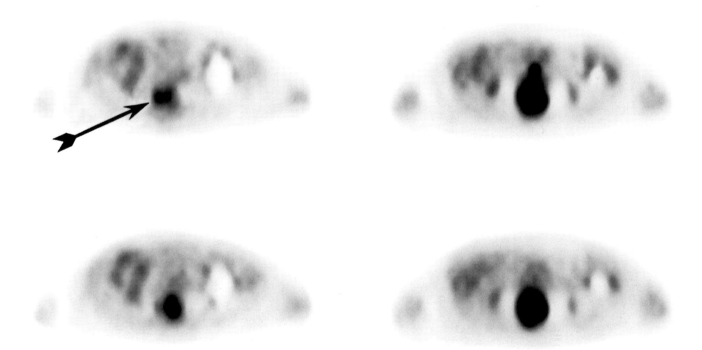

FIGURE 3. Axial PET sections through the pelvis show the intense hypermetabolism of the in situ rectal carcinoma mass and at the highest level (*upper left*) in the right perirectal lymph node (*arrow*). The urinary bladder has been evacuated by a Foley catheter. Photopenia is noted at the site of the replaced left hip. Note the markedly increased bone marrow activity of the right hip.

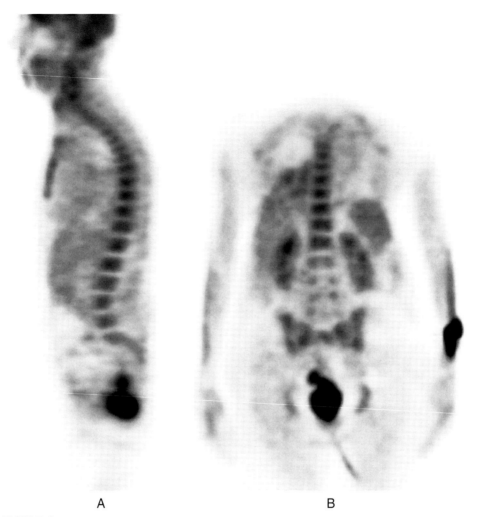

A   B

FIGURE 4. Sagittal (**A**) and coronal (**B**) PET sections show the marked rectal mass activity. The abnormally increased bone marrow activity is also well seen, particularly on the sagittal section (note ease of visualization of the sternum). The increased bone marrow activity is homogeneous. Subsequent MRI spine survey showed normal marrow signal, effectively excluding osseous metastatic disease as the etiology of this activity. The patient was anemic, secondary to ongoing gastrointestinal bleeding, which presumably accounts for these findings.

CASE 3 | *Initial staging, distant metastases*

A 76-year-old woman presented with anorexia, nausea, and abdominal pain. The patient underwent a transverse colectomy after a colon carcinoma was identified on work-up. The pathology was a poorly to moderately differentiated adenocarcinoma, with two of five pericolonic lymph nodes positive. Penetration of the muscularis was noted, with tumor extension into pericolonic fat. Three mesenteric tumor masses, possibly completely replaced lymph nodes, were also excised. PET scan was requested for staging before initiation of chemotherapy. It demonstrated extensive disease, both nodal and osseous (Figures 1 to 3). Hypermetabolic activity was found in nodal distributions of the mediastinum and hila, as well as extensively in the retroperitoneum.

Patchy, diffusely increased bone marrow activity was also noted, indicative of advanced bone metastases. The patient initially had a promising response to chemotherapy but quickly relapsed, dying 5 months after diagnosis.

TEACHING POINTS

This patient underwent no preoperative imaging staging before colon carcinoma surgery. The pathology demonstrated locally advanced disease, and PET was requested to complete staging. Distant metastases were demonstrated, including advanced bone and extensive nodal metastases, both in the retroperitoneum and in the chest.

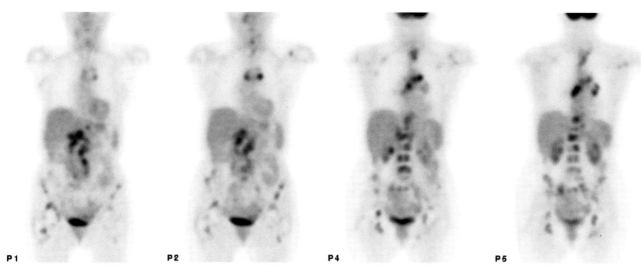

P 1   P 2   P 4   P 5

FIGURE 1. Coronal PET scan images show multiple nodules of increased metabolic activity, localizing to nodal regions of the mediastinum, hila, and retroperitoneum. There also are multiple scattered foci of abnormally increased bone marrow activity, consistent with bone metastases, best seen on these coronal images in the lumbar spine and pelvis.

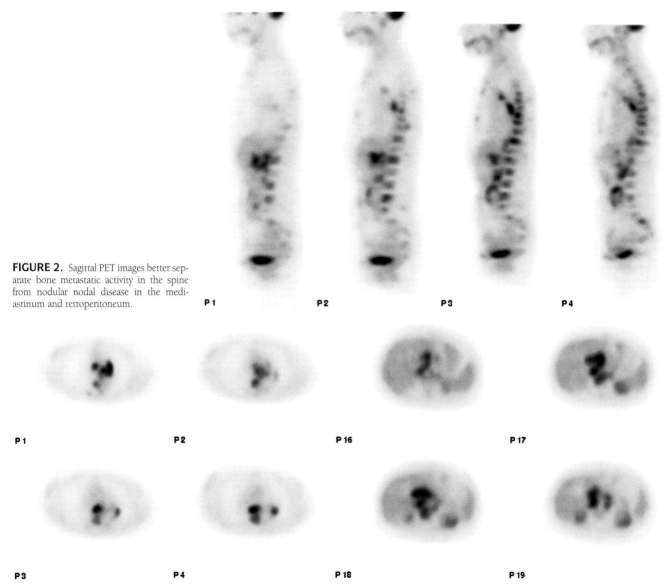

FIGURE 2. Sagittal PET images better separate bone metastatic activity in the spine from nodular nodal disease in the mediastinum and retroperitoneum.

P 1   P 2   P 3   P 4

P 1   P 2   P 16   P 17

P 3   P 4   P 18   P 19

FIGURE 3. Two sets of axial PET images depicting the nodal metastases. The left set of four images is through the chest and shows mediastinal and hilar nodal metastases. The right set of four images is through the abdomen and depicts retroperitoneal foci of metastatic nodal activity.

CASE 4 | *Restaging, solitary liver metastasis*

A 67-year-old man was 8 years post surgery and chemotherapy for colon carcinoma when a rising CEA level raised concern for recurrence. A work-up with CT identified a solitary pulmonary nodule, which was thought to be the site of recurrence and the source of the rising CEA value. This was surgically excised and proved to be benign. PET scan was then requested to search for an occult recurrence. At the time, the patient was feeling well except for RUQ pain.

The PET scan identified an intensely hypermetabolic right lobe liver mass (Figure 1). This was subsequently excised and proven to represent metastasis from colon carcinoma.

TEACHING POINTS

This clinical scenario is one in which PET has well-documented utility. Preoperative performance of PET in this patient may have spared him an unnecessary thoracotomy for what proved to be a benign lung nodule. PET identified the source of recurrence in this case in the liver, which had not demonstrated an abnormality on CT.

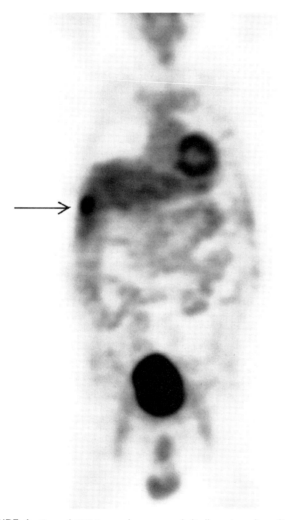

P7

FIGURE 1. Coronal PET image shows a metabolically active solitary liver mass (*arrow*), which proved to be a colon carcinoma metastasis.

CASE 5 | *Restaging, recurrent hepatic metastasis*

A 56-year-old woman underwent surgery for colon carcinoma 18 months before being referred for PET scanning. At the time of surgery, a solitary liver metastasis was excised. The patient was subsequently treated with 6 months of chemotherapy. An increasing CEA level prompted referral for PET imaging and MRI (Figures 1 to 3).

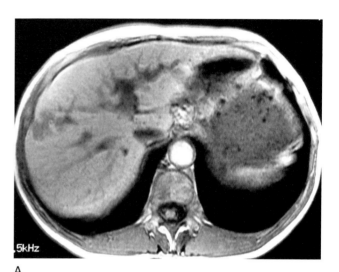

A

B

FIGURE 1. Axial unenhanced fast spoiled gradient recalled (FSPGR) (**A**) and fat-saturated enhanced fast multiplanar spoiled gradient recalled (FMPSPGR) (gradient echo) (**B**) sequences show an irregularly marginated, hypointense, peripherally enhancing lesion in the anterior segment of the right lobe of the liver, suggesting another liver metastasis.

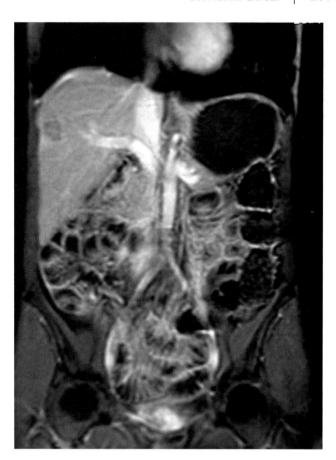

FIGURE 2. Enhanced fat-saturated coronal FMPSPGR sequence shows the same finding in another plane.

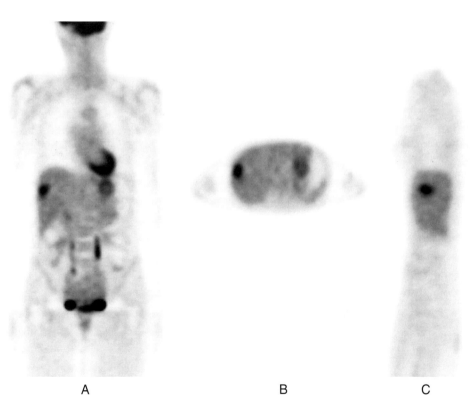

A   B   C

FIGURE 3. PET scan images through the right lobe of the liver show the lesion to be hypermetabolic and consistent with a metastasis. Paraspinal ureteral activity is included on the coronal section (**A**). Transaxial (**B**) and sagittal (**C**) views are also shown.

CASE 6 | *Restaging, solitary liver metastasis*

A 67-year-old man was evaluated with PET for suspicion of recurrent colon carcinoma, based on a rising CEA level. He had been treated surgically for colon carcinoma less than 2 years before. Three lymph nodes were positive at the time of resection, and postoperative chemotherapy was also given. The patient was initially evaluated for the increasing CEA level with CT, which was negative. PET was recommended as the next step in the evaluation and identified a solitary hypermetabolic liver lesion in the inferior tip of the right lobe of the liver (posterior segment) (Figure 1). Even on retrospective re-review of the CT, no corresponding lesion could be found (Figure 2), and so MRI was recommended to pursue this abnormality. Enhanced, breath-hold technique MRI identified a solitary mass at the expected site (Figure 3). Based on the location of the lesion and absence of additional abnormalities, the patient was referred for expected surgical excision.

However, preoperative work-up showed he had coronary ischemia, and he ultimately underwent coronary artery bypass grafting. Chemotherapy was later begun, but follow-up MRIs showed growth of the liver metastasis despite treatment.

TEACHING POINTS

In the evaluation of suspected recurrent colon carcinoma, particularly when heralded by a rising CEA level, CT, MRI, and PET scans are complementary imaging modalities. Because CT is more sensitive for small lung metastases, it probably should be the first imaging modality to be utilized in the work-up of such patients. PET is a very appropriate next step if CT does not identify lung or liver metastases or local recurrence to account for the serologic abnormality. The PET findings can then direct the further imaging needed for correlation to the area(s) of interest. In this case, PET identified the etiology to be a liver metastasis that CT

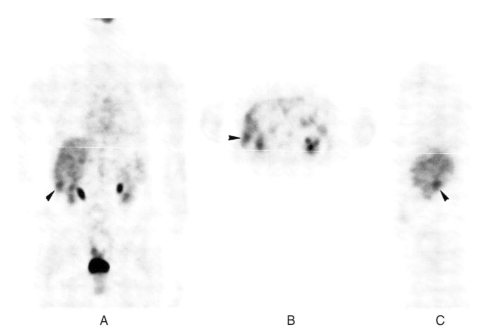

A   B   C

FIGURE 1. PET images show a solitary focus of increased activity at the inferior tip of the right lobe of the liver (posterior segment), suggesting a liver metastasis as the etiology of the patient's rising CEA level and presumed recurrent colon cancer (*arrowheads*). Coronal (**A**), transaxial (**B**), and sagittal (**C**) views are shown.

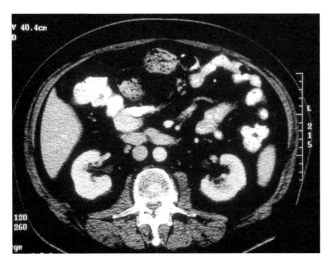

FIGURE 2. Enhanced abdominal CT image (liver window) through the expected level of the lesion shows no abnormality.

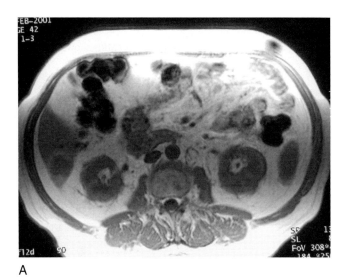

A

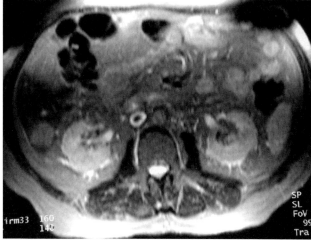

B

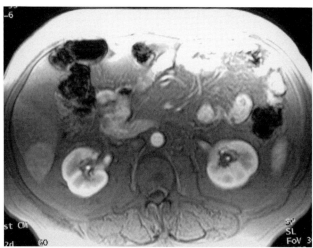

C

FIGURE 3. T1-weighted (**A**), STIR (**B**), and fat-saturated, enhanced T1-weighted (**C**) breath-hold axial MR images through the same level show an enhancing focal liver lesion, consistent with a metastasis.

did not demonstrate. The abnormality was confirmed on MRI, which is more sensitive than CT for liver lesions.

PET is also useful for assessing the significance of confusing CT findings in the follow-up of colon carcinoma, such as postoperative presacral masses or post-radiofrequency ablation liver findings. See Cases 7, 9, 12, and 13 for examples.

CASE 7 | Restaging, retroperitoneal nodal recurrence, assessment of post-treatment presacral mass

A 68-year-old man was evaluated with PET for a presacral mass post treatment for recurrent rectal carcinoma. His past medical history was significant for a T3N2 rectal adenocarcinoma, treated with low anterior resection and sigmoid colostomy. His original pathology revealed poorly differentiated adenocarcinoma with invasion through the full bowel wall thickness into mesenteric fat. Tumor was noted at surgery to be extremely low lying, below the peritoneal reflection. Multiple rectal excision specimens were submitted, with the final margin showing tumor emboli within vascular channels of bowel wall beneath

glandular mucosa. Twelve of 22 mesenteric lymph nodes were positive for metastatic adenocarcinoma, with multiple additional deposits of solid tumor within mesenteric fat. The patient then underwent postoperative chemotherapy and radiation therapy. About 10 months after surgery, a rectal biopsy showed residual or recurrent tumor, and the patient underwent rectal resection. Chemotherapy was again initiated. A follow-up abdomen and pelvis CT showed mild retroperitoneal adenopathy (Figure 1) and new presacral soft tissue changes, thought most likely to be post surgical (Figure 2).

PET scan showed multiple retroperitoneal foci of activity, correlating with the retroperitoneal adenopathy on CT (Figure 3). The presacral findings were scintigraphically inactive, consistent with post-surgical scarring (Figure 4). Follow-up images are shown in Figures 5 and 6.

The patient was unable to tolerate chemotherapy and developed a brain metastasis 6 months after the PET scan. He declined radiation therapy and died several weeks later.

TEACHING POINTS

The presacral findings seen after rectal surgery are a frequent source of diagnostic and clinical uncertainty in the imaging follow-up of these patients. PET can aid in the differentiation between recurrent tumor

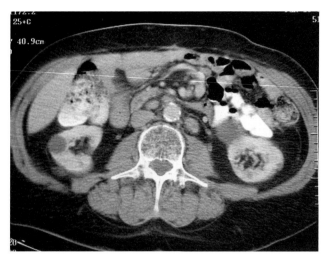

FIGURE 1. Enhanced abdominal CT image shows mildly enlarged retroperitoneal lymph nodes, as well as multiple renal cysts.

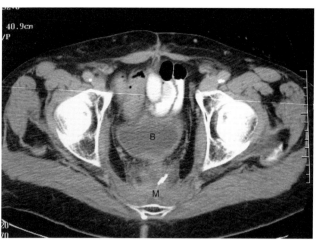

FIGURE 2. Pelvic CT obtained at the same time shows presacral soft tissue and surgical clips, thought most likely to represent postoperative scarring. Recognition of recurrent tumor in the midst of such changes can be problematic (M, mass; B, bladder).

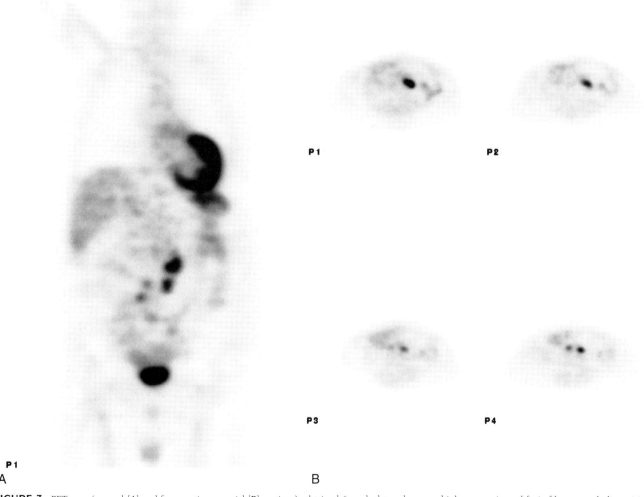

P1   P2

P3   P4

P1

A   B

FIGURE 3. PET scan (coronal [A] and four contiguous axial [B] sections), obtained 6 weeks later, shows multiple retroperitoneal foci of hypermetabolic activity, indicating the CT retroperitoneal findings represent metastatic lymph nodes.

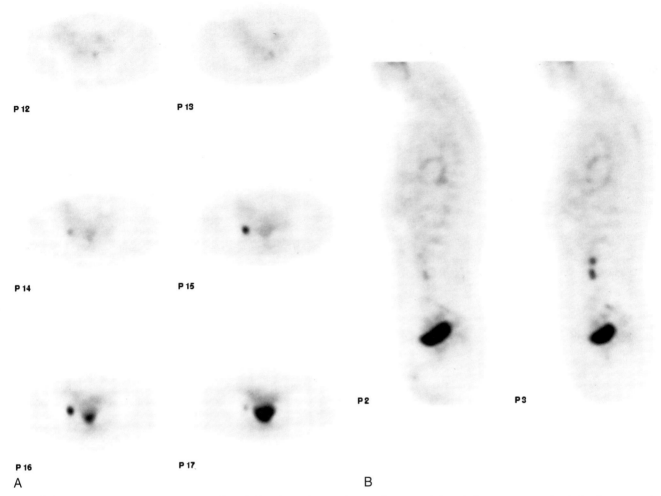

FIGURE 4. Axial (**A**) and sagittal (**B**) PET images through the pelvis and presacral region show no pathologic findings to correspond with CT. The scintigraphic inactivity is consistent with post-surgical changes. The inferiormost axial images show a hypermetabolic focus to the right of the bladder, representing excreted FDG in the right distal ureter. The sagittal images show the prespinal location of the hypermetabolic retroperitoneal lymph nodes.

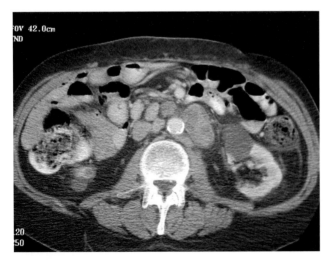

FIGURE 5. Enhanced abdominal image from a follow-up CT study, 7 months later, shows progressive growth of the retroperitoneal adenopathy.

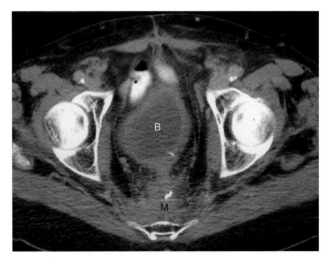

FIGURE 6. Pelvis CT image from the same study shows contraction of the presacral post-surgical scar (M, mass; B, bladder).

and post-surgical scarring in this setting. In this case, PET also served to clarify the significance of the mildly enlarged retroperitoneal lymph nodes. Up to that point, these nodes had not been clearly defined as metastatic lymph nodes, as their subsequent growth confirmed.

CASE 8 | *Restaging, pelvic recurrence*

A 75-year-old woman was found to have a rising CEA level 4 years after sigmoidectomy and chemotherapy for colon carcinoma. Imaging studies, including CT, did not identify a recurrence. PET scanning identified several foci of hypermetabolic activity in the pelvis, above and separate from the bladder (Figure 1). Correlation of the patient's CT with the PET demonstrated soft tissue masses that corresponded, indicating local regional recurrence of colon cancer (Figure 2).

TEACHING POINTS

One contribution of PET is its ability to identify abnormalities that have not been appreciated on other imaging studies. Conversely, equivocal or confusing PET findings are often clarified by careful correlation with CT or MRI. Hence, in most oncologic imaging circumstances, the use of PET should be complementary to anatomic imaging modalities.

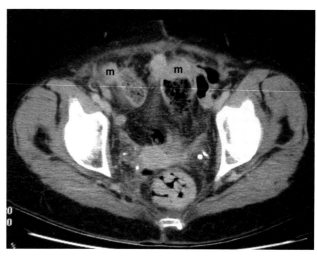

FIGURE 2. CT section through the pelvis, just above the bladder, shows soft tissue masses (m) that correspond to the PET and are consistent with local regional recurrence of colon carcinoma. These were not recognized prospectively to be pathologic. Their identification may have been hampered by the lack of oral contrast medium, which might have helped differentiate recurrent tumor from normal adjacent bowel.

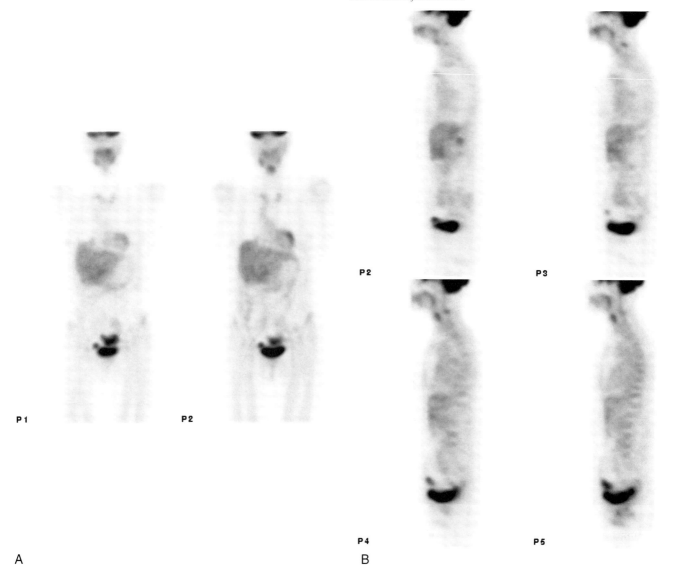

A   B

FIGURE 1. Coronal (**A**) and sagittal (**B**) PET images show two discrete foci of increased activity in the pelvis, above and separate from the bladder.

CASE 9 | *Restaging, presacral recurrence*

An 83-year-old man, 3 years after a low anterior resection for rectal adenocarcinoma, developed right-sided sciatica. His CEA level was rising. CT evaluation showed right hydroureteronephrosis, secondary to a right presacral mass of recurrent tumor, with sacral osseous erosion (Figures 1 and 2). His original diagnosis was of B1 disease, moderately differentiated, with 19 negative lymph nodes. No additional therapy had been performed after surgery.

PET scan confirmed a solitary, corresponding presacral site of hypermetabolic activity, with no additional disease (Figure 3). The patient was treated with combined chemotherapy (5-fluorouracil and leucovorin) and localized radiation, as well as percutaneous nephrostomy.

The patient remained relatively stable on maintenance chemotherapy for about a year and a half before developing left groin and hip pain. MRI showed a left inferior pubic ramus bone metastasis. His chemotherapy regimen was changed to gemcitabine (Gemzar) and irinotecan (CPT-11), and he was treated with radiation with palliation of his symptoms.

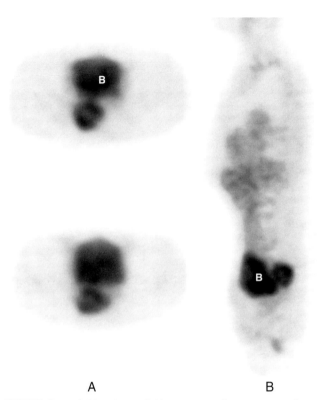

A   B

FIGURE 3. Axial (**A**) and sagittal (**B**) PET images show a retrovesical, presacral mass, corresponding to the mass on CT and consistent with recurrent colon cancer. Central photopenia indicates necrosis of the tumor (B, bladder).

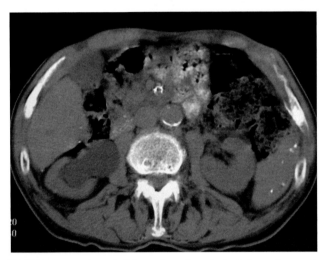

FIGURE 1. Unenhanced abdominal CT through the kidneys shows right hydronephrosis of moderate severity. The dilated ureter was traceable distally to the pelvis.

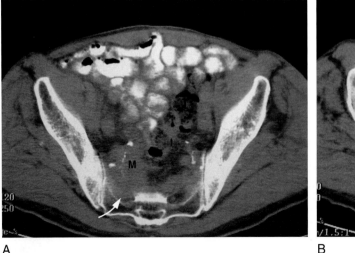

A

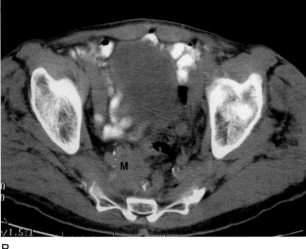

B

FIGURE 2. **A** and **B,** The obstructing mass (M) is a stellate soft tissue density in the right presacral region. Extension into a sacral foramen presumably contributed to the patient's presenting symptom of right-sided sciatica (*arrow*).

TEACHING POINTS

A solitary site of recurrence was identified by CT in this patient, and PET was used both to confirm the malignant nature of the CT finding and to confirm it was solitary. With this information, treatment planning could be effectively directed to address the recurrence, with local radiation therapy administered, in addition to systemic chemotherapy. It is always desirable to histologically confirm suspected recurrence with biopsy. However, in this case, the PET information was used as presumptive confirmation of recurrence.

CASE 10 | Restaging, pulmonary parenchymal and pleural recurrences

A 72-year-old man, 8 years post surgery and proton beam irradiation for rectal carcinoma, was evaluated for a rising CEA level. A lingular lung nodule was identified on CXR (Figure 1) and demonstrated to be metabolically active on PET (Figure 2). Surgical excision confirmed a colon carcinoma metastasis. Within a few months, the patient's CEA level again rose, and he developed a left pleural

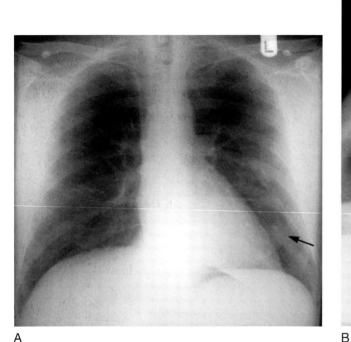
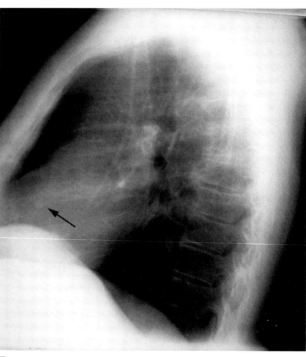

A   B

FIGURE 1. Posteroanterior (**A**) and lateral (**B**) CXR views show a 1-cm lingular solitary nodule (*arrows*).

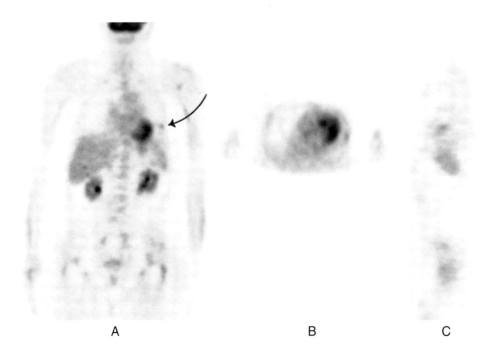

A   B   C

FIGURE 2. PET scan obtained for evaluation of the nodule and for a rising CEA level demonstrates the nodule to be metabolically active (*arrow*). It is not frankly hypermetabolic visually or by standardized uptake value. No other notable findings were seen. Coronal (**A**), transaxial (**B**), and sagittal (**C**) views are shown.

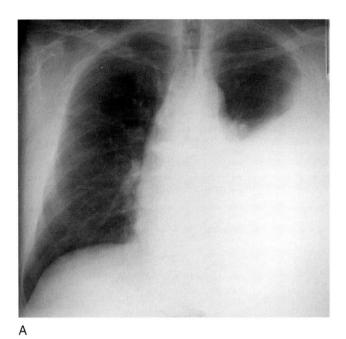

A

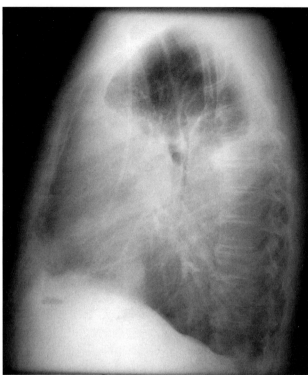

B

FIGURE 3. Posteroanterior (**A**) and lateral (**B**) CXR views show a new large left pleural effusion, filling two thirds of the left hemithorax.

effusion (Figure 3). Chest CT showed lobular pleural masses, consistent with metastases, in addition to fluid (Figure 4). Subsequent PET scan showed corresponding hypermetabolic pleural neoplasia (Figure 5), and the patient was then begun on chemotherapy.

TEACHING POINTS

This case illustrates several different manifestations of colon carcinoma metastatic to the thorax. In the case of the solitary lung metastasis, PET essentially performed a noninvasive biopsy by demonstrating the nodule in question to be metabolically active, if not intensely so. Its relatively small size (about 1 cm) would have made it difficult to sample percutaneously.

In utilizing PET scan data, it is important to put the information gained in context with all other available information to make the best possible assessment of the finding's significance. Too strict reliance on the PET scan activity level of a nodule or other lesion, whether qualitatively assessed or quantified by standardized uptake value (SUV), at the expense of morphologic data, can be misleading. As illustrated here, ready demonstration of metabolic activity in a small new lung nodule should be regarded as suspicious, even if the absolute value of the activity does not reach accepted criteria for malignancy.

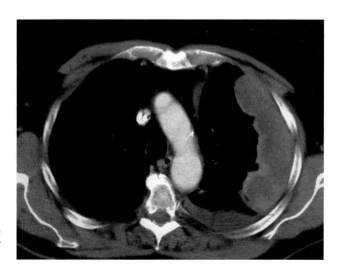

FIGURE 4. Enhanced chest CT shows left pleural fluid, but much of the pleural disease shown on CXR consists of lobular, necrotic, soft tissue density pleural masses, consistent with metastases.

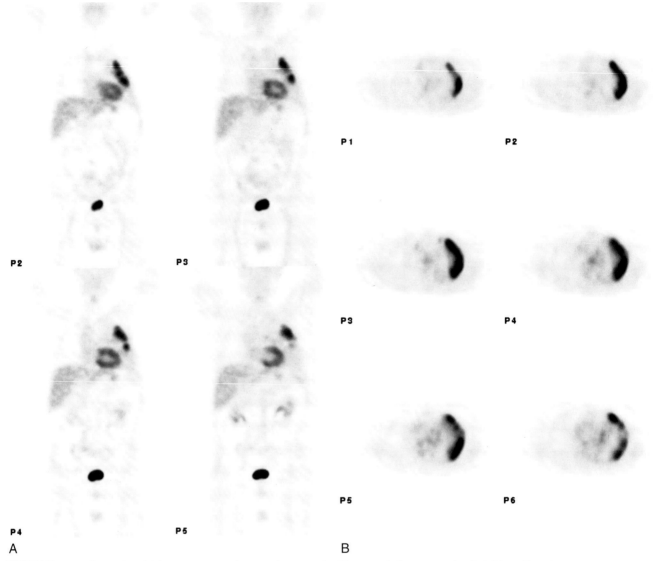

P2   P3

P1   P2

P3   P4

P4   P5   P5   P6

A   B

FIGURE 5. Coronal (**A**) and axial (**B**) PET scan images show curvilinear, peripheral hypermetabolic activity within the left lateral hemithorax, corresponding to the pleural disease on CT.

CASE 11 | *Recurrent colorectal carcinoma, rising CEA level, bone metastases*

A 64-year-old man with a rising CEA level and suspicion of recurrent colorectal carcinoma was referred for PET imaging. He had been diagnosed with colon carcinoma 6 years previously and had undergone a left hemicolectomy and a year of chemotherapy with 5-fluorouracil and levamisole. Imaging evaluations with CT and CEA scan did not identify an etiology for the tumor marker elevation. PET scan was the first imaging study to identify bone metastases, showing foci of increased activity in the left hemipelvis and the right posterior chest wall (Figures 1 and 2). Subsequently, a pelvis CT was obtained and showed soft tissue replacement and lytic change of the left ischium, corresponding to the left hip PET scan abnormality (Figure 3).

Later bone scans, after radiation therapy to the left ischial metastasis, showed findings of progressive osseous metastatic disease (Figures 4 and 5).

TEACHING POINTS

A rising CEA level in a patient post therapy for colorectal carcinoma is a strong indication of recurrent disease. CT is generally the first imaging study to be utilized in the search for occult metastases, because it affords the ability to identify lung nodules, liver lesions, local recurrences, and, occasionally, bone metastases. PET scanning is an excellent complement and next step in the imaging evaluation of suspected recurrences, particularly when no etiology is found on CT, or to confirm noninvasively the suspected malignant nature of abnormalities identified on CT.

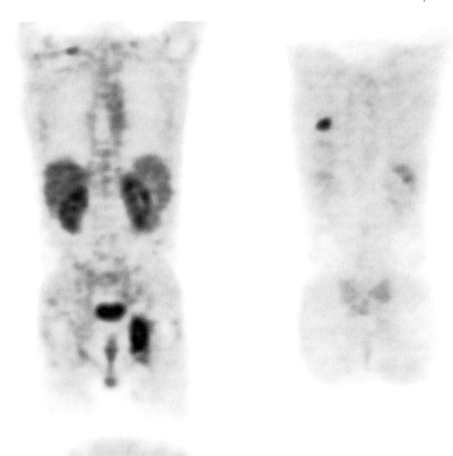

FIGURE 1. Coronal PET images show a large, previously unsuspected left hemipelvic focus of hypermetabolism, most consistent with a bone metastasis. A second focus of pathologically increased activity in the right posterior chest wall also suggested bone metastasis in a rib.

FIGURE 2. Axial PET sections allow more precise localization of the findings in Figure 1. Section shown in **A** is through the chest and shows the right posterior chest wall focus to be very peripheral, suggesting pathologic rib activity. Section shown in **B** is through the pelvis and localizes the abnormal activity to the ischium.

A   B

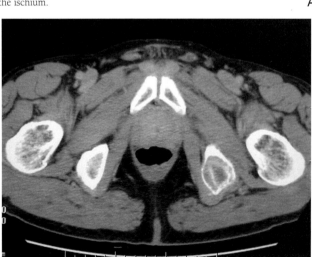

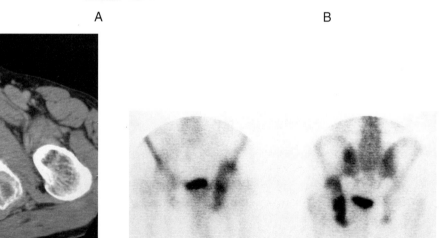

FIGURE 3. Pelvis CT, 1 month later, shows soft tissue replacement and lytic change of the left ischium, correlating with the pelvic PET abnormality and consistent with a bone metastasis.

FIGURE 4. Anterior and posterior pelvic images from a bone scan, 4 months after irradiation to the left hip, show persistent increased activity of the left ischium and acetabulum.

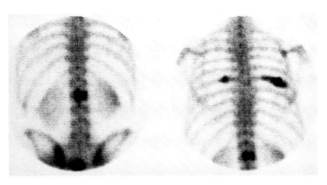

FIGURE 5. Posterior thoracolumbar views from the same bone scan show additional sites of bone metastases, including ribs and the L2 vertebral body. The largest and longest segment of abnormal rib activity at the right posterior seventh rib level corresponds with the abnormality initially noted on PET.

CASE 12 | *Colon cancer, liver metastasis, treatment effect (radiofrequency ablation)*

A 54-year-old man, status post surgery and chemotherapy for a splenic flexure colon carcinoma with one positive lymph node, had a rising CEA level. An outside CT from 1 month before was reportedly negative. PET scan evaluation showed the cause of the CEA level elevation

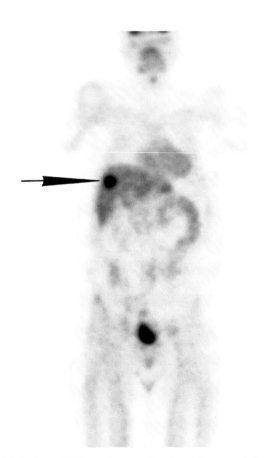

FIGURE 1. Coronal PET scan shows a solitary hepatic hypermetabolic metastasis (*arrow*).

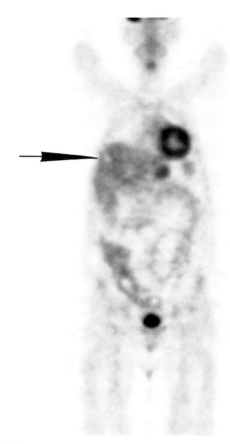

FIGURE 2. PET scan 6 months later shows a photopenic defect at the site of the treated liver metastasis, with no indication of residual tumor or recurrence elsewhere (*arrow*). Note normal variation in myocardial and LUQ gastric activity between the two studies.

to be a solitary hypermetabolic liver metastasis (Figure 1). He was treated with radiofrequency ablation and intrahepatic chemotherapy and returned for repeat PET scan 6 months later (Figure 2).

TEACHING POINTS

Treated liver metastases can be difficult to follow based on morphology, with follow-up CT appearances potentially bizarre and confusing. PET offers an elegant alternative. Contrast this case to Case 13, in which PET showed radiofrequency ablation therapy to be less successful.

CASE 13 | *Liver metastasis, assessment of radiofrequency ablation efficacy*

A 57-year-old man with rectosigmoid carcinoma metastatic to liver was followed with PET scans while undergoing radiofrequency ablation of a solitary metastasis. At the first PET scan evaluation, performed about 3 months after ablation, a photopenic defect could be seen at the site (Figure 1). However, a rim of hypermetabolic activity at the lateral aspect of the defect was suggestive of residual tumor.

The patient was reexamined with PET imaging 3 months later, after re-treatment with radiofrequency ablation. Persistent abnormal activity was again seen at the lateral margin of the lesion (Figure 2). A new rib focus of activity was also noted and initially thought of

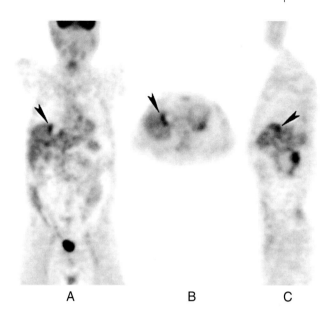

FIGURE 1. First of a series of three PET scans in this 57-year-old man, 3 months post radiofrequency ablation of a solitary colorectal carcinoma liver metastasis, shows a photopenic defect at the site of the treated lesion. Increased metabolic activity is seen at the lateral edge of the defect, consistent with persistent tumor (*arrowheads*). Coronal (**A**), transaxial (**B**), and sagittal (**C**) views are shown.

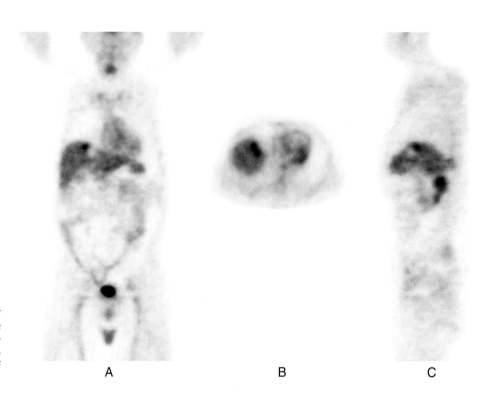

FIGURE 2. Three months later, repeat PET scan shows very similar findings, despite repeat radiofrequency ablation and concurrent systemic chemotherapy. Coronal (**A**), transaxial (**B**), and sagittal (**C**) views are shown.

concern for a bone metastasis. However, the patient had a clear trauma history that was subsequently elicited and the rib lesion resolved on follow-up.

The patient then underwent more "aggressive" radiofrequency ablation and was re-imaged with PET 3 months later. Concurrent systemic chemotherapy, on which he had been maintained throughout this period, concluded 1 month before this PET scan. His liver function tests and CEA level reportedly were normal. The PET scan now showed a larger photopenic defect at the site of the treated lesion, with resolution of the lateral marginal activity noted previously (Figure 3). However, two discrete new marginal foci of activity were now seen, at the medial and posterosuperior margins of the defect, suggestive again

of tumor activity. In addition, new right hilar activity was seen. The right rib focus noted previously had resolved, consistent with the trauma and presumed fracture history.

TEACHING POINTS

Anatomic imaging of treated lesions, like this solitary liver metastasis, not infrequently results in findings that are ambiguous and difficult to interpret. This patient by report had a hyperdense lesion on CT when he was initially evaluated with PET. In such cases, PET provides a useful adjunct to assess the effectiveness of local therapies such as radiofrequency ablation.

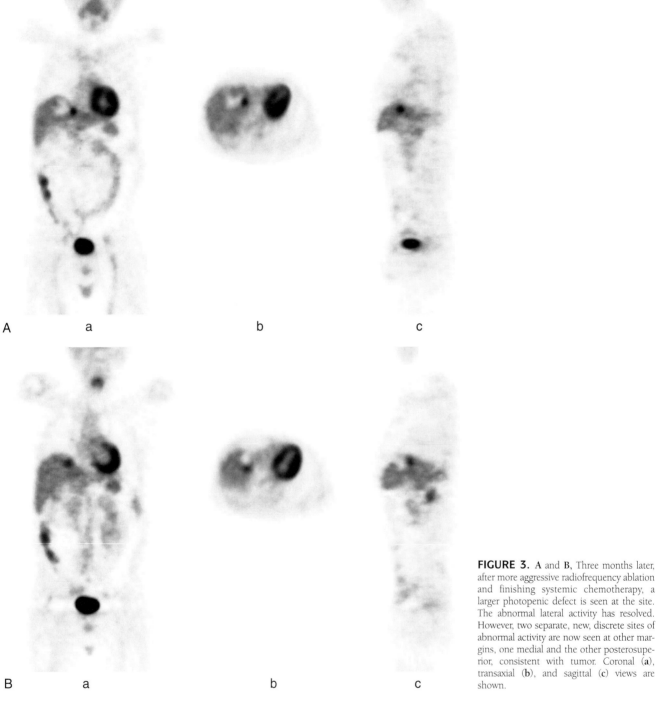

A   a   b   c

B   a   b   c

FIGURE 3. **A** and **B**, Three months later, after more aggressive radiofrequency ablation and finishing systemic chemotherapy, a larger photopenic defect is seen at the site. The abnormal lateral activity has resolved. However, two separate, new, discrete sites of abnormal activity are now seen at other margins, one medial and the other posterosuperior, consistent with tumor. Coronal (**a**), transaxial (**b**), and sagittal (**c**) views are shown.

CASE 14 | *Liver metastases, surgical and interventional treatment effects*

A 54-year-old man, status post sigmoid resection for colon carcinoma with one positive lymph node, was treated with 6 months of chemotherapy. Fourteen months after diagnosis, a rising CEA level led to CT identification of two liver metastases. He was evaluated with PET scan 2 days before scheduled resection of the liver lesions. PET identified five hypermetabolic liver foci, consistent with multiple metastases (Figure 1). At surgery, six metastases were found. He was treated with a left lobectomy, wedge excision of a portion of the right lobe, as well as intraoperative radiofrequency ablation of a metastasis and cryotherapy of an additional lesion. Repeat PET scan 4 months later was essentially negative (Figure 2). Figures 3 and 4 show other images relating to liver metastases.

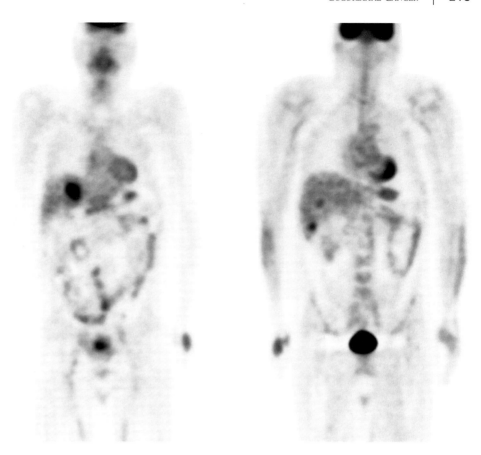

FIGURE 1. Two coronal PET images show three of the five liver metastases identified on this study, which were subsequently confirmed at surgery.

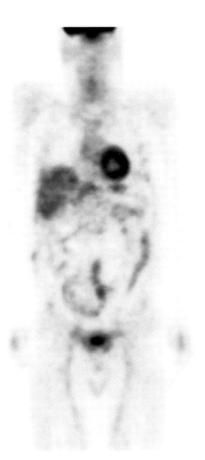

FIGURE 2. Follow-up PET scan, 4 months after surgery, radiofrequency ablation, and cryotherapy, as well as systemic and intra-arterial chemotherapy, shows no hypermetabolic liver metastases.

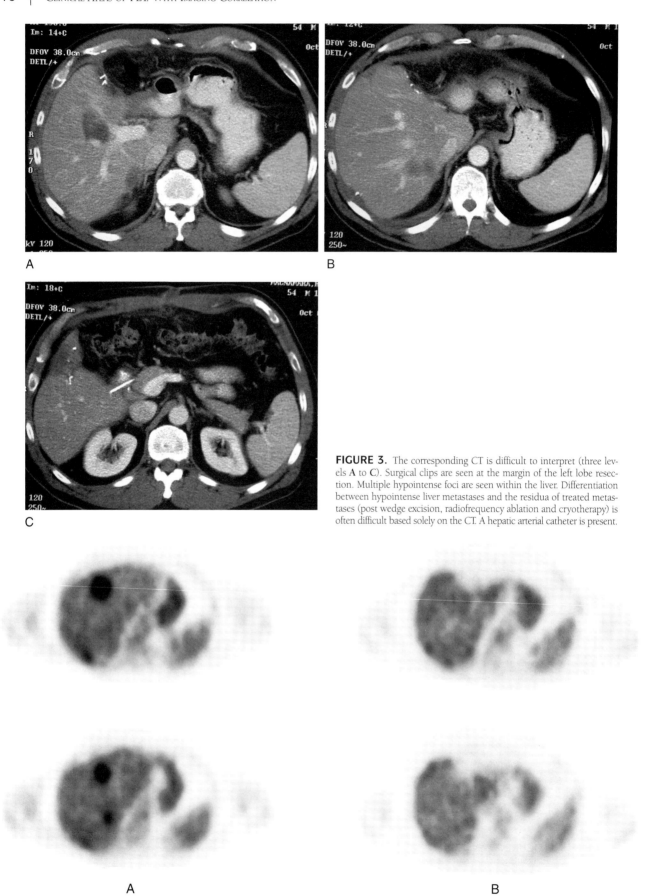

FIGURE 3. The corresponding CT is difficult to interpret (three levels **A** to **C**). Surgical clips are seen at the margin of the left lobe resection. Multiple hypointense foci are seen within the liver. Differentiation between hypointense liver metastases and the residua of treated metastases (post wedge excision, radiofrequency ablation and cryotherapy) is often difficult based solely on the CT. A hepatic arterial catheter is present.

FIGURE 4. Axial PET images, juxtaposing the pretreatment study (**A**) with post-treatment PET study (**B**), show three of the liver metastases on the left and no discernible lesions on the follow-up study on the right.

TEACHING POINTS

PET scan identified more liver metastases than CT in this patient (five compared with two by CT; six were found at surgery), providing a more accurate gauge of the tumor burden and distribution before surgery.

Assessing the efficacy of surgical and interventional therapies for colon carcinoma liver metastases can be difficult on CT. Focal hypodense and sometimes heterogeneous regions frequently persist at the site of successfully treated lesions. PET imaging offers a functional, noninvasive and complementary means of evaluating the success of such treatments.

CASE 15 | *Liver metastases, chemotherapy efficacy*

A 68-year-old man with colon carcinoma presented with liver metastases. The patient was first evaluated with PET scanning for suspicion of liver metastases 2 weeks after surgery for a cecal carcinoma, with negative lymph nodes. Four discrete hypermetabolic foci were confirmed in the liver, consistent with metastases (Figure 1).

After treatment with chemotherapy, the patient was re-imaged with PET scanning 7 months later. The liver metastases were no longer evident, indicating a favorable response (Figure 2).

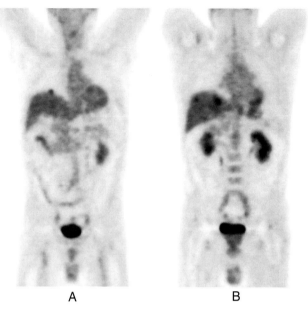

A   B

FIGURE 1. Coronal PET sections from the first PET scan, 2 weeks after cecal carcinoma surgery, confirming suspected liver metastases. A tiny punctate lesion is noted at the dome of the liver on the more anterior section (**A**), with two additional lesions seen on the more posterior section (**B**).

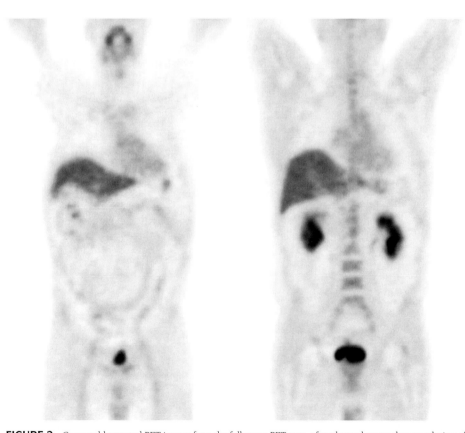

FIGURE 2. Comparable coronal PET images from the follow-up PET scan, after chemotherapy, show resolution of all evidence of liver metastases.

The patient's chemotherapy was continued for an additional 3 months, and the PET scan was repeated. It showed recurrent liver metastases, with two new lesions identified in sites remote from those previously involved (Figure 3). The patient then resumed oral chemotherapy.

TEACHING POINTS

PET imaging helped to confirm liver metastases suspected by palpation at the time of the patient's cecal carcinoma surgery and served as a useful gauge of the effectiveness of this patient's various chemotherapy regimens.

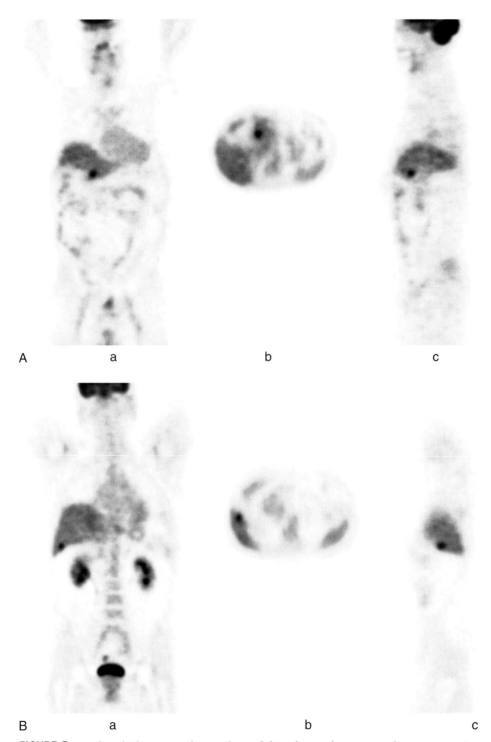

A a   b   c

B a   b   c

FIGURE 3. A and **B,** Third PET scan, after completion of chemotherapy, shows two new liver metastases. One localizes to the left lobe and the other to the posterior segment of the right lobe. The lesions do not represent the same foci noted previously but appear to be entirely new lesions. Coronal (**a**), transaxial (**b**), and sagittal (**c**) views are shown.

CASE 16 | *Pitfall: recurrence, sub-centimeter lung metastases*

A 76-year-old man, 2 years post surgery and chemotherapy for a hepatic flexure colon carcinoma, was evaluated with CT for a rising CEA level. The CT did not identify a recurrence. PET scanning was then performed, which was also negative (Figure 1). A repeat CT scan 4 months later identified multiple small (sub-centimeter) pulmonary parenchymal metastases as the etiology of the rising CEA (Figure 2).

TEACHING POINTS

The sensitivity of PET scanning is dependent on multiple factors. One of the most important is lesion size. In this case, pulmonary metastases were likely present at the time of PET imaging but were too small to visualize on CT, much less PET. Other factors contributing to sensitivity are the metabolic rate of the tumor, location in the body, patient factors such as serum glucose level, and temporal relationship to therapy. When the clinical index of suspicion is high, PET should not be relied on as the sole imaging modality, because there clearly are scenarios in which tumor recurrences may be more readily identified by anatomic imaging than PET. This case is one such example. Another is peritoneal carcinomatosis, such as seen with ovarian carcinoma. Tiny tumor nodules studding peritoneal surfaces may not be identifiable with CT and can be severely underestimated, but there are circumstances (e.g., enough confluent disease to produce omental caking and ascites) in

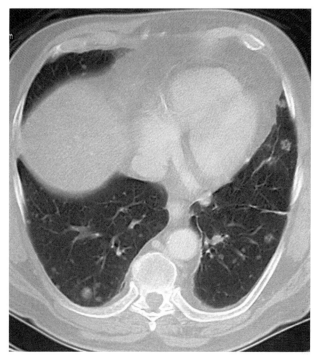

FIGURE 2. Chest CT lung window shows multiple, scattered, small (sub-centimeter) pulmonary nodules, consistent with metastases. These were new compared with CT 5 months earlier.

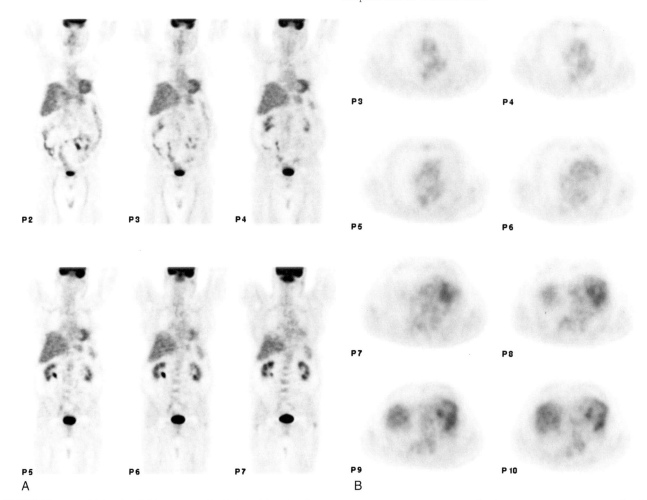

A   B

FIGURE 1. Coronal (**A**) and axial (**B**) PET images (axials through lung bases) are negative, even on retrospective review after the pulmonary metastases were identified.

which a large burden of peritoneal tumor may be much more readily recognized by CT or MRI than PET (see Case 7 in Chapter 7).

CASE 17 | *Pitfall: locally recurrent rectal carcinoma, low scintigraphic activity*

A 75-year-old man developed perineal pain 5 years post colectomy for rectal carcinoma. A CT scan through the pelvis showed a left pararectal mass at the anastomotic level, suspicious for locally recurrent colorectal carcinoma (Figure 1). This was confirmed by biopsy. A concurrent PET scan identified a hypermetabolic RUL lung focus not previously suspected but subsequently confirmed on chest CT. Biopsy confirmed a metastasis. The left pararectal mass displayed only modest metabolic activity and prospectively would likely not have been regarded as pathologic on PET imaging (Figure 2). The presumptive explanation for the absence of hypermetabolism in a biopsy-proven colorectal recurrence is a relatively low metabolic rate, high mucinous content carcinoma variant.

TEACHING POINTS

This case illustrates a potential PET pitfall, peculiar to colorectal carcinoma, that could be encountered in other malignancies. Carcinomas with a high mucinous content, such as colorectal and other gastrointestinal malignancies and ovarian carcinoma, may be relatively low in activity level, hampering PET detection. Presumably this is caused by

a paucity of malignant cells relative to mucinous content. The corresponding focus noted here is identifiable only with CT foreknowledge of the abnormality, is indistinguishable from normal bowel, and would certainly have escaped detection prospectively.

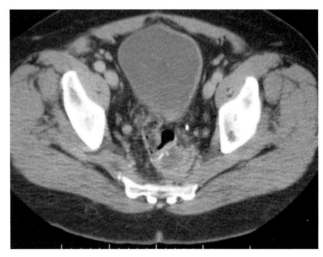

FIGURE 1. Enhanced CT image through the pelvis shows a presacral, left pararectal mass that is of relatively low density centrally. The mass is at the level of the anastomotic staples and extends posterolaterally to muscle. The CT appearance is consistent with a local recurrence.

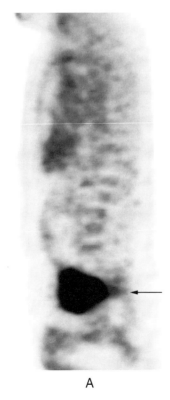

A

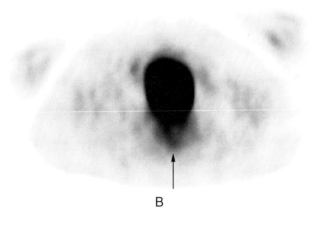

B

FIGURE 2. Corresponding sagittal (**A**) and axial (**B**) PET scan images show only modest metabolic activity at the expected level, posterior to the bladder (*arrows*). This activity level is well within normal limits for physiologic bowel uptake and prospectively would be called negative.

CHAPTER

7

Other Gastrointestinal Malignancies

For gastrointestinal tumors, the largest body of data exists in the diagnosis and monitoring of colorectal carcinomas. PET has been applied in other gastrointestinal malignancies with variable degrees of success. Esophageal tumors are routinely FDG avid with hepatocellular carcinoma at the other end of the sensitivity spectrum. Patients with pancreatic carcinoma, gastric carcinoma, and cholangiocarcinoma may benefit from PET in specific circumstances. This chapter reviews the use of FDG-PET in these tumors with emphasis on the role PET can play as a problem-solving tool.

ESOPHAGEAL CANCER

In the United States, carcinoma of the esophagus accounts for less than 2% of all malignancies.[1] However, it has a very high mortality rate, with 5-year survival in the 5% to 10% range. Even in patients with apparently resectable disease, the 5-year survival is less than 50%.[2] These statistics suggest both late initial diagnosis and inadequate staging. The lack of symptoms in early esophageal cancer may help explain the delay in diagnosis, whereas suboptimal sensitivity for conventional imaging modalities (primarily CT) contributes to inadequate staging.

At present, CT is the most commonly utilized modality for staging. Endoscopic ultrasonography is the most accurate method for T and N staging.[1] MRI and minimally invasive surgery (i.e., thoracoscopy and laparoscopy) are also used, with variable success. PET has been used for staging, restaging, and monitoring response to therapy. Although PET shows a sensitivity of more than 95% at the primary site,[1,3,4] it does not offer any significant advantage over standard modalities. With respect to locoregional nodal involvement, PET has been shown to be as insensitive as CT, averaging approximately 50%.[1,4-6] It is of interest that specificity appears to be improved compared with CT in locoregional nodes.

The major advantage of PET is its ability to recognize distant (i.e., stage IV) disease.[3,4,7] The value of accurately and reliably upstaging disease is in reducing noncurative surgeries. PET has also been proposed to monitor response to neoadjuvant therapy (e.g., chemotherapy ± radiation therapy). A reduction in tumor FDG uptake allows differentiation between responders and non-responders.[8,9] Assessment can be qualitative or quantitative, using standardized uptake values (SUVs). Of interest, esophageal carcinoma has a very high SUV in the untreated person, with a mean greater than 10.[1] Finally, there are preliminary data to support the use of PET for investigating suspected recurrence.[10] The combination of whole-body imaging capability, high tumor SUV, and suboptimal results from conventional studies should secure a place for PET in the longitudinal assessment of patients with esophageal carcinoma. This will assume even greater importance once more effective therapies are developed.

REFERENCES

1. Yeung HWD, Macapinlac HA, Mazudar M, et al: FDG-PET in esophageal cancer: Incremental value over computed tomography. Clin Pos Imag 1999;2:255-260.
2. Choi JY, Lee KH, Shim YM, et al: Improved detection of individual nodal involvement in squamous cell carcinoma of the esophagus by FDG-PET. J Nucl Med 2000;41:808-815.
3. Couper GW, McAteer D, Wallis F, et al: Detection of response to chemotherapy using positron emission tomography in patients with esophageal and gastric cancer. Br J Surg 1998;85:1403-1406.
4. Block MI, Patterson GA, Sundaresan RS, et al: Improvement in staging of esophageal cancer with the addition of positron emission tomography. Ann Thorac Surg 1997;64:770-776.
5. Luketich JD, Shauer PR, Meltzer CC, et al: Role of positron emission tomography in staging esophageal cancer. Ann Thorac Surg 1997;64: 765-769.
6. Kim K, Park SJ, Kim BT, et al: Evaluation of lymph node metastases in squamous cell carcinoma of the esophagus with positron emission tomography. Ann Thorac Surg 2001;71:290-294.
7. Flanagan FL, Dehdashti F, Siegel BA, et al: Staging of esophageal cancer with ^{18}F-fluorodeoxyglucose positron emission tomography. AJR Am J Roentgenol 1997;168:417-424.
8. Weber WA, Ott K, Becker K, et al: Prediction of response to preoperative chemotherapy in adenocarcinomas of the esophagogastric junction by metabolic imaging. J Clin Oncol 2001;19:3058-3065.
9. Brucher BL, Weber W, Bauer M, et al: Neoadjuvant therapy of esophageal squamous cell carcinoma: Response evaluation by positron emission tomography. Ann Surg 2001;233:320-321.
10. Flamen P, Lerut A, Van Cutsem E, et al: The utility of positron emission tomography for the diagnosis and staging of recurrent esophageal cancer. J Thorac Cardiovasc Surg 2000;120:1085-1092.

CASE 1 | *Proximal esophageal squamous cell carcinoma*

A 52-year-old woman with a recent endoscopic diagnosis of proximal esophageal squamous cell carcinoma was referred for PET scan and CT for staging (Figures 1 and 2). The patient was treated with chemotherapy and radiation, in advance of surgical treatment with a gastric pull-through.

TEACHING POINTS

Esophageal carcinoma primary tumors are typically intensely hypermetabolic. PET is no better than CT in identifying paraesophageal nodal involvement, because the activity of involved nodes generally cannot be distinguished from the primary lesion activity with which it is usually confluent. However, PET is useful in identifying distant metastases, which would render a patient incurable by surgery.

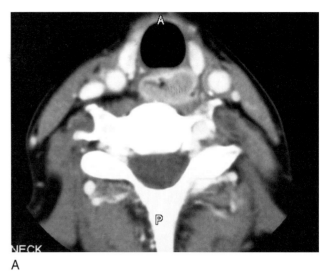

A

B

FIGURE 2. Corresponding neck soft tissue CT images show marked mass-like enlargement of the cervical esophagus at the same level. **A,** Anterior. **B,** Posterior.

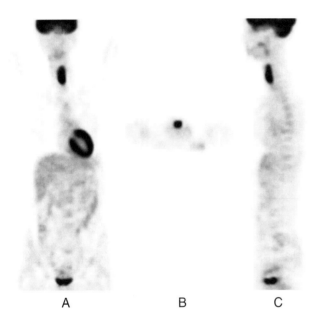

A   B   C

FIGURE 1. Intense linear hypermetabolic activity identifies the extent of the patient's proximal esophageal primary lesion. No additional sites of abnormal activity are seen. Coronal (**A**), transaxial (**B**), and sagittal (**C**) views are shown.

CASE 2 | *Distal esophageal adenocarcinoma, with gastrohepatic nodal involvement*

A 65-year-old man presented with dysphagia. A barium swallow showed a concentric narrowing, with shouldering and mucosal irregularity, at the distal esophageal level (Figure 1). A diagnosis of esophageal adenocarcinoma was made by endoscopic biopsy. Chest CT showed a 3-cm distal esophageal mass and sub-centimeter paraesophageal and gastrohepatic ligament lymph nodes (Figures 2 and 3). Lucent liver lesions were noted, thought most likely to be small volume-averaged cysts. PET was obtained during staging. It showed intense linear distal esophageal activity, corresponding to the primary lesion, as well as a faint, tiny focus of activity at the level of the gastrohepatic lymphadenopathy (Figure 4). The patient was treated with concurrent irradiation and chemotherapy in anticipation of esophagectomy, but he ultimately declined surgery.

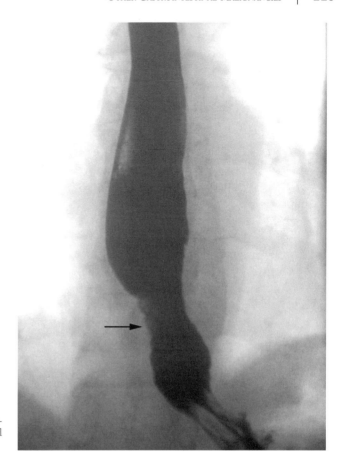

FIGURE 1. A frontal view from a barium swallow shows a concentric narrowing of the distal esophagus, several centimeters above the gastroesophageal junction (*arrow*). The lesion displays mucosal irregularity and shouldering.

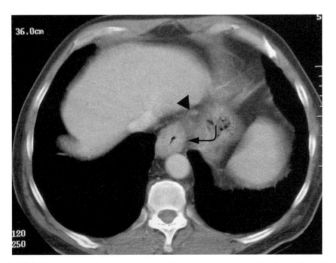

FIGURE 2. Image from an enhanced chest CT shows a distal esophageal mass (*arrow*), manifested by circumferential thickening, corresponding to the barium swallow. A paraesophageal lymph node is noted (*arrowhead*).

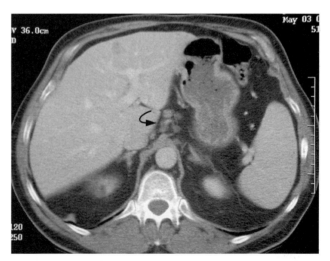

FIGURE 3. A more inferior CT section shows four, sub-centimeter gastrohepatic ligament lymph nodes (*arrow*), suggesting nodal esophageal carcinoma. Both CT images (compare with Figure 2) show faint, small liver lucencies, thought to be volume-averaged cysts.

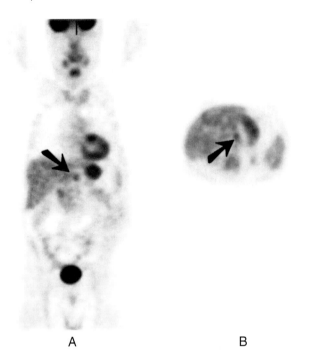

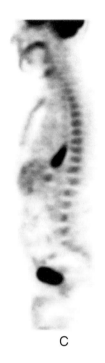

A   B   C

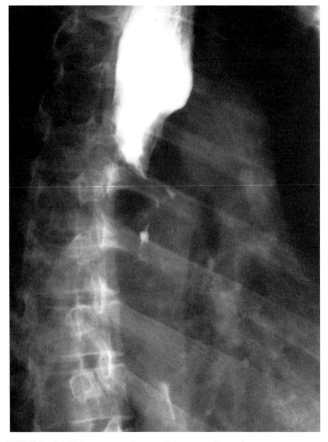

FIGURE 4. Sagittal (**C**) PET scan image shows linear hypermetabolic activity at the level of the distal esophageal primary carcinoma. Coronal (**A**) and axial (**B**) PET images show a small focus of less intense activity in the upper mid abdomen corresponding to the abnormal gastrohepatic ligament adenopathy on CT (*arrows*). No pathologic liver or distant activity was seen.

TEACHING POINTS

CT evaluation suggested local nodal involvement of perigastric lymph nodes. Although still small (6 to 8 mm), identifying any lymph nodes at this location in this clinical setting is suspicious. PET served to confirm the CT impression of gastrohepatic ligament nodal involvement, as well as the impression of benign liver lesions.

CASE 3 | Esophageal carcinoma, superior mediastinal paraesophageal nodal involvement

A 37-year-old woman presented with progressive dysphagia, including liquid intolerance, and a 15-pound weight loss over 2 months. Attempts to eat resulted in gagging and vomiting blood. Endoscopy and biopsy identified a malignancy of epidermal origin, poorly differentiated. An esophagram showed an extensive, obstructing lesion of the mid to distal esophagus, with only a trickle of barium outlining the severely narrowed lumen (Figure 1). CT confirmed a circumferentially thickened and enlarged mid to distal esophagus (Figure 2). PET scanning was requested to complete the patient's initial staging (Figures 3, 4, and 6). There was intense hypermetabolic activity of the distal two thirds of the esophagus, corresponding to the extensive primary demonstrated on barium swallow and CT. In addition, two small, punctate, discrete additional sites of activity were noted in the right paraesophageal plexus above the primary lesion. One was at the level of the uppermost lesion margin, whereas the second focus was higher, just below the thoracic inlet. Additional review of the CT in conjunction with PET showed a corresponding 1 cm right paraesophageal lymph node in the superior mediastinum, at the level of the clavicular heads (Figure 5). The patient was treated with combination irradiation and chemotherapy.

FIGURE 1. Oblique view from a barium swallow shows an extensive, obstructing mass of the mid to distal esophagus. The uppermost margin is above the level of the carina, with polypoid mucosal shouldering. Only a trickle of barium outlines the severely narrowed, virtually occluded lumen.

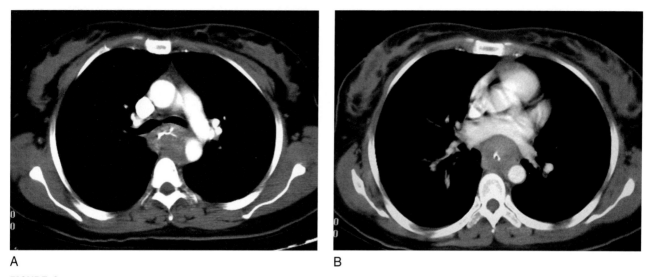

FIGURE 2. Two enhanced chest CT images (upper section [A] is through carina, lower section [B] is at left atrial level) show the markedly thickened esophageal mass. Barium outlines the severely narrowed lumen.

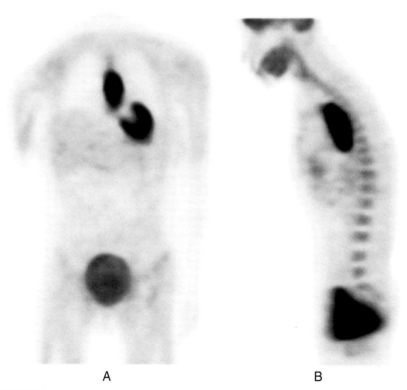

FIGURE 3. Coronal (A) and sagittal (B) PET images through the primary lesion show markedly increased metabolic activity of the mass, involving the distal two thirds of the esophagus.

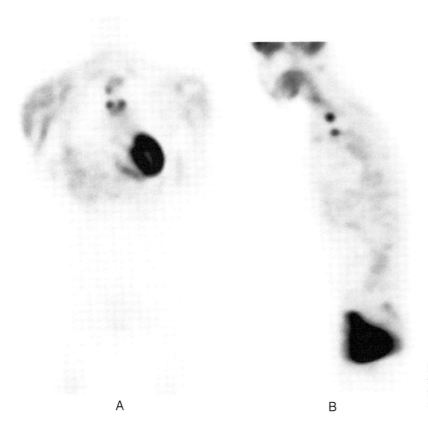

A   B

FIGURE 4. Additional coronal (**A**) and sagittal (**B**) PET images show two separate, punctate, additional foci of activity along the course of the paraesophageal plexus on the right, consistent with nodal activity.

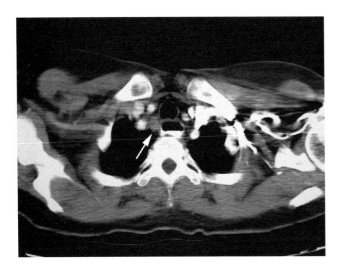

FIGURE 5. A higher chest CT section (note clavicular heads) shows a 1-cm right paraesophageal lymph node (*arrow*), corresponding to the superiormost focus above.

FIGURE 6. Axial PET images (left, through superior mediastinum and at same level as Figure 5, and, right, at superior margin of primary lesion) show counterpart transverse sections to Figure 4.

TEACHING POINTS

FDG-PET is quite accurate in depiction of primary esophageal cancer lesions, with reported sensitivities of 95% and greater. Neither CT nor PET supplants endoscopic ultrasonography for detection of para-esophageal lymph node involvement. Enlarged paraesophageal lymph nodes at the level of the primary lesion cannot accurately be separated from the lesion itself with either CT or PET. Both CT and PET fare better in identifying proximal (cervical) and distal (paragastric) nodal involvement, above or below the primary lesion level. PET more accurately identifies distant metastases than CT.

CASE 4 | *Distal esophageal squamous cell carcinoma*

A 68-year-old man was evaluated with a barium swallow for complaints of severe dysphagia. This showed a mid-distal polypoid esophageal mass (Figure 1). Endoscopic biopsy identified moderately differentiated squamous cell carcinoma. PET scan showed an ovoid focus of intense hypermetabolic activity in the mid-distal esophagus, corresponding to the known primary tumor (Figure 2). Preoperative evaluation with endoscopic ultrasonography showed a T3N1 tumor with one positive paraesophageal lymph node. The patient underwent esophagectomy. The moderately differentiated squamous cell carcinoma was

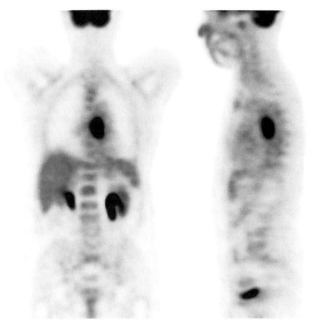

FIGURE 2. PET scan images show intense activity in an ovoid focus at the mid-distal esophageal level, at the site of the known primary lesion.

ulcerated and measured 6.5 × 4 cm. Transmural extension into paraesophageal tissues was noted. Metastatic carcinoma was identified in 2 of 22 paraesophageal lymph nodes, 1 of 4 perigastric lymph nodes, and 1 of 2 pulmonary ligament lymph nodes.

Approximately 3 months after surgery, the patient developed left hip pain. Work-up with x-rays and bone scan suggested metastatic disease. His carcinoembryonic antigen (CEA) level was elevated, and the patient was referred for palliative radiation therapy to the left hip for presumed osseous metastasis. He declined chemotherapy and died 9 months after diagnosis.

TEACHING POINTS

Pooling data from multiple series, the reported sensitivity of PET for identification of primary esophageal carcinoma lesions is 97%, which is significantly greater than the sensitivity reported for CT. Both PET and CT are insensitive for detection of perigastric and paraesophageal lymph node involvement. Specificity is high for both: 99% for PET and 98% for CT. Endoscopic ultrasonography is the most sensitive modality for assessing local lymph node involvement.

CASE 5 | *Distal esophageal adenocarcinoma, with gastric cardia extension and paragastric nodal involvement*

A 49-year-old previously healthy man noted recent onset of dysphagia, associated with a 20+-pound weight loss. Endoscopy showed a malignant-appearing stricture in the distal esophagus, with a hard, nodular surface. A small, submucosal gastric mass was noted in the cardia. Biopsy of the lesion proved moderate to poorly differentiated adenocarcinoma, with features suggesting invasion. PET and CT were performed for staging (Figures 1 to 5).

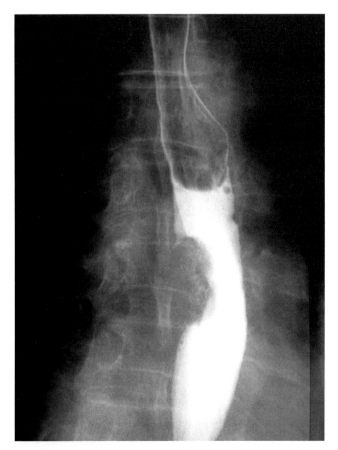

FIGURE 1. Frontal view from a barium swallow shows a polypoid, lobulated mass of the mid-distal esophagus, consistent with an esophageal carcinoma. This diagnosis was subsequently confirmed endoscopically.

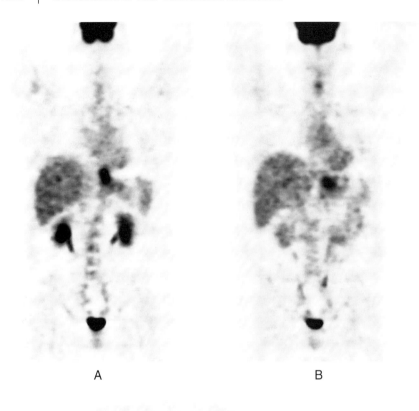

FIGURE 1. Coronal PET images show an intense distal esophageal focus of activity (**A**), extending distally and confluently to the gastric cardia level (**B**).

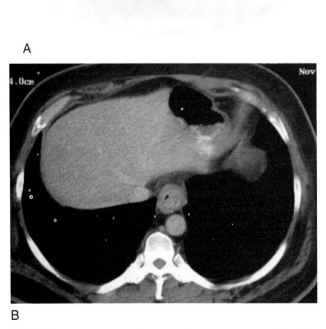

FIGURE 2. Precise correspondence is seen between PET images (**A**) and CT (**B**). Intense gastroesophageal junction activity on PET corresponds to the abnormally thickened gastroesophageal junction on CT.

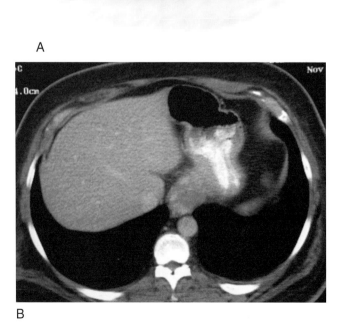

FIGURE 3. Inferiorly, the hypermetabolic mass extends confluently into the contiguous gastric cardia mass (**A**), well seen on CT (**B**).

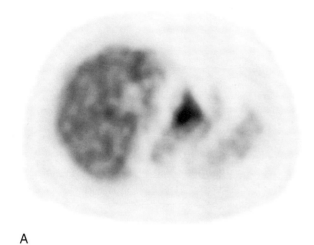

A

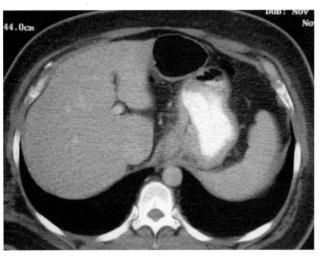

B

FIGURE 4. Again, the gastric cardia mass on CT (**B**) is abnormally increased in metabolic activity on PET (**A**).

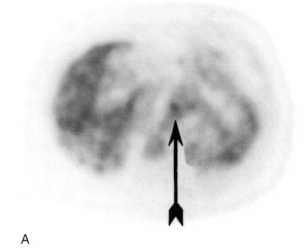

A

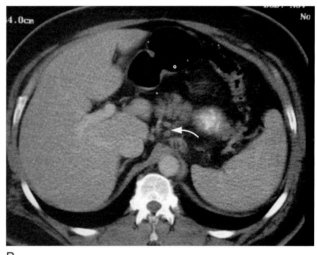

B

FIGURE 5. Only stepwise correlation of the above sections allows confident identification of the tiny focus of increased activity on PET (**A**, *arrow*) as corresponding to celiac axis adenopathy on CT (**B**, *curved arrow*).

TEACHING POINTS

The primary lesion is readily identifiable, both above the diaphragm at the distal esophageal and gastroesophageal level and in the proximal stomach. The regional nodal involvement at the celiac axis is readily recognizable by CT, even at sub-centimeter size, because lymph nodes of any size are not normally seen here. However, only stepwise correlation with the CT, level by level, allows one to identify the same small finding on PET. Lymph nodes on the order of 6 mm are generally too small to be identified on PET.

GASTRIC CANCER

Worldwide, gastric cancer is the second leading cause of cancer-related death.[1] In the United States, the incidence of cancer of the upper stomach has been rising, while at the same time the diagnosis of early stage disease accounts for less than 20% of new cases.[2] Overall, the 5-year survival is poor and better diagnostic tests are clearly needed. Very few well-done studies utilizing PET are available in the literature and are primarily focused on recurrence. These studies tend to show low sensitivity and negative predictive value as a screening test.[1,3] Explanations for the low sensitivity include low FDG avidity in

signet cell tumors, reduced FDG concentration in mucinous adenocarcinomas, and relative reduction of Glut-1 transporters. These factors contribute to sensitivity of approximately 60%, suboptimal for cost-effectiveness. However, in selected patients, PET can be quite valuable. The preoperative identification of distant metastases will prevent noncurative surgery, PET can clarify postoperative findings on CT and serve as a whole-body screen, and studies are under way to assess the utility of FDG-PET for monitoring therapy.

There are two additional areas of caution: primary site evaluation may be problematic because normal gastric uptake of FDG may be quite intense and peritumoral lymph nodes in close proximity and small peritoneal metastases may be missed.

REFERENCES

1. Stahl A, Ott K, Weber WA, et al: FDG PET imaging of locally advanced gastric carcinomas: Correlation with endoscopic and histopathological findings. Eur J Nucl Med Mol Imaging 2003;30:288-295.
2. Gamhir SS, Czernin J, Schwimmer J, et al: A tabulated summary of the FDG PET literature. J Nucl Med 2001;42:40S.
3. De Potter T, Flamen P, Van Custen E, et al: Whole-body PET with FDG for the diagnosis of recurrent gastric cancer. Eur J Nucl Med 2002;29:525-529.

CASE 6 | *Gastric carcinoma, with retroperitoneal nodal metastases*

A 52-year-old man with metastatic, poorly differentiated gastric adenocarcinoma on maintenance chemotherapy for retroperitoneal nodal disease was followed with CT. When CT showed growth of previously stable lymph nodes, PET scan was requested.

At the time of the patient's partial gastrectomy 2 years earlier, his 4.5-cm invasive, poorly differentiated adenocarcinoma extended through the full gastric wall thickness into fat and was accompanied by solid tumor deposits in the perigastric soft tissue. Nine of 18 lymph nodes were positive for metastatic disease. Retroperitoneal adenopathy had been noted on a presurgical staging CT. He underwent four cycles of adjuvant chemotherapy postoperatively, with a reduction in adenopathy noted on CT. Continued CT follow-up of the adenopathy was stable until 6 months later, when an increase was noted. The patient was then started on weekly gemcitabine (Gemzar), with a decline noted on CT in the size of his retroperitoneal disease. He was evaluated with PET after an endoscopic gastric biopsy demonstrated adenocarcinoma 2 years after initial diagnosis and surgery. PET scan showed nodular and confluent prevertebral foci of activity, corresponding to pathologic retroperitoneal adenopathy on CT (Figures 1 to 3).

TEACHING POINTS

Macroscopic gastric carcinoma, metastatic to retroperitoneal lymph nodes, is well demonstrated on this PET, in contrast to the gastric carcinomatosis seen in Case 7.

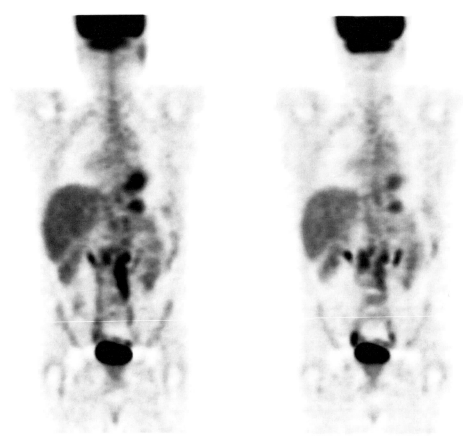

FIGURE 1. Coronal PET scan images show prevertebral foci of increased metabolic activity. The left para-aortic activity is linear and confluent and could be mistaken for a dilated ureter. In this case, the normal-caliber ureters can be visualized separately in the paraspinal regions.

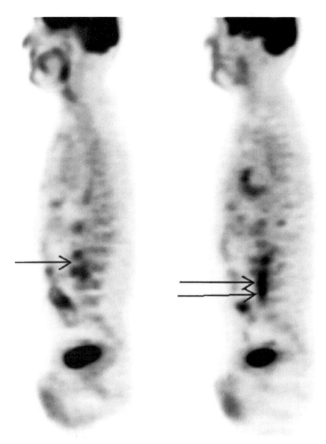

FIGURE 2. Sagittal PET images corresponding to those in Figure 1. The prevertebral foci on the left are "lumpy-bumpy," typical of adenopathy. The nodal chain of activity in the image on the right corresponds to left para-aortic adenopathy and is surprisingly linear and confluent, simulating a dilated ureter (*arrows*, adenopathy).

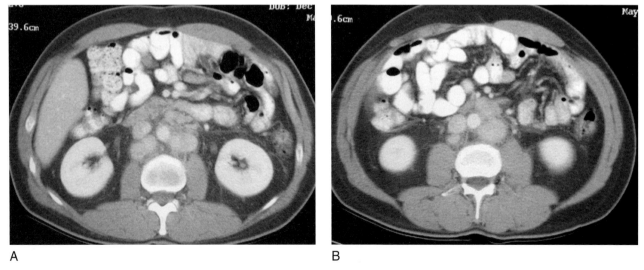

A   B

FIGURE 3. Enhanced abdominal CT images (two sections, **A** and **B**) show pathologically enlarged retroperitoneal lymph nodes, corresponding to the PET abnormalities.

CASE 7 | Gastric carcinoma, with peritoneal carcinomatosis

A 44-year-old man with gastric carcinoma presented with diffuse peritoneal carcinomatosis. The patient had abdominal pain and weight loss. Upper gastrointestinal series (Figure 1) and abdominal CT showed circumferential wall thickening of the distal body and antrum of the stomach (Figure 2). CT also demonstrated ascites and diffuse stippling of the omentum, consistent with peritoneal carcinomatosis. This was confirmed at exploratory laparotomy. PET scanning was performed before initiation of chemotherapy. It showed an abnormal appearance of the stomach, corresponding to the CT findings (Figure 3). In addition, subtle, mild, diffuse increase in activity was seen within the abdomen, corresponding to the omental "cake" (Figure 4).

TEACHING POINTS

Gastric activity is frequently seen as a normal finding on PET. The stomach should not be distended, because the patient should have been NPO a minimum of 4 hours. The lumen is not usually visualized in the empty stomach. The stomach can be recognized as abnormal here by correlation with the imaging studies and history, but to identify this prospectively as pathologic seems unlikely.

Similarly, recognition of peritoneal carcinomatosis is a known pitfall of PET. Clearly, because peritoneal metastases may be tiny, innumerable, and severely underestimated by CT, this is a potent source of error for PET. Again, correlation with imaging (generally CT) is the most reliable means for avoiding this mistake. The counterpart PET findings correlate well with CT but are subtle and would be difficult to recognize prospectively and independent of imaging.

PANCREAS

The overall 5-year survival of patients with newly diagnosed pancreatic cancer is approximately 3%. When discovered early, pancreaticoduodenectomy (Whipple procedure) can improve survival to more than 20%.[1] Challenges in the evaluation of patients with a pancreatic mass include differentiation of benign from malignant disease, accurate staging for the 30,000 patients found to have pancreatic cancer annually, and assessment of response to therapy. Available pancreatic imaging techniques include CT, ultrasonography, MRI, endoscopic retrograde cholangiopancreatography (ERCP), and PET.

The use of PET in the evaluation of pancreatic disease goes back more than 2 decades. The first studies utilized carbon-11–labeled amino acids.[2,3] Although these studies were encouraging, it was recognized that PET imaging with these agents could not reliably separate cancer from pancreatitis. As investigators turned to FDG, more data appeared on the use of PET for diagnosis. Review of this data is complicated, because some studies do not clearly separate diagnosis from staging. A recent literature review of diagnosis found a sensitivity of 94% and specificity of 90% in more than 350 patients.[4] Sperti and colleagues specifically looked at patients with cystic tumors of the pancreas and found a significantly better sensitivity, specificity, and overall accuracy for PET as compared with CT and/or measurement of CA 19-9.[5] Causes for reduced sensitivity include lesions smaller than 1 cm and coexisting hyperglycemia. Reduced specificity is often caused by active inflammation, including acute and chronic pancreatitis.[1,6-8]

Data on staging are more extensive than for primary site diagnosis and show higher PET sensitivity and specificity

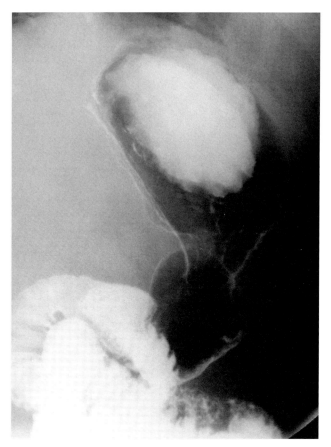

FIGURE 1. View from an air contrast upper gastrointestinal series shows a constricted, indistensible "waist" to the distal stomach body, with mucosal shouldering and an apple-core type appearance.

than CT.[4] PET sensitivity and specificities average in the low 80% range, whereas CT is in the low 60% range. PET cannot evaluate local extension or the relationship of tumor to surrounding blood vessels. Although there are little data focused on hepatic evaluation, one study of 168 patients concluded that PET was reliable for hepatic staging with lesions greater than 1 cm.[9] However, there were six patients with false-positive studies due to intrahepatic cholestasis. PET can significantly influence surgical decision making and may serve a complementary role in staging the disease in these patients.

Monitoring therapy in pancreatic cancer is still in its infancy. Maisey and associates reported encouraging results on the use of PET in patients undergoing chemotherapy,[10] whereas Higashi and coworkers found PET useful in monitoring patients after intraoperative radiation therapy.[11] They confirmed the well-recognized phenomenon of reduction in metabolism before size regression.

The use of PET in pancreatic cancer evaluation is increasing. For diagnosis, equivocal CT findings may be clarified by PET. For staging, PET appears to be more accurate than other available modalities. Importantly, even though overall prognosis is poor, PET findings alter decision making, often sparing a patient noncurative surgery or redirecting therapy.

REFERENCES

1. Delbeke D, Rose DM, Chapman WC, et al: Optimal interpretation of FDG PET in the diagnosis, staging, and management of pancreatic carcinoma. J Nucl Med 1999;40:1784-1791.

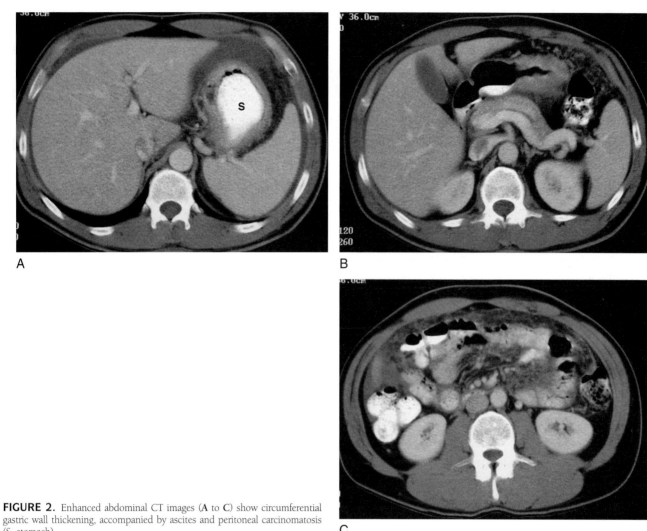

FIGURE 2. Enhanced abdominal CT images (**A** to **C**) show circumferential gastric wall thickening, accompanied by ascites and peritoneal carcinomatosis (S, stomach).

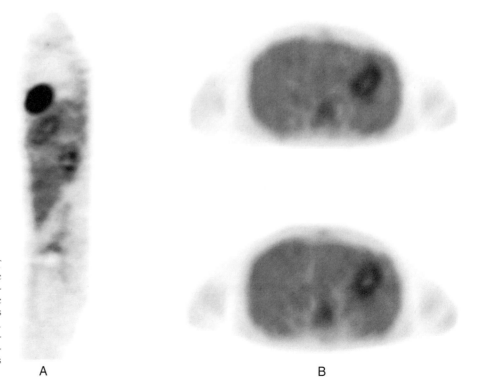

FIGURE 3. Sagittal (**A**) and axial (**B**) PET images show an unusual, abnormal appearance of the stomach, the PET equivalent of linitis plastica. Although the level of activity seen in the gastric walls is not unusual, to see the walls and the lumen of the stomach so distinctly is. Normally, the lumen of the stomach is not visualized, unless the stomach is abnormally distended or the walls are indistensible, as in this case.

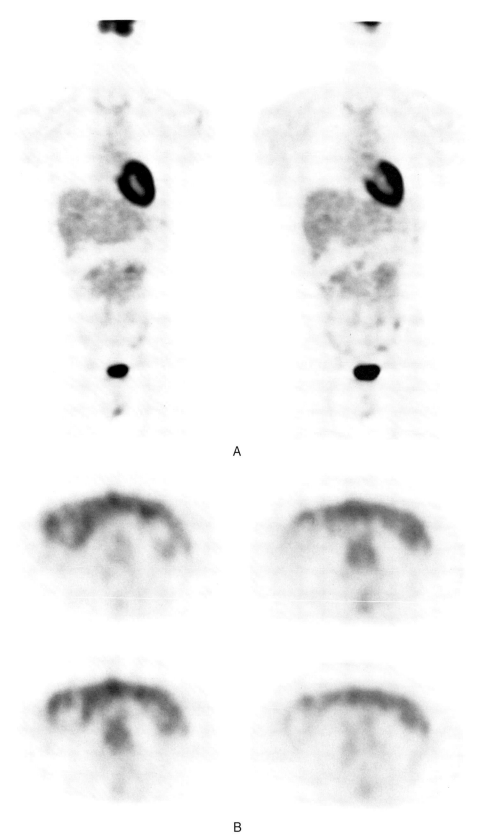

A

B

FIGURE 4. Coronal (**A**) and axial (**B**) PET images of a follow-up PET scan, after chemotherapy, show persistent findings corresponding to "omental cake" on CT. On coronal PET, this is manifested by cloud-like low-level diffuse increased activity within the abdomen, distinct from the usual serpiginous pattern of bowel activity. The axial images show the activity to be nondependent, under the anterior abdominal wall, in contrast to normal bowel activity.

2. Syrota A, Duquesnoy N, Paraf A, et al: The role of positron emission tomography in the detection of pancreatic disease. Radiology 1982;143:249-253.
3. Kirchner PT, Ryan J, Zalutsky M, et al: Positron emission tomography for the evaluation of pancreatic disease. Senin Nucl Med 1980;10:374-391.
4. Gambhir SS, Czernin J, Schwimmer J, et al: A tabulated summary of the FDG PET literature. J Nucl Med 2001;42:50S-52S.
5. Sperti C, Pasquali C, Chierichetti F, et al: Value of 18-fluorodeoxyglucose positron emission tomography in the management of patients with cystic tumors of the pancreas. Ann Surg 2001;234:675-680.
6. Keogan MT, Tyler D, Clark L, et al: Diagnosis of pancreatic carcinoma: role of FDG PET. AJR Am J Roentgenol 1998;171:1565-1570.
7. Zimny M, Schumpelick V: Fluorodeoxyglucose positron emission tomography (FDG-PET) in the differential diagnosis of pancreatic lesions. Chirug 2001;72:989-994.
8. Bares R, Klever P, Hauptmann S, et al: F-18 fluorodeoxyglucose PET in vivo evaluation of pancreatic glucose metabolism for detection of pancreatic cancer. Radiology 1994;192:79-86.
9. Frohlich A, Diederichs CG, Staib L, et al: Detection of liver metastases from pancreatic cancer using FDG PET. J Nucl Med 1999;40:250-255.
10. Maisey NR, Webb A, Flux GD, et al: FDG-PET in the prediction of survival of patients with cancer of the pancreas: A pilot study. Br J Cancer 2000;83:287-293.
11. Higashi T, Sakahara H, Torizuka T, et al: Evaluation of intraoperative radiation therapy for unresectable pancreatic cancer with FDG-PET. J Nucl Med 1999;40:1424-1433.

CASE 8 | *Pancreatic adenocarcinoma*

A 75-year-old woman presented with painless obstructive jaundice developing over several weeks, without weight loss or other symptoms. Initial evaluation was with MRI, which demonstrated dilated bile and pancreatic ducts, secondary to a mass in the head of the pancreas (Figures 1 to 3). An attempt at ERCP was unsuccessful, and transhepatic cholangiography and biliary drainage were accomplished percutaneously. Enhanced CT was performed after biliary decompression and showed a hypodense obstructing pancreatic head mass, typical in appearance for a pancreatic carcinoma (Figures 4 and 5). Without evidence from these studies of unresectability, PET imaging was requested for further evaluation. It showed only focal hyperintensity at the primary site, with no evidence of distant metastases (Figure 6). Exploratory laparotomy before an attempt at a Whipple procedure showed chronic bile congestion of the liver, without evidence of metastases. Soft porta hepatis lymph nodes were sampled, and frozen section analysis was negative for malignancy. No enlarged lymph nodes were encountered near the superior mesenteric vessels or celiac axis. The plane between the portal vein and pancreas was free, and the tumor was believed to be resectable. Pancreaticoduodenectomy and cholecystectomy were performed. At pathology, the mass proved to be a 3.5-cm, invasive, moderate to poorly differentiated adenocarcinoma, extensively involving the head of the pancreas and extending to adjacent fat, with nerve invasion. A portal lymph node, which had been negative at frozen section, showed metastatic adenocarcinoma on permanent section.

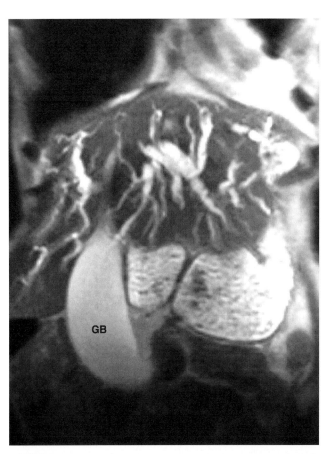

FIGURE 1. T2-weighted fast spin echo coronal MR image shows markedly dilated intrahepatic bile ducts, as well as distention of the gallbladder (GB).

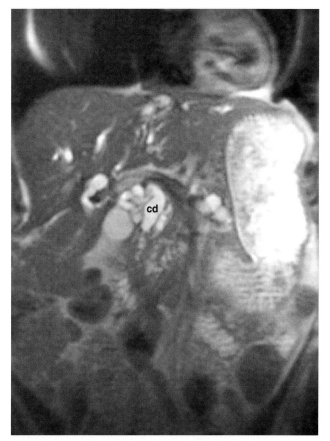

FIGURE 2. Another T2-weighted fast spin echo coronal MR section shows dilatation of the extrahepatic common duct (cd) and the distal pancreatic duct. The distal common bile duct changes caliber abruptly.

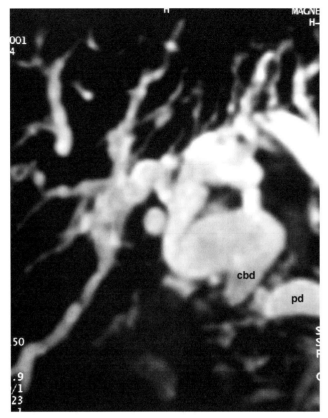

FIGURE 3. Magnetic resonance cholangiopancreatography (MRCP) shows dilatation and abrupt truncation of the distal common bile (cbd) and pancreatic ducts (pd), suggestive of an obstructing pancreatic head mass.

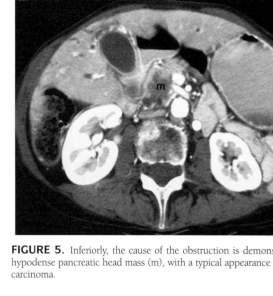

FIGURE 5. Inferiorly, the cause of the obstruction is demonstrated to be a hypodense pancreatic head mass (m), with a typical appearance of a pancreatic carcinoma.

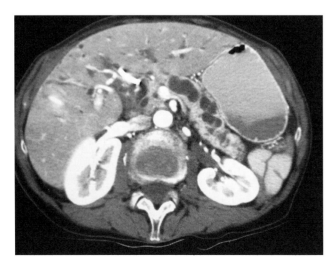

FIGURE 4. Enhanced abdominal CT, obtained after percutaneous biliary drainage, shows a portion of the drainage tube and relief of the intrahepatic biliary dilatation. The extreme pancreatic ductal dilatation is well seen on this section.

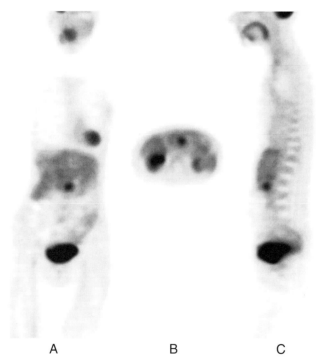

A   B   C

FIGURE 6. PET scan images show localized hyperintensity at the site of the pancreatic mass. No evidence of distant metastatic disease is seen in the liver or elsewhere. Coronal (**A**), transaxial (**B**), and sagittal (**C**) views are shown.

TEACHING POINTS

PET imaging can demonstrate pancreatic carcinomas and may be helpful in selected cases in differentiating between benign and malignant pancreatic masses. However, caution is advised, because there can be increased activity at the site of active pancreatitis. PET's major utility at staging of a suspected pancreatic carcinoma is the noninvasive assessment for metastases, particularly in the liver. Its major limitation in staging is its suboptimal ability to assess nodal involvement separate from activity of the primary tumor. PET has little to offer in the assessment of involvement of adjacent structures, such as vessels.

CASE 9 | *Locally recurrent pancreatic carcinoma*

A 75-year-old woman, 3 months post a Whipple procedure for pancreatic carcinoma, had abdominal pain and an elevated CA 19-9 level (>3000). Margins were not clear at the time of Whipple resection. Outside imaging tests reportedly did not confirm recurrence. PET scan was requested to differentiate between suspected local versus disseminated recurrence. This distinction would influence further treatment decision making. The plan was to treat the patient with irradiation and single-agent chemotherapy for local recurrence, versus an alternative chemotherapeutic regimen for disseminated disease. An intense midabdominal focus of activity, at the pancreatic bed level, confirmed suspected local disease (Figure 1).

TEACHING POINTS

PET scanning in this case enabled confirmation of local recurrence that had eluded conventional imaging modalities. The post-Whipple pancreatic bed can be difficult to evaluate on post-surgical CT scans, and PET provides a noninvasive, complementary approach to the examination of such problems areas.

CASE 10 | *Recurrent pancreatic carcinoma, metastatic to liver and brain*

An 81-year-old woman was referred for PET imaging for suspicion of recurrent pancreatic carcinoma. She had been treated with irradiation and chemotherapy at initial diagnosis, which concluded 2 years before. She had a subsequent negative whole-body PET scan evaluation. Later that year, she developed mental status changes and was found to have intracranial presumed metastatic lesions, one in the left parietal region and another in the right temporal lobe. These were treated with radiation therapy, followed by gamma knife therapy. At the time of referral for PET scanning, the patient's CA19-9 level had risen to 860.

PET imaging showed new hypermetabolic liver lesions, consistent with metastases (Figures 1 and 2). A dedicated brain PET study was also performed, which showed hypermetabolic activity at the posterior margin of the persistent ring-enhancing left parietal lesion seen on CT and MRI (Figures 3 to 5).

TEACHING POINTS

The question of the use of PET in the evaluation of oncology patients for brain metastases arises frequently. Clinicians often assume the brain can be included in a whole-body PET study and is an adequate evaluation for intracranial metastases. In fact, even dedicated brain PET studies are no substitute for enhanced, high-field MRI in the search for intracranial metastases. The high intrinsic metabolic activity of the brain parenchyma and inherent size limitations in lesion detectability on PET are factors operating against PET for diagnosis of brain metastases. High-quality head MRI, obtained with thin sections and contrast media enhancement, can detect tiny lesions, on the order of millimeters, as well as identifying leptomeningeal disease. Such metastases would typically escape detection on dedicated brain PET, much less be identifiable on a head stop included with a whole-body study.

That said, the addition of a dedicated brain PET study to whole-body studies in selected patients with lesions of sufficient size may

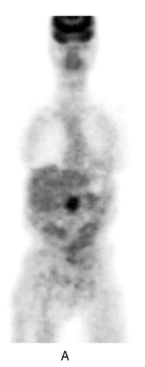

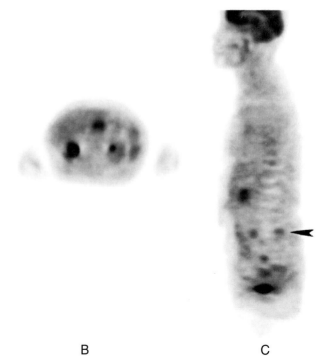

FIGURE 1. PET scan images in coronal (**A**), axial (**B**), and sagittal (**C**) planes show an intense focus of midabdominal activity, in the pancreatic bed, consistent with locally recurrent pancreatic carcinoma. Foci of lower intensity in the pelvis (seen on sagittal section) are normal variant bowel activity. Note also a more posterior focus of activity, at the level of the lumbar spinous processes (*arrowhead*). This probably represents inflammatory, joint-centered arthritic activity between articulating spinous processes or Baastrup's disease.

A   B   C

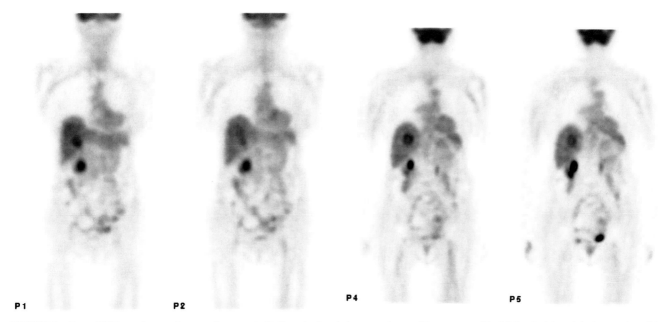

FIGURE 1. Coronal PET scan images show two large metabolically active liver lesions, consistent with metastases. The left hemipelvic activity is a portion of the bladder.

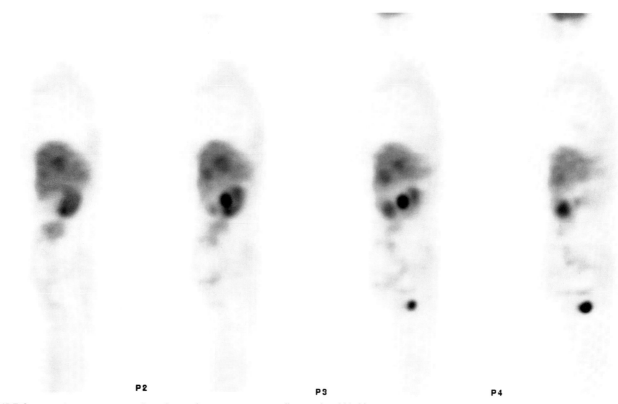

FIGURE 2. Sagittal PET scan images show the two liver metastases, as well as renal and bladder activity.

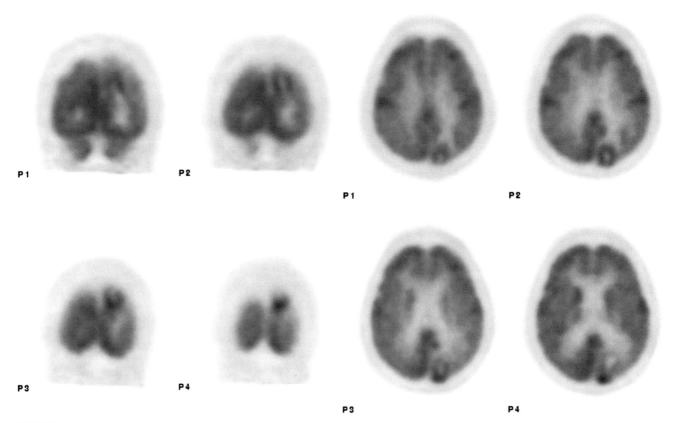

FIGURE 3. Dedicated brain PET images show a metabolically active ring in the left parietal lobe, with focal hyperintensity at the posterior margin of the lesion.

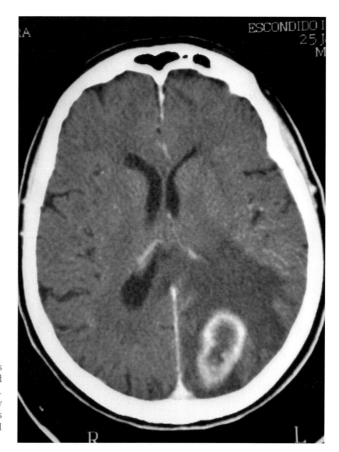

FIGURE 4. Enhanced CT image corresponding to the brain PET images shows a ring-enhancing left parietal treated metastasis. The lesion is associated with a large amount of edema and effaces the atrium of the left lateral ventricle. Most of the enhancing ring is isointense to normal brain parenchymal activity on PET. However, the posterior margin is clearly hypermetabolic and suggests persistent tumor activity. There had been essentially no change on CT and MRI in the appearance of the lesion after radiation and gamma knife therapies.

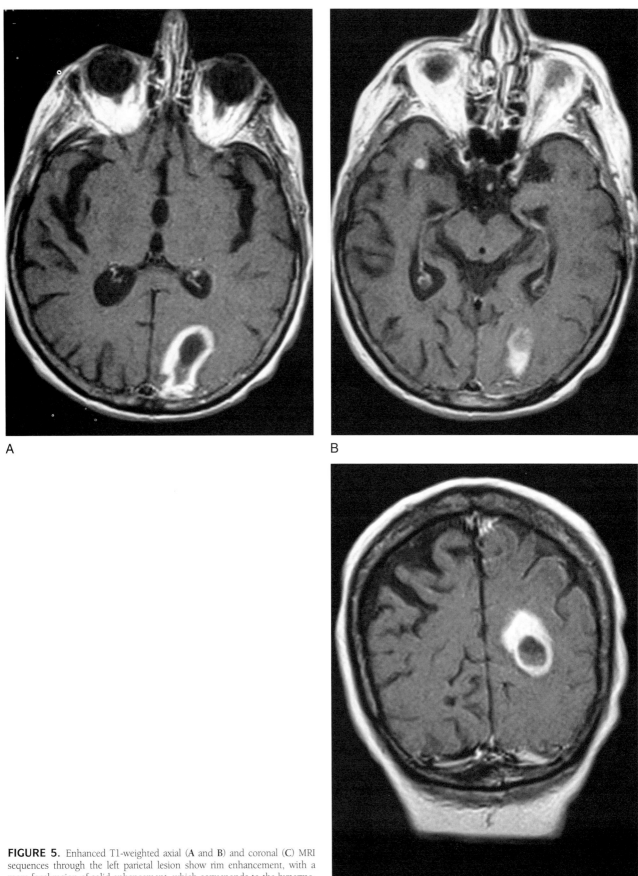

A

B

C

FIGURE 5. Enhanced T1-weighted axial (**A** and **B**) and coronal (**C**) MRI sequences through the left parietal lesion show rim enhancement, with a more focal region of solid enhancement, which corresponds to the hypermetabolism on PET. The tiny second right temporal lesion is too small to be visualized on PET imaging.

provide useful information, such as the tumor activity status of treated lesions. See Case 3 in Chapter 11 and Case 20 in Chapter 10 for additional examples.

CHOLANGIOCARCINOMA

Cholangiocarcinoma is a highly malignant tumor with poor long-term survival. Chronic inflammation of the biliary tract increases the risk for cholangiocarcinoma.[1] MRI, ERCP, and CT may be suboptimal, and therefore interest has been shown in PET.[2-5] Although early results have been encouraging, some caveats are noted: false-positive studies have been reported in benign lesions, false-negative studies occur with mucinous adenocarcinomas, and regional and hepatoduodenal lymph node metastases are frequently missed. In a small number of patients, PET has proven to be very helpful in identifying distant metastases.

REFERENCES

1. Torok N, Gores GJ: Cholangiocarcinoma. Semin Gastrointest Dis 2001; 12:125-132.
2. Fritscher-Ravens A, Bohuslavizki KH, Broering DC, et al: FDG PET in the diagnosis of hilar cholangiocarcinoma. Nucl Med Commun 2001; 22:1277-1285.
3. Kluge R, Schmidt F, Caca K, et al: Positron emission tomography with [(18)] fluoro-2-deoxy-D-glucose for diagnosis and staging of bile duct cancer.
4. Keiding S, Hansen SB, Rasmussen HH, et al: Detection of cholangiocarcinoma in primary sclerosing cholangitis by positron emission tomography. Ugeskr Laeger 2000;162:782-785.
5. Kato T, Tsukamoto E, Shiga T, et al: Preliminary results of whole body FDG PET in biliary carcinoma. J Nucl Med 2000;298P.

CASE 11 | *Ampullary adenocarcinoma, with local nodal involvement*

A 74-year-old man presented with painless jaundice. CT evaluation showed intrahepatic and extrahepatic biliary ductal dilatation, with thickening at the ampulla level, suggesting an ampullary carcinoma. Mildly enlarged periceliac and retroperitoneal lymph nodes were noted (Figures 1 to 4). ERCP confirmed an ampullary lesion and bile duct

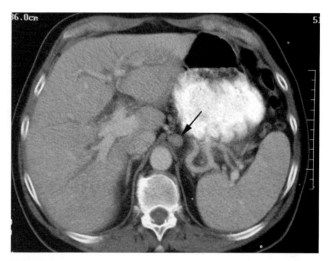

FIGURE 2. A more inferior section shows an enlarged periceliac lymph node (*arrow*).

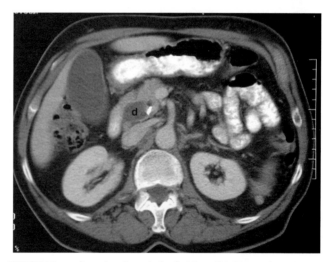

FIGURE 3. Farther inferiorly, at the level of the gallbladder, marked dilatation of the common bile duct (d) is seen in the head of the pancreas. A focus of calcification is seen in the pancreas adjacent to the duct. Evidence of pancreatitis was found at pathology.

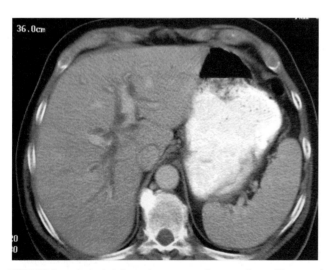

FIGURE 1. Enhanced abdominal CT section shows moderate dilatation of intrahepatic bile ducts.

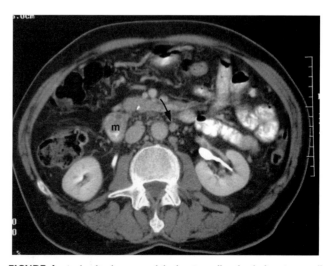

FIGURE 4. At the distal common bile duct/ampullary level, there is a small soft tissue density, inhomogeneous mass (m). A mildly prominent left para-aortic lymph node is noted (*arrow*).

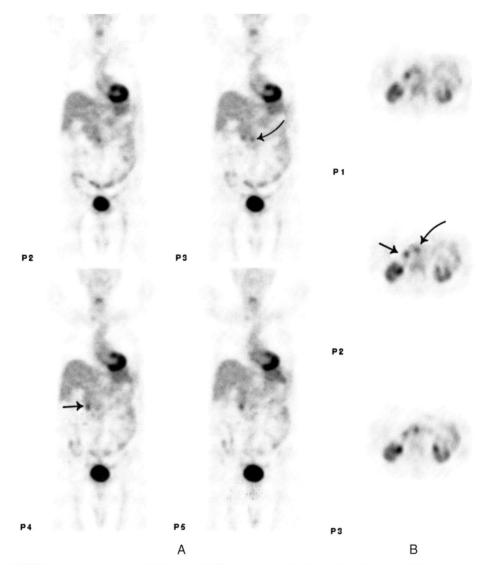

FIGURE 5. PET scans (coronal [A] and axial [B]) show two, small, discrete foci of hypermetabolic activity in the region. The larger and more intense focus (*to the right*) appears to correlate with the ampullary tumor mass itself (*straight arrow*), whereas the other focus (*curved arrow*) suggests local nodal involvement, as was confirmed pathologically.

narrowing. Brushings confirmed poorly differentiated adenocarcinoma, and the patient was stented. PET scan showed two small foci of increased metabolic activity in the region (Figure 5). The patient was treated with a Whipple procedure, with pathology reported as a 1-cm poorly differentiated, diffusely infiltrating adenocarcinoma, arising from the common duct/ampulla, with extensive angiolymphatic tumor involvement. Nine of 12 periampullary and peripancreatic lymph nodes showed metastatic carcinoma. Six perigastric lymph nodes were negative. Because of the high risk of local recurrence, the patient was treated with weekly carboplatin and gemcitabine (Gemzar) but soon showed progression, dying 9 months after diagnosis.

TEACHING POINTS

Based on imaging, this patient was suspected to have locally advanced disease and to have a poor prognosis. PET served to confirm the impression of local nodal involvement.

CASE 12 | *Cholangiocarcinoma, with liver metastasis*

A 78-year-old man developed fatigue, pruritus, and painless jaundice. Abdominal CT showed intrahepatic and extrahepatic biliary ductal dilatation, secondary to a subtle lobulated mass at the level of the pancreas (Figures 1 to 4). ERCP was performed, as well as MRI (Figure 5), revealing cholangiocarcinoma, and a temporary stent was placed. The patient was being simulated for palliative radiotherapy when he developed stent obstruction and cholangitis. PET scanning was requested to better assess the extent of disease. This showed a hypermetabolic midabdominal focus, corresponding to the primary lesion (Figure 6). An additional metabolically active focus was seen in the right lobe of the liver, suggesting a liver metastasis. MRI of the liver was obtained for confirmation, which showed a corresponding 2-cm lesion (Figure 7). Accordingly, plans for radiation therapy were abandoned, and the

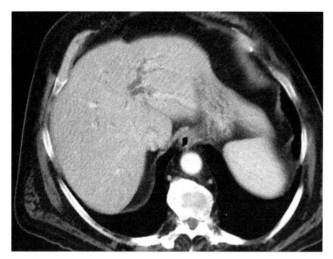

FIGURE 1. Enhanced abdominal CT shows intrahepatic biliary ductal dilatation.

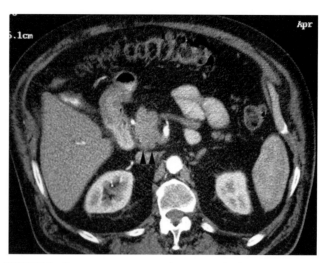

FIGURE 4. Thin section, pancreatic technique image at the same level shows similar findings. Posterior pancreatic head margin shows subtle posterior bulging.

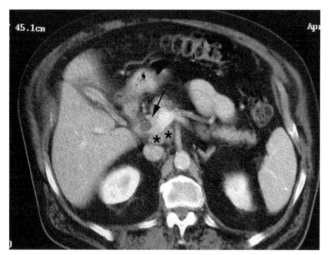

FIGURE 2. A more inferior section shows the common bile duct to be dilated (*arrow*). Two enlarged portocaval lymph nodes are noted posterior to the pancreatic head (*asterisks*).

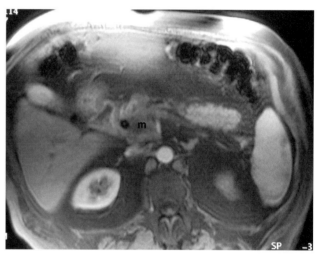

FIGURE 5. Fat-saturated, enhanced T1-weighted axial breathhold image shows an uncinate process level mass (m). The CBD is delimited by the hypointense stent.

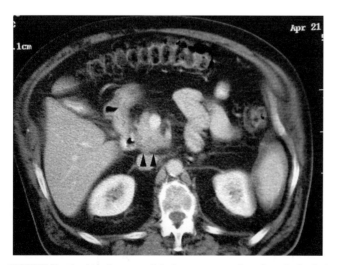

FIGURE 3. The dilated common bile duct terminates abruptly at the level of subtle hypodensity and bulging posterior contour of the uncinate process of the pancreas (*arrowheads*).

patient was started on a trial of gemcitabine (Gemzar) chemotherapy. He died 7 months after diagnosis.

TEACHING POINTS

This patient was not an operative candidate, owing to coexisting medical conditions. The planned palliative therapy was modified when it became apparent he had liver metastatic disease, not evident on CT and first identified by PET imaging.

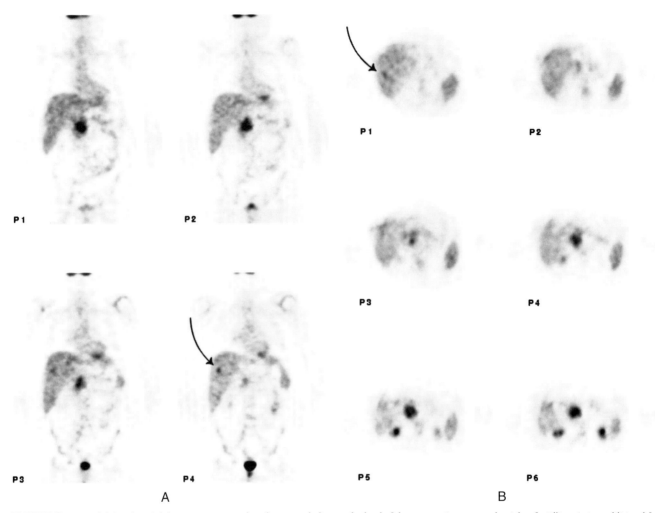

FIGURE 6. Coronal (**A**) and axial (**B**) PET scan images show hypermetabolism at the level of the pancreatic mass, to the right of midline. A tiny, additional focus of increased activity is seen in the right lobe of the liver, suggesting a liver metastasis (*arrow*).

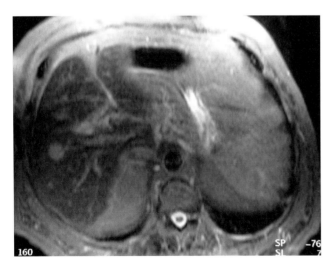

FIGURE 7. Short tau inversion recovery (STIR) axial image through the right lobe of the liver shows a small mass, corresponding to the abnormal PET scan finding and consistent with a liver metastasis.

CASE 13 | Recurrent cholangiocarcinoma, drop metastasis

A 34-year-old man with a past history of cystic duct cholangiocarcinoma developed postprandial abdominal pain and weight loss. His cholangiocarcinoma was unexpectedly diagnosed on a laparoscopic cholecystectomy specimen 3 years previous. He underwent a second surgical procedure at that time after a negative metastatic work-up, including common bile duct resection, lymph node dissection, and hepaticojejunostomy, followed by irradiation and chemotherapy.

When the patient developed new symptoms of abdominal pain and weight loss, he was thoroughly evaluated with a battery of imaging tests, including abdomen and pelvis CT, upper gastrointestinal studies, esophagogastroduodenoscopy, and magnetic resonance cholangiopancreatography (MRCP), all essentially negative. Colonoscopy showed a near obstructing mass effect, but biopsies showed only adenomatous changes without malignancy. The colonoscopic findings prompted repeat pelvic CT evaluation, which showed a large mass in the cul-de-sac, extrinsically compressing the colon, new from the prior CT examination 3 months earlier (Figure 1). The mass was scinitigraphically

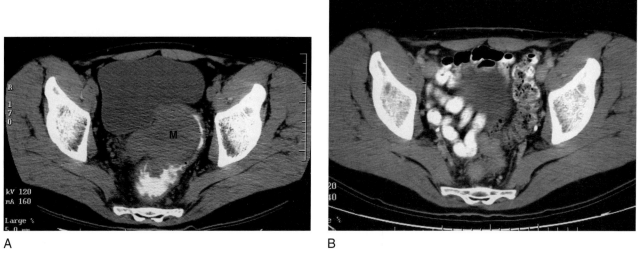

A

B

FIGURE 1. Pelvis CT (**A**), with rectal contrast only, shows a large soft tissue density mass (M) in the cul-de-sac, narrowing the lumen of the rectosigmoid colon. Epicenter of the mass appears extrinsic to the colon or in the wall of bowel, but at least a portion extends intraluminally. The mass represented a dramatic change from a normal enhanced CT at the same level 3 months before (**B**).

active on PET (Figure 2). The location of the lesion represented a drop metastasis. CT-guided biopsy revealed large cell carcinoma, not otherwise classified. The patient underwent operative rebiopsy, revealing undifferentiated carcinoma. The patient's subsequent course was complicated by development of gastrointestinal bleeding, apparently caused by continued erosion of the mass into the colon.

TEACHING POINTS

This mass was initially overlooked on PET imaging and represents a location pitfall where activity may be mistakenly ascribed to normal variant rectal or pelvic bowel activity. In this case, the reader was probably also misled by the normal CT from 2 months before, which was available for correlation. Occasionally, normal variant rectal or bowel

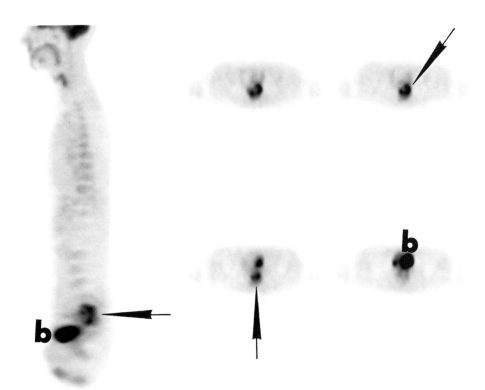

FIGURE 2. PET shows focally hyperintense pelvic activity at the same level, above and behind the urinary bladder (b, *arrows*).

activity is disturbingly focal, but it usually still retains its tubular, ser-piginous configuration. Activity within the abdomen or pelvis that differs significantly from the overall level of bowel activity in intensity, configuration, or focality should be carefully scrutinized as potentially pathologic.

CASE 14 | *Suspected residual gallbladder carcinoma*

A 52-year-old woman was diagnosed with gallbladder carcinoma after laparoscopic cholecystectomy. Her past medical history was significant for a high-risk left breast cancer diagnosed 2 years previously, with 21 involved lymph nodes. The patient was treated with mastectomy, chemotherapy, and chest wall irradiation. When she reported abdominal wall numbness to her oncologist, she was sent for CT, which showed a gallbladder mass (Figure 1). The gallbladder was surrounded by a hyperdense rim, raising a differential of extension of the mass into the liver, versus sparing in a fatty liver. Ultrasonography also identified a soft tissue mass within the gallbladder (Figure 2). Ultrasound-guided biopsy

of the mass showed atypical glandular epithelium, thought most likely to be reactive and related to chronic cholecystitis. No immuno-histochemical evidence to support a diagnosis of metastatic breast cancer was identified. A laparoscopic cholecystectomy was performed. Gallstone erosion into the liver was noted at surgery. Pathology demonstrated a 3 × 3.5-cm well-differentiated adenocarcinoma arising in an adenoma, with tumor extending into but not through the muscle layer.

PET scanning was performed 2 weeks after surgery and showed activity in the gallbladder fossa, suggestive of residual tumor in the surgical bed (Figure 3). Biopsy of the gallbladder fossa was performed and showed no evidence of malignancy. Fatty metamorphosis of the liver was noted. The patient was treated with systemic chemotherapy for cholangiocarcinoma. Follow-up CT, 2 months later, showed new ascites and omental stippling, suggesting carcinomatosis. These findings had progressed to omental cake on another CT 4 months later.

TEACHING POINTS

Activity is not normally seen in or around the gallbladder, although metabolically active processes, including cholecystitis or gallbladder

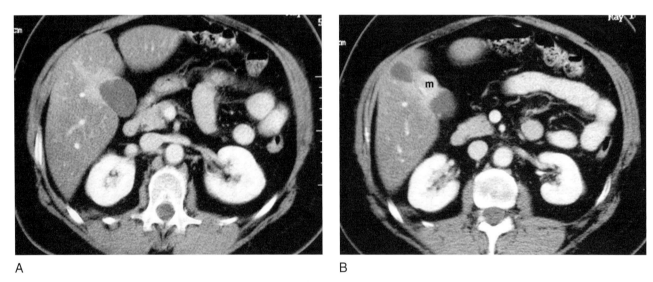

A   B

FIGURE 1. Contrast medium–enhanced abdominal CT images (**A** and **B**) through the gallbladder show diffuse fatty change of the liver, except for a higher density rim surrounding the gallbladder. Within the gallbladder, an enhancing mass (m) is seen, associated with localized gallbladder wall thickening.

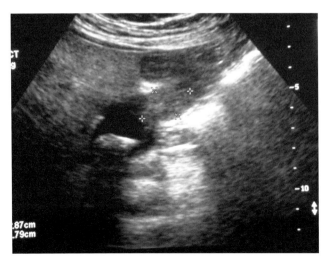

FIGURE 2. Ultrasound image shows a hyperechoic fatty liver and gallstones. Calipers outline an intraluminal mass.

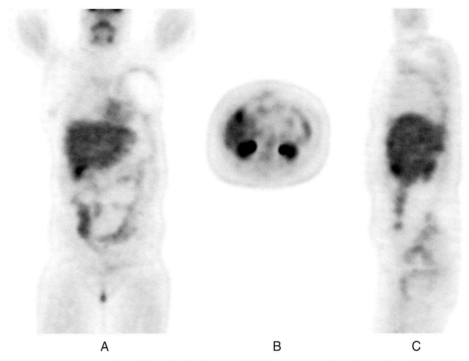

A   B   C

FIGURE 3. PET scan, performed 2 weeks after laparoscopic cholecystectomy, shows increased metabolic activity in the gallbladder fossa, suggestive of residual tumor in the surgical bed. Coronal (**A**), transaxial (**B**), and sagittal (**C**) views are shown.

carcinoma, could produce gallbladder fossa activity. Significance of the gallbladder fossa activity in this case, obtained only 2 weeks after laparoscopic cholecystectomy, was uncertain. It was regarded as suggestive of persistent tumor activity, but the recent surgery certainly complicates the assessment. The duration of FDG uptake can be variable in the post-surgical setting depending on the nature and extent of the surgery and the subsequent postoperative inflammatory response. The subsequent development of omental cake and peritoneal carcinomatosis suggests the gallbladder fossa activity noted in this case probably was pathologic and not just postoperative.

Head and Neck Cancer

Approximately 5% of all malignancies are head and neck tumors. Squamous cell cancers (SCCs) account for 90% of these. Major risk factors are prolonged tobacco and alcohol abuse, and there is a possible environmental association with viruses.[1] A major prognostic factor is the presence of lymph node metastasis, necessitating an accurate assessment of nodal spread. Currently, most physicians use the TNM system for staging head and neck tumors. T corresponds to the primary site, N refers to regional lymphatic metastases, and M to distant metastases. At the time of initial diagnosis, 10% of patients have distant metastases whereas 50% have locally advanced disease. This contributes to reduced long-term survival, and the reliable identification of these patients may have significant prognostic as well as therapeutic implications.[2]

Initial evaluation is traditionally performed with physical examination, endoscopy, biopsy, and anatomic imaging modalities such as CT, MR, and ultrasonography. Although PET has been shown to be extremely accurate in identifying the primary tumor site, it offers no real advantage over standard imaging and physical examination for T evaluation. In selected cases, FDG-PET may help determine the site or extent of the primary lesion. PET has a much more important role to play in staging N and M disease, detecting recurrence, and perhaps assessing response to therapy.

STAGING LYMPH NODE STATUS

In a large series, it was shown that the 5-year actuarial survival of 455 patients with head and neck carcinomas was 65% for patients without cervical metastasis but only 29% for patients with cervical metastasis.[3] Combining multiple studies reveals a sensitivity and specificity for PET detection of 87% and 89%, respectively. Sensitivity and specificity for CT in the same patients were 62% and 73%.[4] Importantly, for diagnosis/staging, an estimated 33% change was noted in management. The overwhelming majority of reported studies have confined their search to the head and neck region; however, it can be predicted that a whole-body survey with PET will more accurately stage the 10% of patients with distant metastases. There are

even data that demonstrate added value of PET in the N0 patient (determined by physical examination and anatomic imaging).[5] PET is not advocated as a replacement for the traditional initial staging evaluation, but strong consideration should be given to its utilization as a complementary study in this patient population. The very high recurrence rate, inherent problems with CT and MR for restaging, and the potential for tumor as well as treatment-related morbidity are reasons to recommend the use of PET.

RECURRENCE

The mainstays of treatment for SCC of the head and neck are surgery and radiation therapy. Recently, chemotherapy has shown some benefit. Both surgery and irradiation can produce edema, scarring, and anatomic distortions that may interfere with the detection of persistent/recurrent disease. The specificity of CT and MR are significantly reduced in the post-treatment setting. PET, which relies on changes in tumor cell metabolic activity rather than structural changes, is much less affected. Summary data on 511 patients showed a statistically significant advantage for PET over CT with respect to specificity (83% versus 74%) and an even greater discrepancy for sensitivity (PET = 93%, CT = 54%).[4] In spite of the evidence pointing to the diagnostic superiority of PET for restaging, caution is advised in the patient who has recently completed radiation therapy. Recommendations in the literature range from waiting 2 months to 6 months or more before performing PET after a course of radiation therapy. Radiation induces inflammatory effects that may lead to increased glucose metabolism by leukocytes. This may result in false-positive PET studies. Guidelines are evolving, but many take the conservative approach of delaying PET for 6 months if possible.

RESPONSE TO THERAPY

There is relatively little in the literature assessing the accuracy of PET in monitoring response to therapy. Although the data that do exist are encouraging for both radiation and chemotherapy, larger studies are needed. One study of 28 patients, using tissue biopsies as the gold standard, found a PET sensitivity of 90% and specificity of 83% (see tabulated data in reference 11). Conversely, there is some suggestion that absent FDG uptake 1 month after radiation therapy may not exclude viable tumor and could result in false-negative studies. This is perhaps another good reason to delay imaging after radiation therapy.[2,6,7]

PET scan interpretation for head and neck tumors is subject to some debate concerning the use of standardized uptake values (SUVs) versus visual, qualitative assessment. A number of authors have identified an SUV cutoff value that maximizes sensitivity and specificity. Unfortunately, these values range from 3 to 7+. Reproducibility from center to center is dependent on many factors, including parameters used (e.g., body weight vs. body surface area, mean SUV vs. maximum SUV, length of uptake phase, serum glucose level/state of fasting, and lesion size [see Chapter 1]). Although in theory, reproducible SUVs should facilitate diagnosis (and possibly therapy response assessment), most centers rely on visual assessment. Because of the cost of PET, some authors point to the use of other, less expensive radionuclides as an adjunct to CT and MRI. The two primary ones are thallium and technetium-99m-sestamibi. Both are nonspecific tumor-avid agents that do show a relatively high sensitivity (lower specificity) for head and neck cancer. They are hampered by their normal distribution and size threshold for lesion detectability (about 2 cm).

Lastly, there are three scenarios in which PET may prove to be of value in head and neck cancer. The first is in the patient with an unknown primary tumor. This patient typically is found to have SCC in a neck node biopsy, and all standard tests prove negative. Before "shotgun" therapy, it is reasonable to perform whole-body PET.[8,9] Although the yield is less than 50%, a positive study can result in more specific, possibly less morbid treatment. The second area is the identification of a second primary lesion, either synchronous or metachronous, which is not uncommon in patients with head and neck malignancies. The third area is the assessment of the patient post therapy. Preliminary studies have shown PET to be useful in evaluating the effects of both chemotherapy and radiotherapy.[10-13]

In studying the cases in this chapter, it may be beneficial to review the preliminary material on normal FDG distribution in the head and neck presented in this chapter as Case 1.

REFERENCES

1. Lowe VJ, Stack BC: PET's role in head and neck cancer. In Freeman LM (ed): Nuclear Medicine Annual, Philadelphia, Lippincott Williams & Wilkins, 2001, pp 1-22.
2. Hubner KF, Thie JA, Smith GT, et al: Clinical utility of FDG-PET in detecting head and neck tumors: A comparison of diagnostic methods and modalities. Clin Pos Imag 2000;3:7-16.
3. Grandi C, Alloisio M, Moglia D: Prognostic significance of lymphatic spread in head and neck carcinomas: Therapeutic implications. Head Neck Surg 1985;8:67-73.
4. Gambhir SS, Czernin J, Schwimmer J, et al: A tabulated summary of the FDG PET literature. J Nucl Med 2001;42:21S-25S.
5. Myers L, Wax MK, Nabi H, et al: Positron emission tomography in the evaluation of the N₀ neck. Laryngoscope 1998;108:232-236.
6. Peng N-J, Yen S-H, Liu W-S, et al: Evaluation of the effect of radiation therapy to nasopharyngeal carcinoma by positron emission tomography with 2-[F-18] fluoro-2-deoxy-D-glucose. Clin Pos Imag 2000;3:51-56.
7. Kas C-H, ChangLai S-P, Chieng P-U, et al: Detection of recurrent or persistent nasopharyngeal carcinomas after radiotherapy with 18-fluoro-2-deoxyglucose positron emission tomography and comparison with computed tomography. J Clin Oncol 1998;16:3550-3555.
8. Laubenbacher C, Saumweber D, Wagner-Manslau C, et al: Comparison of fluorine-18-fluorodeoxyglucose PET, MRI, and endoscopy for staging head and neck squamous-cell carcinomas. J Nucl Med 1995;36:1747-1757.
9. Regelink G, Brouiver J, de Bree R, et al: Detection of unknown primary tumors and distant metastases in patients with cervical metastases: Value of FDG-PET versus conventional modalities. Eur J Nucl Med 2002;29:1024-1030.
10. Kitagawa Y, Sadato N, Azuma H, et al: FDG-PET to evaluate combined intra-arterial chemotherapy and radiotherapy of head and neck neoplasms. J Nucl Med 1999;40:1132-1137.
11. Lowe VJ, Dunphy FR, Varvares M, et al: Evaluation of chemotherapy response in patients with advanced head and neck cancer using [F-18] fluorodeoxyglucose positron emission tomography. Head Neck 1997;19:666-674.
12. Lowe VJ, Boyd JH, Dunphy FR, et al: Surveillance for recurrent head and neck cancer using positron emission tomography. J Clin Oncol 2000;18:651-658.
13. Cheon GJ, Chung J-K So Y, et al: Diagnostic accuracy of F-18 FDG-PET in the assessment of post therapeutic recurrence of head and neck cancer. Clin Pos Imag 1999;2:197-204.

CASE 1 | *Normal head and neck anatomy example*

Normally on PET imaging of the neck there is a variable amount of physiologic activity (Figure 1).

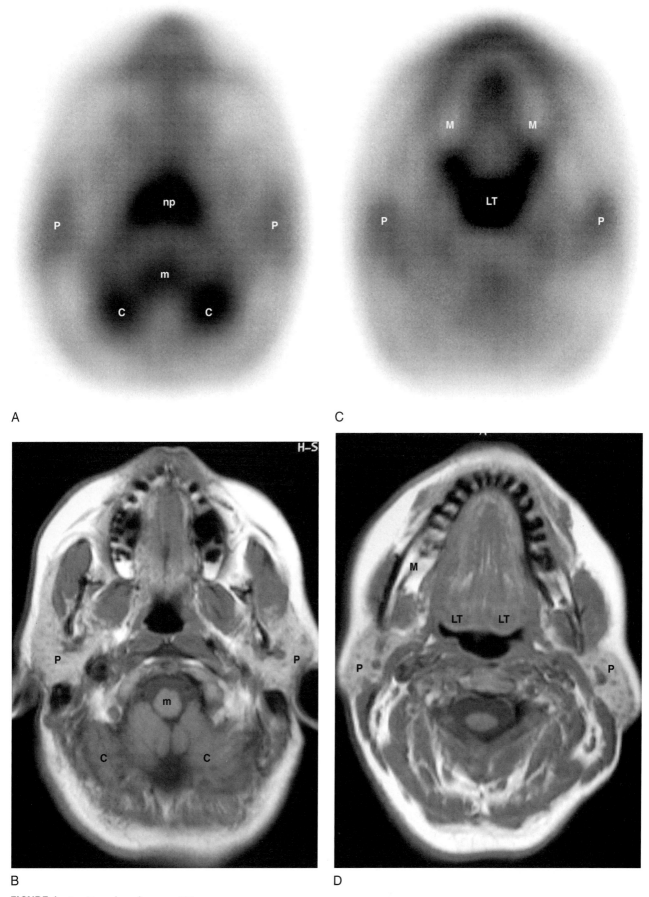

A

C

B

D

FIGURE 1. **A** to **D**, see legend on page 253.

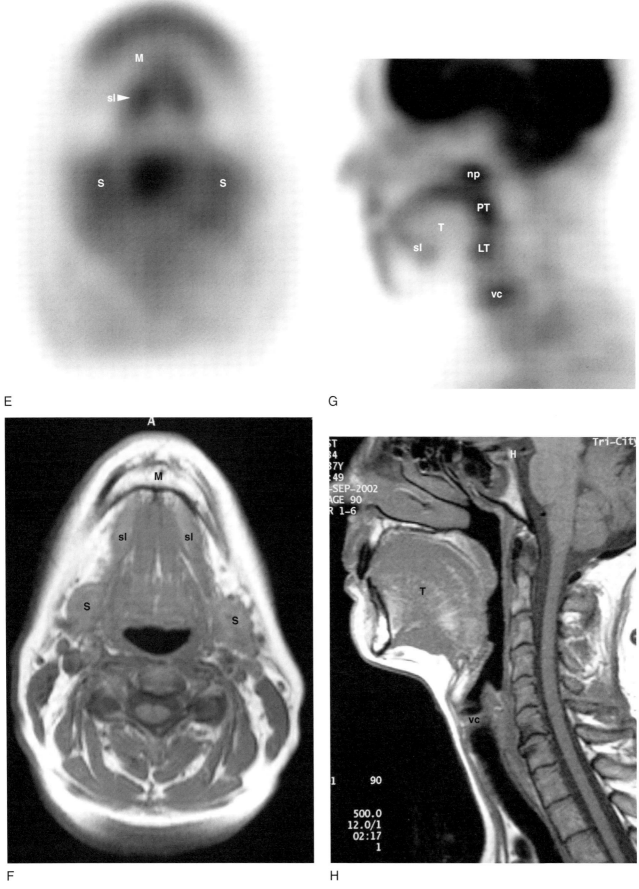

FIGURE 1. cont'd E to H, see legend on opposite page.

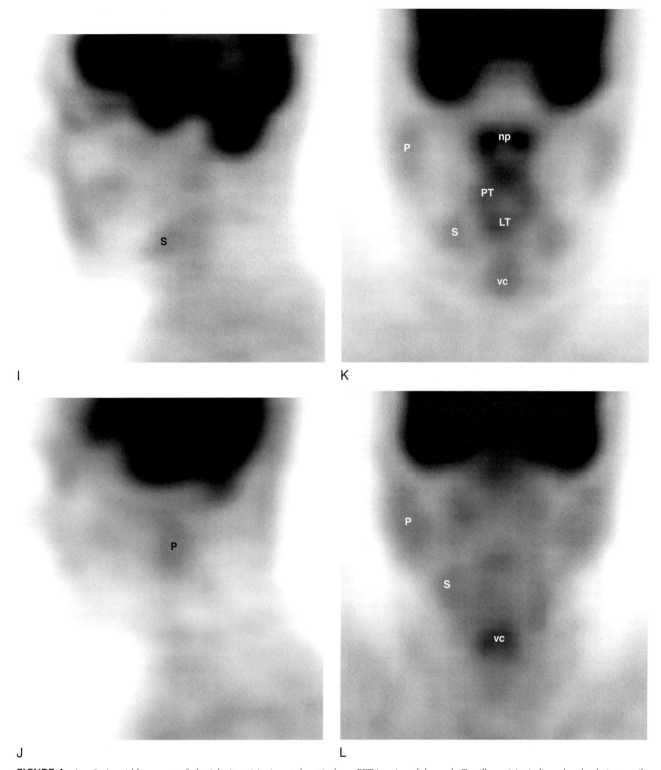

FIGURE 1. A to L, A variable amount of physiologic activity is noted routinely on PET imaging of the neck. Tonsillar activity in lingual and palatine tonsils is frequently seen. Nasopharyngeal tonsillar activity is seen less often but is illustrated in this normal example. Salivary gland activity is usually modest and symmetrical but can vary considerably. Vocal cord activity results from patient speech during the uptake period. C, cerebellar hemisphere; M, mandible; m, medulla; P, parotid gland; np, nasopharyngeal tonsillar tissue; PT, palatine tonsil; sl, sublingual gland; LT, lingual tonsil; vc, vocal cords; S, submandibular gland; T, tongue.

CASE 2 | *Glottic squamous cell carcinoma, initial diagnosis*

A 66-year-old man was evaluated with MRI and PET for suspicion of occult head and neck carcinoma. He had been hoarse for over 4 years, when he developed a persistent sore throat. Laryngoscopic examination showed swelling and mucosal fullness of the right false cord, obscuring a paralyzed right vocal cord. Operative panendoscopy was performed. Superficial and deep biopsies of the right false cord showed only chronic inflammation. Enhanced MRI of the neck soft tissues was obtained, seeking an occult malignancy (Figures 1 to 4). MRI showed the vocal cord paralysis by the abnormal paramedian position of the right arytenoid cartilage and showed evidence of destruction of the cartilage by a 1.5-cm submucosal mass. Thickening and edema were noted of the overlying strap muscles (Figure 8). PET scan was also obtained and showed asymmetrical, mass-like hypermetabolic activity

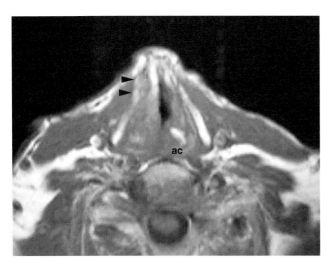

FIGURE 1. T1-weighted axial MR section at the level of the thyroid cartilage shows right vocal cord paralysis. The right vocal cord is fixed in a paramedian position. (Note normal position of left vocal cord and normal fatty marrow signal of the left arytenoid cartilage [ac]). The right arytenoid cartilage normal fatty marrow signal is lost, and the cartilage is not discretely identifiable. Note also loss of normal fatty marrow signal and soft tissue expansion in the anterior portion of the right thyroid cartilage, in contrast to the normal appearance on the left (*arrowheads*).

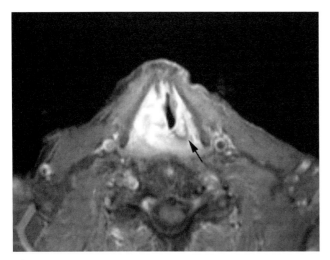

FIGURE 2. Enhanced, fat-saturated T1-weighted axial MR section at the same level shows the swelling and enhancement of the edematous right false vocal cord. The right arytenoid cartilage is not identified. The left arytenoid cartilage (*arrow*) is delineated by the hypointense bone cortex.

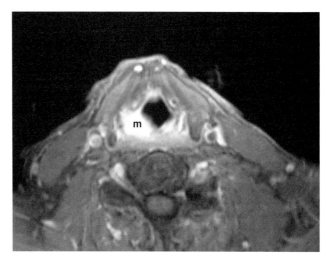

FIGURE 3. At a level just below Figure 2, an enhancing mass (m) is seen on the right at the glottic level.

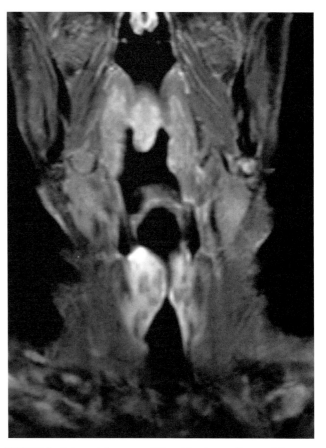

FIGURE 4. Enhanced, fat-saturated T1-weighted coronal image of the airway shows the asymmetry and mass of the right glottis.

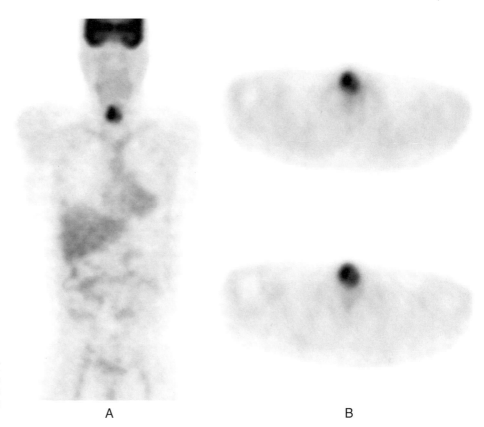

FIGURE 5. Coronal (**A**) and axial (**B**) PET images show intense vocal cord activity. The activity is asymmetrical and mass-like on the right. Left-sided activity is within the range seen with normal phonation.

A   B

of the right vocal cord, corresponding to the MRI findings (Figure 5). No evidence of nodal or distant metastatic disease was seen by PET imaging.

Based on these findings, an operative microlaryngoscopy with biopsies and laser excision of the false cord was performed. Well-differentiated SCC was confirmed from biopsy material of the right false and true cords and ventricle.

Once the diagnosis was established, treatment options were considered for this patient. Because of the strap muscle thickening and question of laryngeal cartilage destruction on MRI, CT was also

obtained in an effort to better address this question. Irregularity of thyroid cartilage mineralization in the area in question suggested probable involvement (Figures 6 and 7). Therapy with laryngectomy and post-operative irradiation was elected. The patient underwent wide field laryngectomy and right thyroid lobectomy. The pathology report showed a 2 × 1-cm right transglottic well-differentiated infiltrating SCC invading underlying cartilage, skeletal muscle, and soft tissue. Although the left vocal cords appeared grossly uninvolved with tumor, invasive SCC was identified in the skeletal muscle of the left true cord.

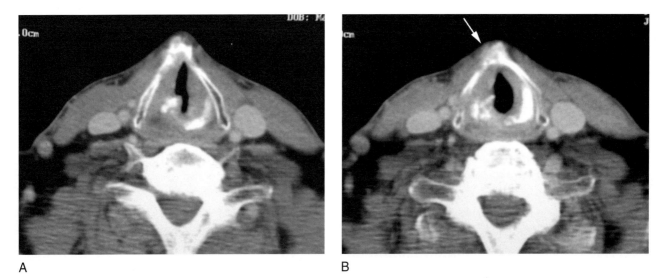

A   B

FIGURE 6. Contrast medium–enhanced soft tissue neck CT sections show disturbed mineralization of the right paramedian anterior thyroid cartilage, with an associated soft tissue mass suggested, extending into subcutaneous fat (arrow). Right arytenoid cartilage is in abnormal paramedian position, indicating vocal cord paralysis.

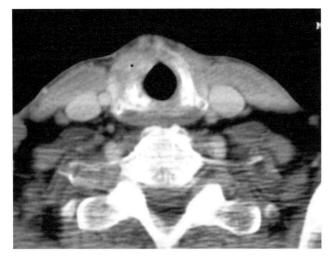

FIGURE 7. Asymmetrical thickening, suggesting infiltration, is noted of right-sided strap muscles, with extension into subcutaneous fat again suggested (*asterisk*).

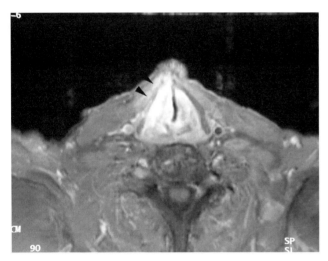

FIGURE 8. Additional enhanced, fat-saturated T1-weighted MR sections show abnormally increased signal of right anterior thyroid cartilage and thickening and abnormal enhancement of adjacent right strap muscles (*arrowheads*). Findings suggest cartilage and strap muscle invasion by tumor.

TEACHING POINTS

Direct inspection was hampered in this patient by the false vocal cord edema, and biopsy yielded only inflammation. Imaging evaluation with MRI and PET was pursued because of high clinical suspicion, and both studies indicated the right glottis to be suggestive of a primary carcinoma site. On PET, the glottic level activity was asymmetrical and mass-like on the right but activity on the left cannot be differentiated from normal vocal cord activity owing to phonation. In these evaluations, an effort is made to minimize the patient's talking during the uptake period, but a chronically hoarse patient may display vocal cord activity from inflammation despite these efforts. When important treatment decisions hinge on involvement of the laryngeal cartilages and strap muscles, anatomic modalities will have to be relied on. PET's primary utility, in addition to identification of primary sites, is in the detection of nodal and distant metastases.

Initial staging, base of tongue squamous cell carcinoma, with nodal metastasis at presentation

A 47-year-old previously healthy man presented with a left upper neck mass. Fine-needle aspiration showed no malignancy. On CT, the mass appeared cystic, suggesting a necrotic lymph node. Left-sided asymmetry was noted at the base of the tongue (Figure 1). Laryngoscopy with biopsy of the base of tongue showed SCC. The stage of the patient's disease based on these evaluations was T3N2M0. PET scan confirmed this, showing intense left base of tongue activity at the primary site, with lesser activity at the left neck level (Figure 2). The patient was treated with chemotherapy combined with irradiation, with an excellent response. Follow-up PET and CT scans, 10 months after the staging study and 6 months after completing chemoradiation, showed no evidence of disease (Figures 3 and 4).

TEACHING POINTS

The patient's disease stage, based on physical and laryngoscopic examinations, biopsy, and CT, was confirmed by PET. The whole-body capability of PET further establishes that disease is confined just to the head and neck. It also complements CT in follow-up of the patient after therapy.

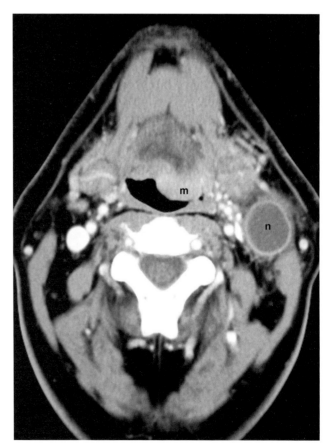

FIGURE 1. Enhanced soft tissue neck CT shows asymmetrical mass and soft tissue at the left base of tongue level, suggesting a primary site (m). This was confirmed by laryngoscopic biopsy. The palpable lump in the left neck with which the patient presented is cystic, suggesting a necrotic lymph node (n).

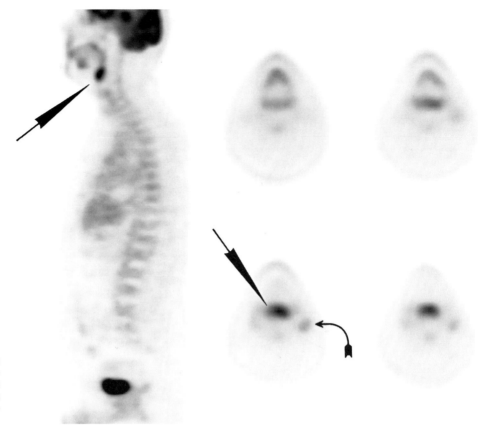

FIGURE 2. Focal, intense activity is seen at the left base of tongue level, corresponding to fullness on CT (*straight arrows*). Less intense activity is noted at the site of the lymph node, presumably due to the extensive necrosis (*curved arrow*).

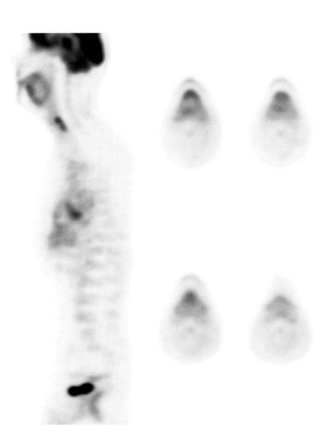

FIGURE 3. Above findings have resolved on follow-up PET, 10 months later and 6 months after completion of chemoradiation. Lower midline cervical activity is vocal cord.

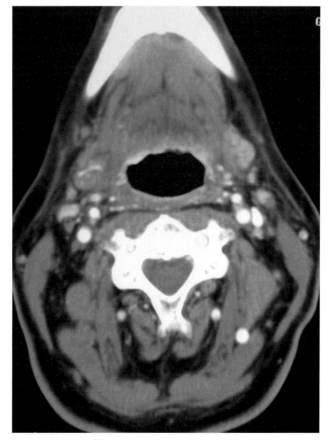

FIGURE 4. Corresponding neck CT also shows resolution of the presenting findings after therapy.

CASE 4 | *Locally advanced base of tongue squamous cell carcinoma, with bilateral necrotic lymph node metastases*

A 58-year-old man presented with hemoptysis, which was thought to be secondary to bronchitis and treated initially with antibiotics.

Subsequently, he developed a sore throat and left neck adenopathy was noted on physical examination. A CT scan showed a 4-cm left base of tongue mass, accompanied by necrotic 4-cm left internal jugular level II-III and 2-cm right internal jugular level III lymph nodes (Figure 1). Laryngoscopy confirmed a large base of tongue mass, and fine-needle aspiration was performed of the left neck node. SCC was diagnosed pathologically. PET imaging was obtained to complete his staging and confirmed the impression of stage IV, T3N2M0 disease (Figures 2 and 3). He underwent intra-arterial cisplatin (Platinol) chemotherapy,

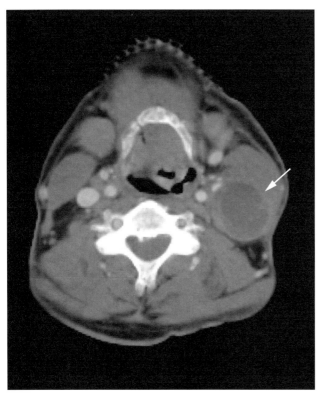

A

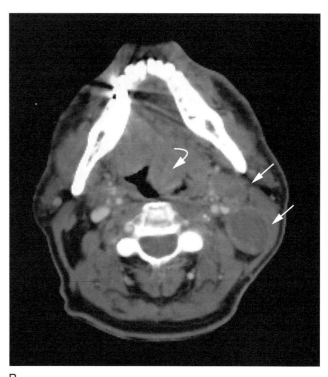

B

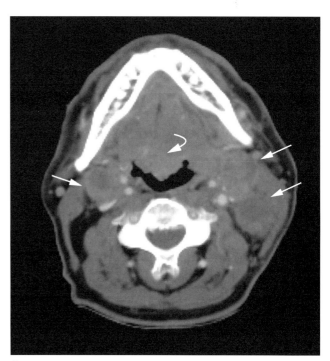

C

FIGURE 1. Enhanced soft tissue neck CT shows a bulky, posteriorly exophytic left base of tongue mass, extending to the midline (*curved arrows,* **B** and **C**). Bilateral necrotic internal jugular chain metastatic lymph nodes are noted, left greater than right (*straight arrows,* **A** to **C**).

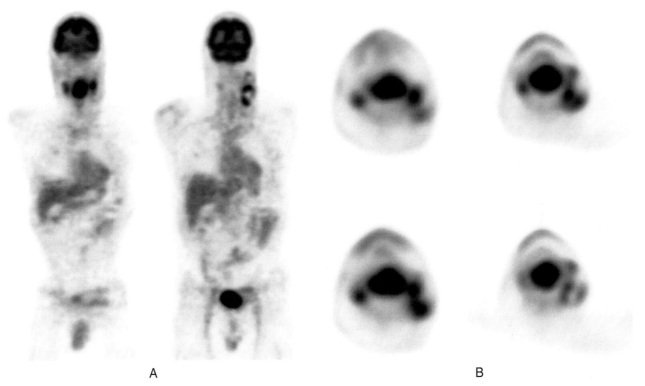

A   B

FIGURE 2. Coronal (**A**) and axial (**B**) PET images show the large base of tongue primary to be intensely hypermetabolic and to extend over the midline. Hypermetabolism is also evident of the metastatic bilateral neck nodes. Central necrosis can be appreciated in left neck lymph nodes. No distant metastases were seen in the lungs or elsewhere.

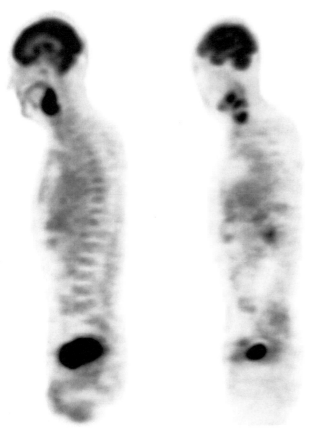

FIGURE 3. Sagittal PET images through the midline and to the left showing the intensely hypermetabolic base of tongue SCC and multiple left neck metastatic nodes.

with simultaneous radiotherapy, with near complete resolution of his bulky base of tongue primary tumor and incomplete, but marked regression of the adenopathy (no palpable residual on the right, but clinical suspicion of persistent left neck disease). Operative endoscopy and therapeutic left neck dissection were then undertaken. The left base of tongue was noted to be firm and fibrotic, but no lesions were visualized. Biopsies were negative for tumor. Left modified neck dissection removed a total of 36 lymph nodes, all negative for malignancy.

CASE 5 | *Metastatic squamous cell carcinoma, cervical lymph node presentation, primary lesion search*

A 63-year-old man presented with a painless right neck lump. After an antibiotic trial without improvement, he was referred for ENT evaluation. A CT scan of the neck showed a necrotic 2.3 cm right internal jugular lymph node (Figures 1 and 2). This was excised and proved to be metastatic SCC. Endoscopic evaluations on two occasions showed an abnormal right base of tongue, but biopsies were unremarkable. PET imaging was requested to search for a head and neck primary lesion. It identified abnormal activity at the right base of tongue region (Figure 3). This was re-sampled and proven to be tumor.

The patient was treated with chemotherapy and irradiation, and 1 month later he was reevaluated with a repeat PET, which showed dramatic improvement. Further PET follow-up after 3 additional months

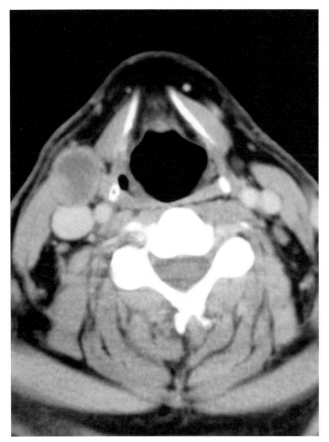

FIGURE 1. Enhanced neck CT shows a necrotic right internal jugular level II lymph node.

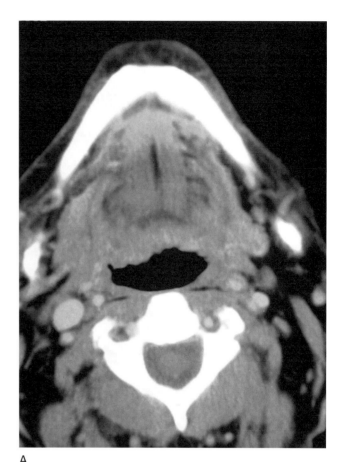

A

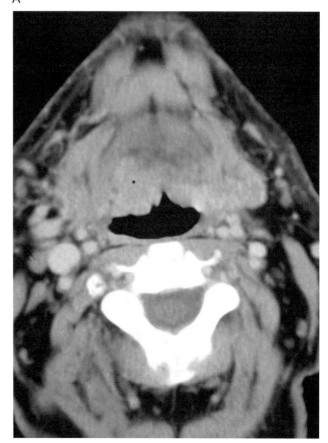

B

FIGURE 2. Enhanced neck CT images (**A** and **B**) through the base of tongue show only mild thickening and asymmetry of the right base of tongue compared with the left (*asterisk*). The patient did not have a preoperative or pretreatment MRI.

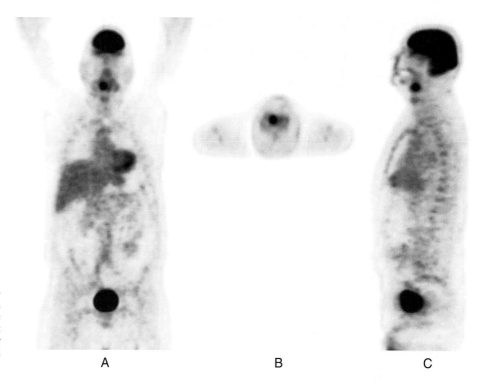

FIGURE 3. PET imaging, after surgical excision of the necrotic metastatic SCC lymph node and inconclusive right base of tongue biopsy, shows abnormal activity at the right base of tongue, highly suggestive of a primary site. Coronal (**A**), transaxial (**B**), and sagittal (**C**) views are shown.

A   B   C

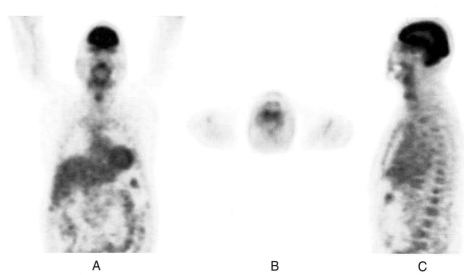

FIGURE 4. Repeat PET scan, 1 month later, after institution of chemotherapy and irradiation, shows normalization of the base of tongue primary findings noted previously. Coronal (**A**), transaxial (**B**), and sagittal (**C**) views are shown.

A   B   C

of chemotherapy and 1 month after finishing irradiation showed resolution of all abnormal PET activity. He remained negative on PET imaging 4 months later (8 months after diagnosis; Figure 4) and on MRI follow-up 2 years later.

TEACHING POINTS

PET imaging can be an important adjunct in the search for an occult primary tumor, as when a patient presents with a metastatic lymph node. Although the right base of tongue was abnormal on inspection, two separate biopsy attempts failed to yield a diagnosis of malignancy. Demonstration of hypermetabolic activity at this level on PET confirmed the impression of the base of tongue as the probable primary site and redirected biopsy efforts to this level. PET was also utilized in this case to assess the efficacy of combined chemotherapy and irradiation.

CASE 6 | *Hard palate squamous cell carcinoma, radiation therapy planning*

An 80-year-old male former smoker and drinker developed a T4 (5.3 cm) hard palate SCC, as demonstrated on MRI (Figures 1 to 3). The preoperative MRI also showed abnormal signal in the right parapharyngeal region and masticator space, of uncertain significance. Preoperative CT confirmed bony involvement of the floor of the nose (Figure 4). The patient opted for radical excision of the tumor and hard palate, including the mucoperiosteum of the floor of the nose. The tumor was exophytic, with a small base of attachment to the palate bone. There was gross invasion of the floor of the nose. Final pathology was reported as invasive well to moderately differentiated hard

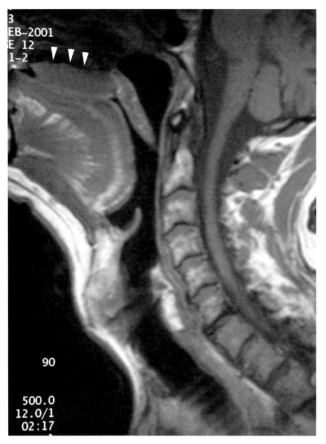

FIGURE 1. T1-weighted sagittal MR image shows the soft tissue SCC mass at the hard palate level (*arrowheads*).

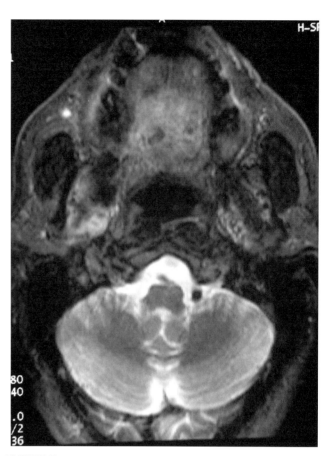

FIGURE 3. Short tau inversion recovery (STIR) axial MR image shows the hyperintense mass at the hard palate level. There is also abnormally increased signal at the right parapharyngeal level, extending to surround the pterygoid muscles of mastication. This latter finding was only demonstrable on STIR sequences.

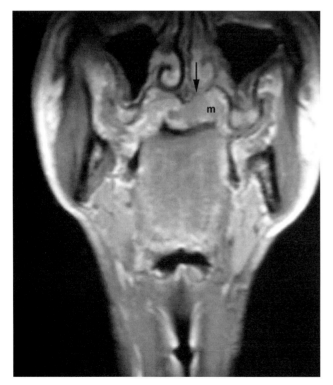

FIGURE 2. Enhanced T1-weighted coronal MR image shows the hard palate SCC mass (m), outlined by enhancing mucosa. The hypointense line of hard palate bone is breeched (*arrow*), suggesting bony erosion or involvement, which was confirmed on CT.

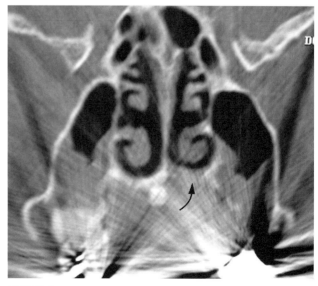

FIGURE 4. Coronal sinus CT confirms the loss of bone at the left hard palate/floor of nose level (*arrow*).

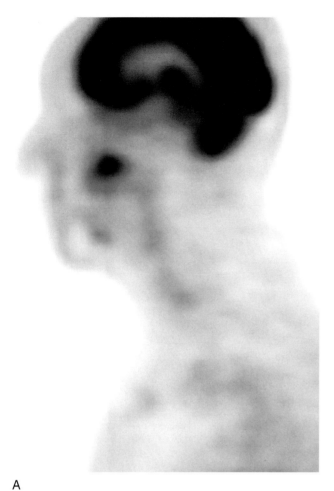

A

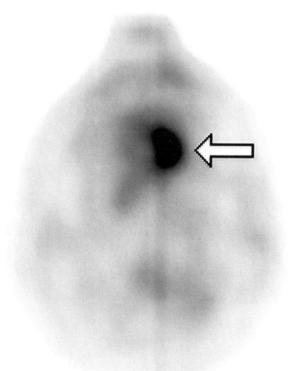

B

FIGURE 5. Sagittal (**A**) and coronal (**B**) PET images, obtained 2 months after surgery, show a hypermetabolic focus at the left hard palate surgical level.

palate SCC, with final soft tissue margins of the palate free of tumor. However, tumor was identified in hard palate bone that clinically was uninvolved and in additional tissue from the left floor of the nose. PET scan was requested about 2 months after surgery, before radiation therapy, to assess the significance of the right parapharyngeal signal abnormality (Figures 5 and 6). The PET scan showed intense focal activity at the site of the palatal excision but no abnormality at the right parapharyngeal level. Radiation therapy was given, with the regimen adjusted during the course of therapy when the tumor was noted to be progressing in size. Follow-up MRI of the region a year later showed the surgical defect, without evidence of local recurrence, and the right parapharyngeal signal abnormality had resolved (Figure 7). Shortly thereafter, a routine chest radiograph obtained for follow-up showed a new 6 cm right upper lobe mass. Fine-needle aspiration of this lesion showed poorly differentiated SCC. It could not be determined whether this was metastatic from the patient's prior palatal primary or a primary bronchogenic carcinoma. It was treated as metastatic, and chemotherapy was given.

TEACHING POINTS

PET was used in this case to follow up on a preoperatively noted finding, to aid radiation therapy planning after surgery. The absence of an abnormality on PET at the site of the right parapharyngeal activity was reassuring regarding probable benignity, which was subsequently validated on follow-up MRI 1 year later. The intensity of activity at the post-surgical site, evaluated with PET 2 months after surgery, was regarded with suspicion for persistent tumor. This seems validated by the clinical progression noted during administration of radiation.

FIGURE 6. Axial PET image also shows the focally intense left palatal activity (*arrow*) but does not identify an abnormality at the right parapharyngeal level in question.

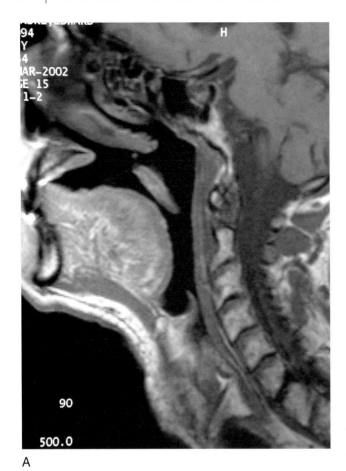

A

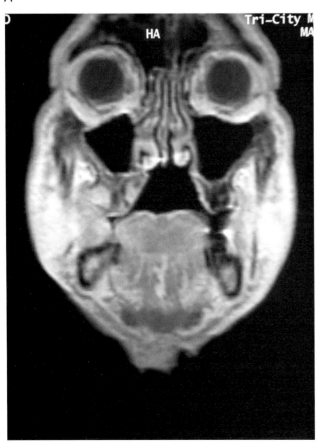

B

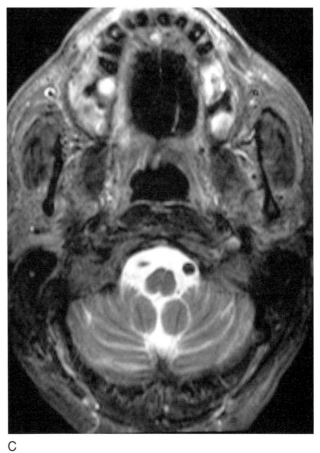

C

FIGURE 7. Follow-up, postoperative MRI, 1 year later: T1-weighted sagittal (**A**), enhanced T1-weighted coronal (**B**), and STIR axial (**C**) MR images, corresponding in levels to the prior study (Figures 1 to 3), show a postsurgical defect of the palate but no evidence of local recurrence. The right parapharyngeal activity noted previously is no longer evident on axial STIR imaging.

CASE 7 | *Recurrent maxillary non–small cell malignancy*

A 76-year-old previously healthy woman noted an irregular area on the intraoral side of her right cheek, which was confirmed on dental examination during denture fitting. A biopsy demonstrated a poorly differentiated non–small cell malignancy. On MRI, a right maxillary sinus mass was confirmed, involving the nasal cavity, right maxilla, inferior orbit, and masticator space (Figures 1 to 3). A right submandibular lymph node was also noted. Ultrasound-guided aspiration of this node was inconclusive for malignancy. The patient was treated with radiation therapy and concomitant cisplatin, with a good clinical response. Planned surgery to follow the chemoradiation was refused. A CT scan was obtained for follow-up about 3 months after completion of radiation. This identified a destructive right maxillary sinus lesion with bone lysis and soft tissue extension into the pterygoid fossa and orbit (Figure 4). Because many of the post-treatment findings had been present before therapy, their precise significance was uncertain.

PET scan was requested for clarification. The PET scan showed intense activity in the right maxillary sinus, consistent with persistent tumor activity (Figure 5). Within a few weeks, the patient's clinical examination showed increased edema and induration, as well as decreased mobility of the skin overlying the right maxilla, clinical evidence of relapse.

TEACHING POINTS

PET scan was used in this case to clarify the nature of the persistent maxillary sinus mass noted after completion of treatment. At the time, the patient clinically was doing very well. In fact, the demonstration on PET of persistent tumor activity at the site predicted the subsequent clinical progression.

Although there was no pre-treatment PET scan performed to allow for comparison, the intensity of the sinus activity and the interval since treatment of 4 months permitted confident interpretation of the activity as tumorous. Less intense activity and/or a shorter interval since treatment might well have yielded a more ambiguous result.

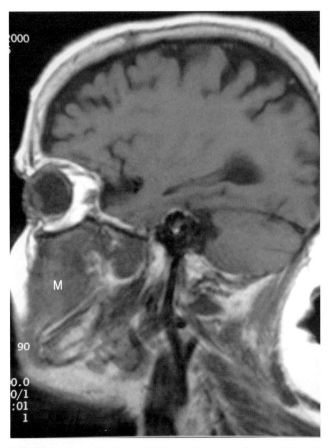

FIGURE 1. T1-weighted sagittal MR image shows opacification of the right maxillary sinus (M, mass).

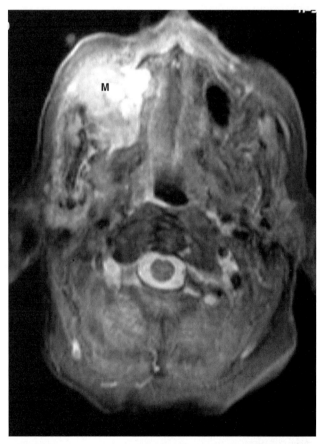

FIGURE 2. Short tau inversion recovery (STIR) axial MR image demonstrates a hyperintense mass (M, mass) filling the right maxillary sinus, with circumferential extension outside the expected bony confines of the sinus into the buccal soft tissues anteriorly, the bony maxilla medially, and the pterygoid fossa posteriorly.

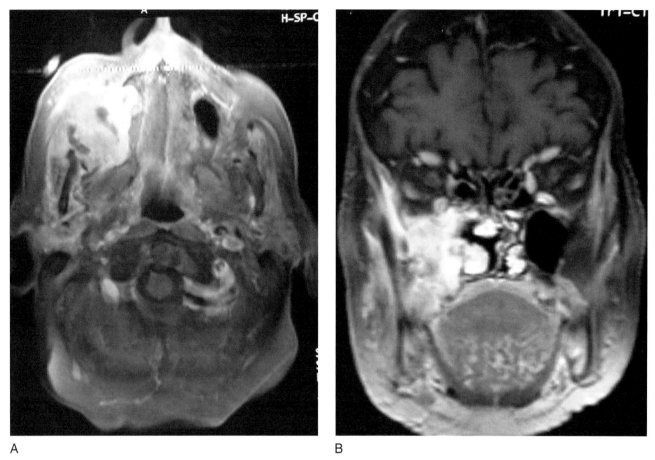

A

B

FIGURE 3. Fat-saturated, enhanced T1-weighted axial (**A**) and coronal (**B**) MR images demonstrate the breach by the mass of the bony contours of the sinus, with extension of the mass into the masticator space musculature and soft tissues, into the inferior orbit, and into the lateral nasal cavity and maxilla.

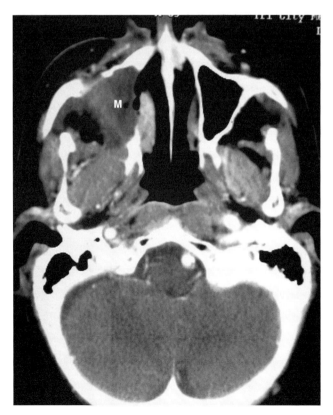

FIGURE 4. Three months post irradiation, enhanced axial CT through the maxillary sinuses shows soft tissue filling the right sinus, with lysis of the surrounding bone. The soft tissue mass (M, mass) in the sinus is smaller than on the pretreatment MRI, and the bone involvement was also evident previously.

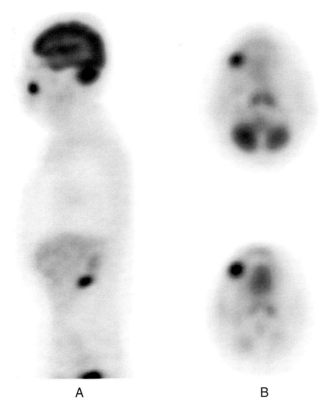

FIGURE 5. Sagittal (**A**) and axial (**B**) PET images show intense hypermetabolic activity in the right maxillary sinus, 4 months after finishing irradiation and chemotherapy. The intensity of the activity indicates that the residual imaging findings represent active tumor. Clinical evidence of relapse developed less than a month after this study.

CASE 8 | *Recurrent and progressive squamous cell carcinoma*

A 58-year-old man developed a persistent sore throat. Upper airway endoscopy under anesthesia did not identify an abnormality, but the examination was considered compromised by radiation therapy–related edema. His past medical history included a right radical neck dissection 7 years before, followed by irradiation, for moderately differentiated metastatic SCC. At the time, 3 of 35 lymph nodes were positive. A primary site was not identified.

With the persistent sore throat and inconclusive endoscopy, a PET scan was requested to evaluate the patient for an unidentified head and neck primary tumor (Figure 1). A right base of tongue hypermetabolic lesion was found that extended toward the epiglottis. These results helped direct the subsequent biopsy. Panendoscopy visualized an ulcerated tumor of the vallecula. An invasive, poorly differentiated SCC was confirmed from the right base of tongue biopsy. Because the newly identified primary lesion was within the field of the prior radiation and the patient declined glossectomy, he was treated with chemotherapy followed by interstitial implant high-dose radiation therapy.

On follow-up, approximately 1 year later, the patient was noted on physical examination to have new neck swelling and firmness in the right anterior submaxillary area and in the right posterior triangle. Needle biopsies were performed of both sites, with seropurulent material obtained from the anterior site and the posterior lesion solid. Aspirates showed no evidence of malignancy. Repeat aspiration of the anterior neck mass showed only necrotic material. Repeat PET scan showed significant change from the prior study, with multiple new hypermetabolic right head and neck foci of activity (Figure 2). Metabolically active foci were noted at the base of tongue (two foci), right submental level, right angle of the jaw, and right posterior triangle. MRI was then obtained for correlation, which showed corresponding findings (Figures 3 to 6). No additional attempts at needle biopsy

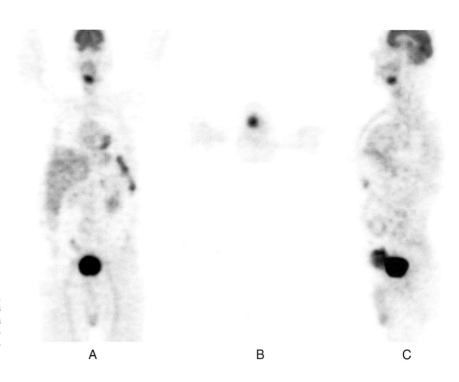

FIGURE 1. PET images in coronal (**A**), axial (**B**), and sagittal (**C**) planes show an isolated active focus in the right base of tongue, highly suggestive of a primary carcinoma site. This study directed a subsequent biopsy, which confirmed a poorly differentiated SCC at this level.

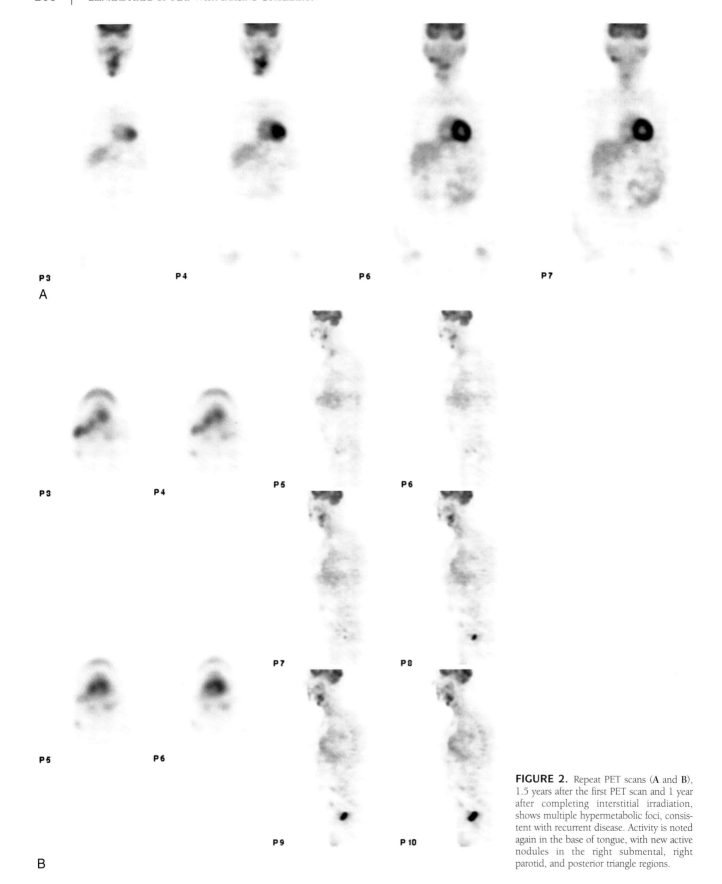

FIGURE 2. Repeat PET scans (**A** and **B**), 1.5 years after the first PET scan and 1 year after completing interstitial irradiation, shows multiple hypermetabolic foci, consistent with recurrent disease. Activity is noted again in the base of tongue, with new active nodules in the right submental, right parotid, and posterior triangle regions.

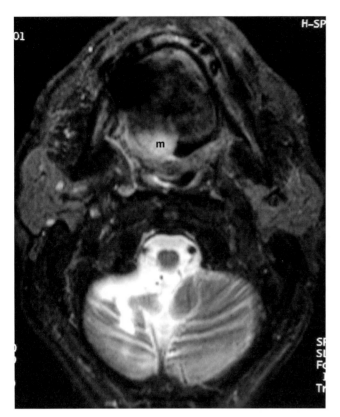

FIGURE 3. Short tau inversion recovery (STIR) axial MR image, after the second PET scan, shows a hyperintense mass (m) at the right base of tongue, which corresponded to abnormal metabolic activity on PET.

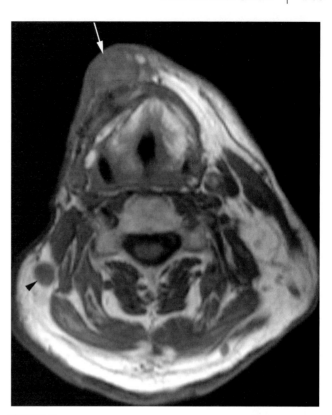

FIGURE 5. T1-weighted axial MR shows changes from prior right neck dissection, with sacrifice of the right sternocleidomastoid muscle. In the right submental region, a mass bulges the overlying skin (*arrow*). A sub-centimeter lymph node in the posterior triangle was hyperintense on PET and consistent with a metastatic lymph node (*arrowhead*).

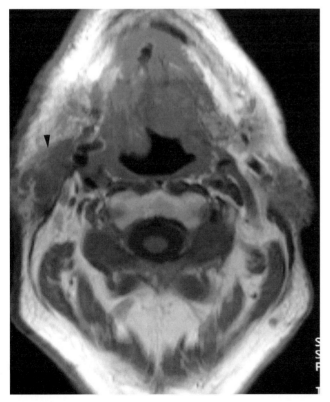

FIGURE 4. T1-weighted axial MR image shows right parotid level nodules, metabolically active on PET and consistent with metastatic lymph nodes (*arrowhead*).

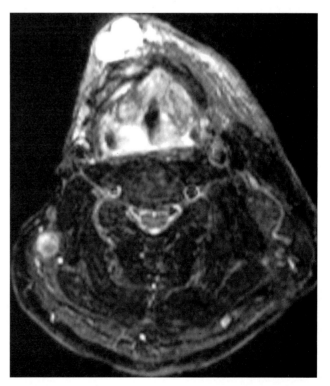

FIGURE 6. STIR axial image at the same level as Figure 5. Both the right submental mass and posterior triangle lymph node are hyperintense. Chronic edema is noted of the aryepiglottic folds from prior radiation.

were made. New and progressive findings on both PET and MRI were considered overwhelming evidence of recurrent malignancy. The patient was restarted on chemotherapy.

TEACHING POINTS

PET scanning served several important functions in the management of this previously treated and difficult to examine patient with head and neck carcinoma. When the patient presented with persistent sore throat and endoscopy proved difficult and inconclusive, PET provided a noninvasive means of evaluating the head and neck region for a suspected occult malignancy. The PET base of tongue abnormality directed a subsequent biopsy, yielding a positive diagnosis of malignancy. When on later follow-up the patient's physical examination suggested relapse, and needle aspirations were inconclusive, PET was then utilized to confirm the impression of recurrent disease. The abnormalities identified on PET were then confirmed anatomically with MRI.

CASE 9 | Nasopharyngeal squamous cell carcinoma, with bone metastases

A 67-year-old woman with locally advanced nasopharyngeal carcinoma was treated with chemoradiation. Histology was poorly differentiated SCC, with disease stage T3N2. Nine months after treatment ended, persistent tumor was identified on MRI (Figures 1 and 2) and confirmed by biopsy. The patient was noted to have progressive weight loss. Head and neck MRI showed a focus of abnormal marrow signal in the T2 vertebral body, suggestive of a bone metastasis (Figure 3). PET scan showed asymmetry in the nasopharynx (Figure 4) and intense activity at T2, confirming the impression of osseous metastasis (Figure 5). This was confirmed by biopsy, which showed metastatic carcinoma, similar in histology to the patient's primary tumor. Follow-up MRI demonstrated progression of thoracic metastatic disease (Figure 6).

TEACHING POINTS

The PET scan in this patient showed moderate activity at the level of her nasopharyngeal primary tumor. The study was performed nearly a year after completion of chemoradiation, a sufficient interval in which most treatment effects would have resolved. The patient was known at the time of PET imaging to have biopsy-proven persistent tumor, and the activity at this level is consistent with this. The more important role played by PET was in clarifying the nature of the T2 lesion previously noted on MRI, at a time when the patient was being considered for aggressive local surgery. The combination of MRI and PET scan

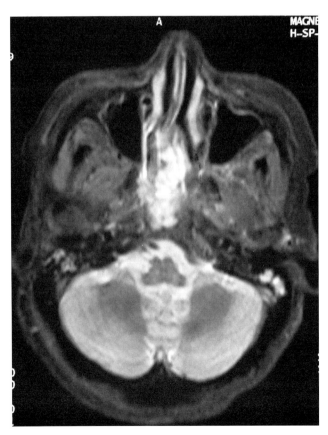

FIGURE 1. Short tau inversion recovery (STIR) axial MR image shows a hyperintense mass filling the nasopharynx, consistent with a nasopharyngeal carcinoma.

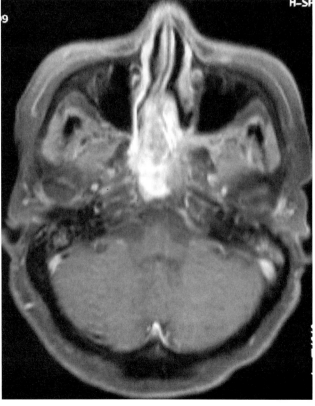

FIGURE 2. Fat-saturated, enhanced T1-weighted axial MR image at the same level shows inhomogeneous enhancement of the nasopharyngeal mass.

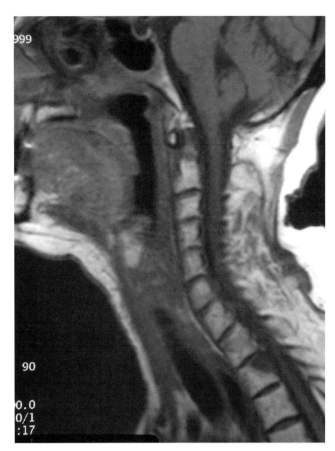

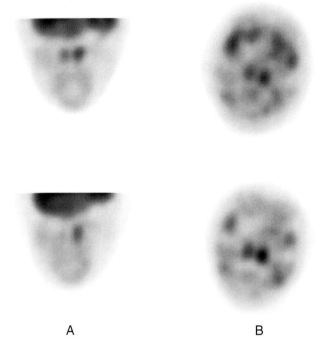

FIGURE 4. PET scan images (coronal [A] and axial [B]) show moderate, asymmetrical activity at the level of the left nasopharynx, corresponding to the persistent mass on MRI.

A   B

FIGURE 3. T1-weighted sagittal image from the same study shows a focus of abnormal marrow signal at the posterosuperior T2 vertebral body, suggesting a metastasis.

FIGURE 5. Coronal (A) and sagittal (B) PET scan images show an intense focus of activity at the upper thoracic spine level, corresponding to the MRI abnormality and most consistent with a bone metastasis. Symmetrical, intense activity on the coronal images in the shoulder girdle regions bilaterally may be muscular or represent activation of brown fat.

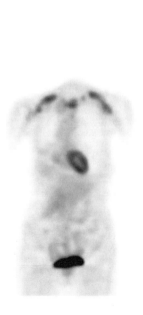

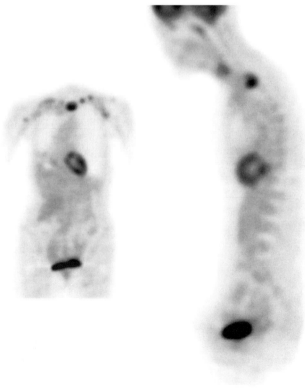

A   B

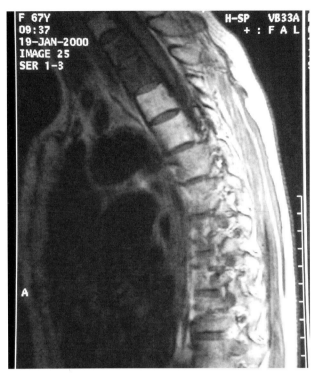

FIGURE 6. A follow-up thoracic spine MRI shows progression of the osseous metastases, now involving the adjacent T2 and T3 vertebral bodies nearly confluently.

findings at T2 suggested overwhelmingly that the patient had osseous metastatic disease (confirmed histologically), redirecting subsequent care.

CASE 10 | *Squamous cell carcinoma, metastatic to thoracic spine, incipient cord compression presentation*

A 60-year-old man with a past history of SCC of the floor of the mouth developed severe interscapular back pain. Four years before, the patient had been diagnosed with diffuse carcinoma in situ of the floor of the mouth, treated with laser. A small focus of recurrent in situ malignancy was excised 6 months later. Subsequently, a left sub-mandibular nodal recurrence was identified, and he underwent neck dissection. One year before the current presentation, a right neck recurrence in a lymph node with extranodal extension was treated surgically and irradiated. He had recently been seen for ENT follow-up, with no evidence of recurrent local disease. He complained of severe interscapular back pain for several months and had been evaluated at another facility with a bone scan, which reportedly was negative for metastases. Because of the persistent and progressive back pain, a PET scan was requested. On the day of the PET scan, the patient noted the onset of new lower extremity numbness and electric shock sensation.

The PET scan showed intense focal hypermetabolism in the upper thoracic spine (Figure 1). The morphology of the activity suggested a

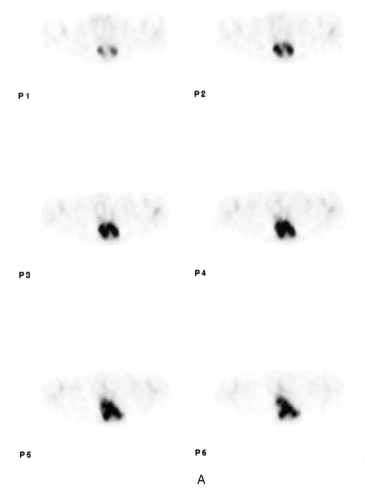

A

B

FIGURE 1. Axial (**A**) and sagittal (**B**) PET scan images show markedly increased activity at the T4 vertebral body level. The sagittal sections show the abnormal activity to involve a vertebral body and enlarged spinous process. The involvement of both the vertebral centrum and posterior elements, coupled with the patient's symptoms, predicted incipient cord compression.

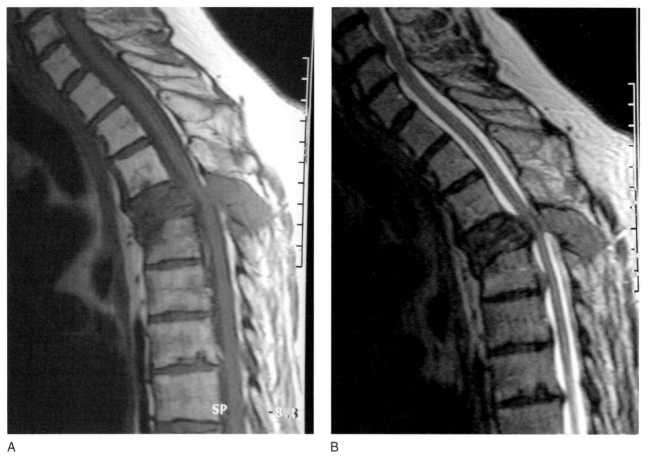

A

B

FIGURE 2. Sagittal T1- (**A**) and T2-weighted (**B**) MR images of the thoracic spine show corresponding findings. The T4 vertebral body and enlarged spinous process are replaced by soft tissue tumor. The body is collapsed, and early cord compression is present.

thoracic vertebral metastasis, with involvement both of the body and the posterior elements. The potential for incipient cord compression was recognized, and the patient was admitted for emergency thoracic spine MRI (Figures 2 and 3). This showed replacement and collapse of the T4 vertebral body. As predicted by the PET scan, the posterior

elements were also replaced. The spinal cord was encircled and compressed. The patient was placed on corticosteroids, and his symptoms inproved. Surgical decompression was performed, with T4 and T5 corpectomies and anterior and posterior fusion. The pathology report showed metastatic poorly differentiated SCC.

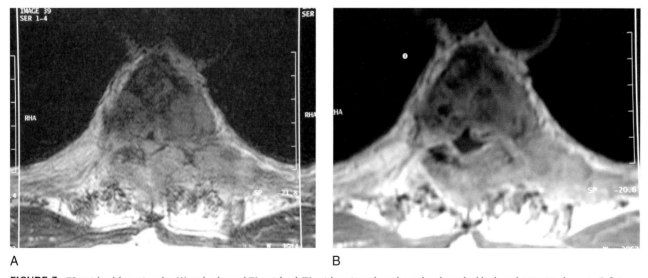

A

B

FIGURE 3. T2-weighted fast spin echo (**A**) and enhanced T1-weighted (**B**) axial sections show the replaced vertebral body and posterior elements. Soft tissue tumor encroaches on the epidural space, and the cord is encircled and compressed. Left lateral extension of the tumor replacing the adjacent rib is noted.

TEACHING POINTS

PET emergencies are rare. This is one of the few we have encountered in a community hospital setting. The key observation is the involvement of both the vertebral body and the posterior elements, accompanied by a subtle gibbous deformity. The PET findings of the enlarged and replaced spinous process predicted the MRI appearance, although the collapse of the vertebral body was not recognized by PET. Because of the known clinical history of back pain and the new leg numbness, incipient cord compression was first suspected based on the PET scan and subsequently confirmed on MRI.

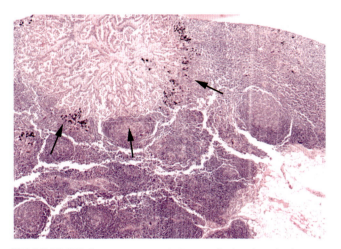

COLOR PLATE 1. Low-power H & E stain of a lymph node showing a 1-mm focus of gland-forming metastic adenocarcinoma (*arrows*).

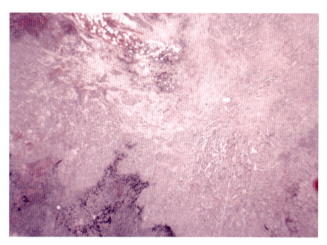

COLOR PLATE 2. Low-power view of an H & E stain from another lymph node depicting the largest nodal focus (7 mm) of metastatic adenocarcinoma. Residual normal lymph node remains at lower left corner of image. (Histopathology images courtesy of Gary Wilcox, MD, Tri City Medical Center, Oceanside, CA).

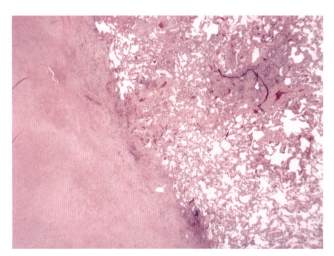

COLOR PLATE 3. Low-power H & E–stained view from the surgical specimen showing lung to the right, and a portion of the necrotic granuloma to the left. The nodule margin is relatively smooth.

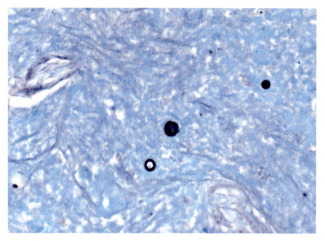

COLOR PLATE 4. High-power view of the methenamine silver stain study of the nodule, showing stainable spherules, both empty and filled with endospores. The fungal organisms are compatible with *Coccidioides immitis* (Histopathology images courtesy of Gary Wilcox, MD, Tri City Medical Center, Oceanside, CA).

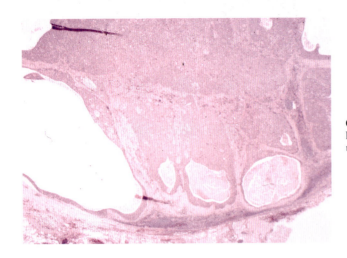

COLOR PLATE 5. Low-power H & E–stained view of the lymph node with the largest focus (1 cm) of metastatic tumor. Cystic degeneration is seen within the tumor. (Courtesy of Gary Wilcox, MD, Tri City Medical Center, Oceanside, CA.)

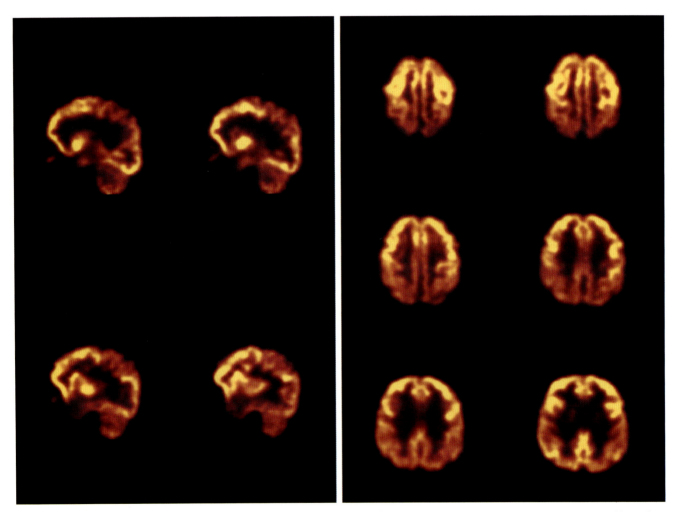

COLOR PLATE 6. Reviewing images with different color scales can be helpful in delineating differential metabolic activity. The parietal and temporal lobes show symmetrically reduced activity, a pattern suggestive of Alzheimer's dementia. The higher metabolic activity is depicted in a greater intensity of yellow.

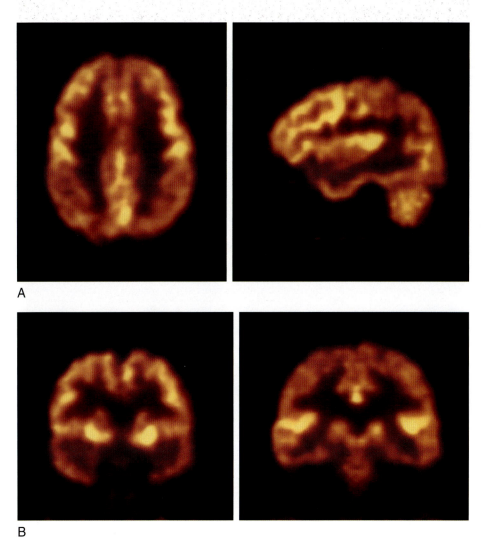

A

B

COLOR PLATE 7. PET sections (**A**, axial and sagittal, and **B**, coronal) show comparatively normal metabolism of the frontal lobes, with reduced metabolism of both parietal and temporal lobes. Patients with advanced cases of Alzheimer's disease frequently show frontal involvement as well.

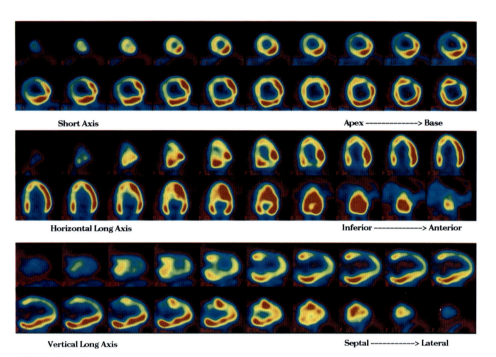

Short Axis   Apex ---------------> Base

Horizontal Long Axis   Inferior -------------> Anterior

Vertical Long Axis   Septal ------------> Lateral

COLOR PLATE 8. PET myocardial viability study, obtained 5 days after admission with a non–Q wave myocardial infarction, shows the inferior and inferolateral walls to be viable. Myocardial metabolic activity at these levels is actually greater than in the anterior wall and septum, presumably reflecting the predilection of ischemic myocardium for glucose as a substrate.

Breast Cancer

Breast cancer is the most common malignancy in women in the United States, with an annual incidence now of more than 180,000. It is second only to lung cancer as a cause of cancer-related death in women. The diagnosis of primary breast cancer most often results from detection of a palpable lump or an abnormal mammogram. Although mammography has a sensitivity of 80% to 90%, its specificity is significantly lower.[1] This results in a large number of biopsies for benign disease. Additionally, mammographic diagnosis may be difficult in patients with dense breasts, implants, or after surgery or irradiation. The role of PET in imaging breast cancer can be assessed with respect to diagnosis of the primary tumor, initial staging, restaging, and monitoring response to therapy.

PRIMARY TUMOR

Several options exist for patients with an inconclusive mammogram. Ultrasonography is of benefit in many of these patients, as is MRI. Unfortunately, although the negative predictive value of MRI approaches 100%, the specificity is similar to that of mammography.[2] Scintimammography is accurate for lesions larger than 1 to 1.5 cm but has not established itself in routine practice. There are data to support the use of PET as a complementary test or in certain subsets of patients.[3] Sensitivities for detecting breast cancer range from 66% to 96%, and specificities range from 83% to 100%.[4] The lower sensitivity is likely caused by a minimum size requirement of approximately 1 cm for detection by PET and a relatively normal to minimally increased metabolic rate for certain tumor types (e.g., lobular carcinomas and ductal carcinoma in situ).[5] PET may be of benefit in identifying an occult primary lesion or in establishing multicentricity. The role of PET in primary diagnosis is relatively minor, and it is best employed for problem solving. Two significant advantages PET offers in the primary or early assessment of these patients are excellent specificity and its whole-body staging capability.

STAGING

Regional lymph node metastases may occur in up to 60% of patients at the time of initial diagnosis.[4] PET has demonstrated very high sensitivity for detection of axillary metastases, related in part to the size of the primary tumor (i.e., larger primary tumors show better sensitivity for PET). An early multicenter survey showed a sensitivity of 96%.[6] Although subsequent results have shown lower sensitivity, PET is still considered very accurate in the axilla. PET can also assess internal mammary and supraclavicular nodes and serve as a whole-body screen. The critical prognostic information obtained from knowledge of axillary nodal status thus far precludes the substitution of PET for axillary dissection. It is also unlikely that PET will replace lymphoscintigraphy for nodal assessment. With extremely high reliability, lymphoscintigraphy can identify the sentinel node(s), which is the first node(s) draining the primary tumor site. This allows surgical sampling and detailed histologic evaluation of this node. PET, with its resolution limitations, cannot delineate microscopic disease in nodes.

RESTAGING

Local or regional recurrence is noted in 7% to 30% of patients after initial diagnosis and treatment.[7] MRI is presently the modality of choice to evaluate the axillary region and brachial plexus. Although sensitivity for detection of recurrence is high, specificity can be reduced by its inability to differentiate tumor infiltration from radiation or surgery-related scarring. PET is especially valuable in this scenario and should be considered complementary to MRI. For distant metastases, PET has shown excellent results. Soft tissue as well as bony metastases can be visualized. It is worth noting that there is variability in uptake in bone metastases, with better visualization of osteolytic than sclerotic lesions.[1] The reverse is true for standard bone scintigraphy, with the majority of purely osteolytic lesions escaping detection.

It is also important to recognize that there is a correlation between FDG uptake and histologic tumor type. Studies have shown greater uptake with invasive ductal breast carcinoma than with invasive lobular breast carcinoma.[8] The reduced standardized uptake value in lobular carcinoma may translate into a lesser sensitivity. However, invasive lobular carcinomas make up only 6% to 10% of breast cancers.[1] The use of PET results in a higher sensitivity than conventional imaging studies for determining the true extent of disease.[9-11]

MONITORING THERAPY

Pooled data indicate an 81% sensitivity and 90% specificity for PET in monitoring response to chemotherapy.[12] In vitro studies have shown that after treatment, tumor FDG uptake reflects the number of viable tumor cells.[13] Therapy response may be determined earlier than with other modalities. The information provided by PET may be used to modify treatment, limiting the use of ineffective, potentially toxic chemotherapy.

To summarize, PET has shown very encouraging results in the evaluation of patients with breast cancer. It may be used as a "problem-solving" tool when other tests are indeterminate and as an accurate method to stage and identify recurrence, and it holds promise for monitoring response to therapy.

REFERENCES

1. Avril N, Schelling M, Dose J, et al: Utility of PET in breast cancer. Clin Pos Imag 1999;2:261-271.
2. Gilles R, Guinebreatiere JM, Lucidarme O, et al: Nonpalpable breast tumors: Diagnosis with contrast-enhanced subtraction dynamic MR imaging. Radiology 1994;191:625-631.
3. Avril N, Dose J, Janicke F, et al: Metabolic characteristics of breast tumors with positron emission tomography using F-18 fluorodeoxyglucose. J Clin Oncol 1996;14:1848-1857.
4. Flanagan FL, Dehdashi F, Siegel BA: PET in breast cancer. Semin Nucl Med 1998;28:290-302.
5. Nieweg OE, Kim EE, Wong WH, et al: Positron emission tomography with fluorine-18-deoxyglucose in the detection and staging of breast cancer. Cancer 1993;71:3920-3925.
6. Adler LP, Cascade E, Crowe J, et al: Axillary lymph node involvement in breast cancer: A retrospective study. Presented at 1994 ICP meeting, San Francisco, CA, October 25-29, 1994.
7. Hathaway PB, Mankoff DA, Maravilla KR, et al: Value of combined FDG PET and MR imaging in the evaluation of suspected recurrent local-regional breast cancer: Preliminary experience. Radiology 1999;210:807-814.
8. Avril N, Menzel M, Dose J, et al: Glucose metabolism of breast cancer assessed by ^{18}F-FDG-PET: Histologic and immunohistochemical tissue analysis. J Nucl Med 2001;42:9-16.
9. Wahl RL, Cody RL, Hutchins GD, et al: Primary and metastatic breast carcinoma: Initial clinical evaluation with PET with the radiolabeled glucose analogue 2-[F-18]-fluoro-2-deoxy-D-glucose. Radiology 1991;179:765-770.
10. Hoh CK, Hawkins RA, Glaspy JA, et al: Cancer detection with whole-body PET using [18F] fluoro-2-deoxy-D-glucose. J Comput Assist Tomogr 1993;17:582-589.
11. Avril N, Dose J, Janicke F, et al: Assessment of axillary lymph node involvement in breast patients with positron emission tomography using radiolabeled 2-(fluorine-18)-fluoro-2-deoxy-D-glucose. J Natl Cancer Inst 1996;88:1204-1209.
12. Gambhir SS, Czernin J, Schwimmer J, et al: A tabulated summary of the FDG PET literature. J Nucl Med 2001;42:26S-31S.
13. Haberkorn U, Reinhardt M, Strauss LG, et al: Metabolic design of combination therapy: Use of enhanced fluorodeoxyglucose uptake caused by chemotherapy. J Nucl Med 1992;33:1981-1987.

CASE 1 | *Focal breast activity due to an unsuspected breast cancer*

A 73-year-old woman was referred for PET imaging for suspicion of recurrent lung cancer. Eighteen months after undergoing RLL resection for lung cancer, she developed shortness of breath and a small right pleural effusion. PET scan demonstrated an unexpected hypermetabolic left breast focus (Figure 1). Subsequent evaluations confirmed breast cancer, which was excised by lumpectomy.

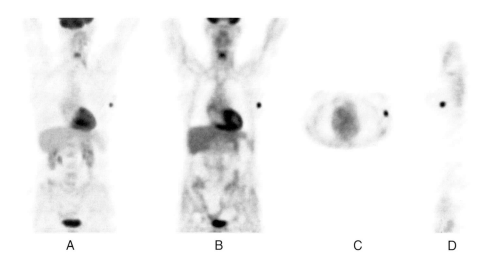

A   B   C   D

FIGURE 1. PET imaging shows an intensely hypermetabolic, unexpected left breast focus, which was subsequently proved to be a breast cancer. Projection image (**A**) and coronal (**B**), transaxial (**C**), and sagittal (**D**) views are shown.

TEACHING POINTS

PET, typically performed as a whole-body examination, affords the occasional opportunity to identify unexpected, but significant findings that are unrelated to a patient's known diagnoses. Focal, intense breast activity such as seen here mandates further evaluation and is generally readily differentiated from the lower-level, more diffuse physiologic activity that can be seen normally in breast tissue. Knowledge of the typical patterns of disease spread for any given histology must also be weighed in assessing the significance of activity encountered in an unexpected location. Not infrequently, investigation of such serendipitous active foci will identify significant additional diagnoses. A series of 68 unsuspected findings (pathologic activity unrelated to a known or suspected malignant process), drawn from a database of 1800 scans performed on 1650 patients at Hackensack University Medical Center, yielded a group of 42 patients for which histopathologic correlation

was available (H. Agress Jr., Academy of Molecular Imaging meeting abstract and personal communication, October 2002). Malignant or premalignant findings were diagnosed in 62% of these patients on subsequent work-up (30 significant findings in 26 patients), with the most common abnormalities being colonic, including villous, tubular, and tubulovillous adenomas and adenocarcinomas. In this series, other unsuspected carcinomas identified as a result of unexpected PET findings included two laryngeal, two breast, one gallbladder, one endometrial, one ovarian, one fallopian tube, and one papillary thyroid carcinoma.

CASE 2 | Breast cancer, initial staging, axillary nodal presentation, primary search, and internal mammary adenopathy

A 44-year-old woman was diagnosed with metastatic right breast carcinoma in the axilla. Three lymph nodes were surgically removed at the time of diagnosis. Mammography did not identify a primary tumor. Chest CT suggested a possible primary site, as well as internal mammary adenopathy (Figures 2 and 4). PET imaging showed three sites of increased metabolic activity in and around the right breast (Figure 1). Two sites were discrete and hypermetabolic and corresponded with the suspected primary lesion within the breast and with the internal mammary adenopathy on CT. Less discrete, lower intensity activity laterally corresponded with the site of recent surgery (Figure 3).

TEACHING POINTS

The role of PET imaging at initial diagnosis of breast cancer is in evolution. It clearly can be useful in selected cases as a diagnostic and problem-solving tool, as exemplified here in the search for a primary lesion in a patient presenting with metastases. PET's role in breast cancer imaging is more firmly established in identifying recurrences and assessing therapy effectiveness.

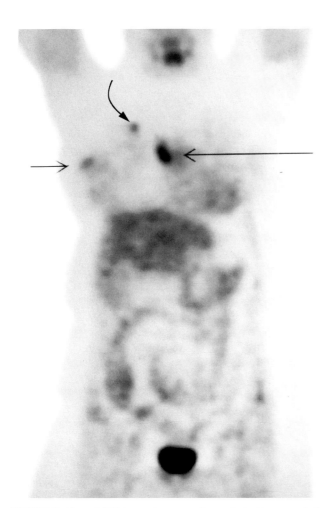

FIGURE 1. Coronal PET image shows two discrete foci of hypermetabolic activity, corresponding to CT abnormalities. The nodular focus in the right superior breast corresponds to a breast mass visualized on CT and is consistent with a primary lesion (curved arrow). The second hypermetabolic focus is right paramedian and corresponds to internal mammary adenopathy on CT (long arrow). Vaguer, less intense right lateral breast/axillary activity corresponds to post-surgical changes (short arrow).

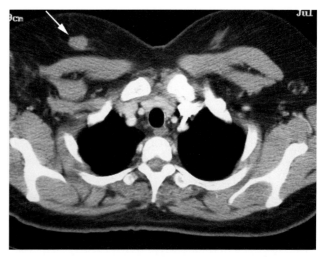

FIGURE 2. Enhanced chest CT through the superior aspect of both breasts shows a right-sided mass (arrow), with irregular margins, differing significantly from the wispy appearance of this patient's normal breast tissue, seen on left.

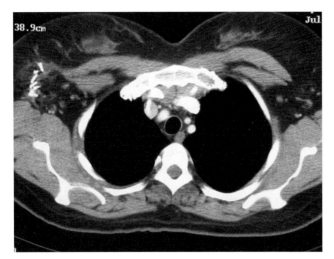

FIGURE 3. Stranding and surgical clips are noted at the right axillary operative site and corresponds to the less intense lateral activity on PET.

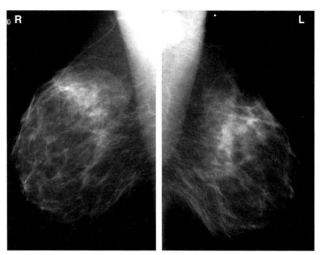

FIGURE 1. MLO mammographic views show a radiopaque marker at the level of the palpably enlarged left axillary lymph nodes. No breast parenchymal abnormality was recognized prospectively (R, right; L, left).

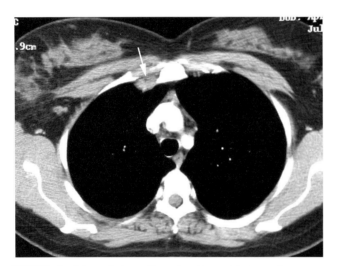

FIGURE 4. Enhanced chest CT section shows right internal mammary adenopathy *(arrow)*.

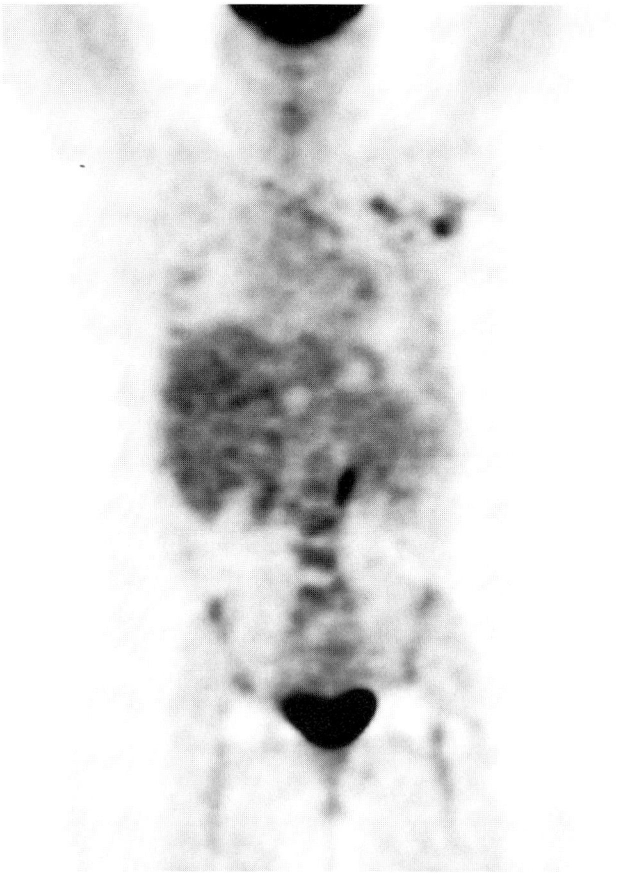

CASE 3 | *Axillary nodal presentation of breast cancer; primary lesion identified by PET*

A 39-year-old woman presented with left breast pain and axillary adenopathy. Mammography noted the enlarged lymph nodes in the axilla but did not identify a source within the breast (Figure 1). The left axilla was sampled, and metastatic carcinoma compatible with a breast primary was confirmed. She was referred for PET imaging to search for an unknown primary lesion.

PET imaging showed three hypermetabolic foci in the left axilla, corresponding to the known residual palpable lymph nodes (Figure 2). In addition, a separate, small, hypermetabolic focus was identified in the upper inner quadrant of the left breast (Figure 3). The mammogram was re-reviewed with this information, and a neodensity was noted in the medial breast compared with the prior year's study (Figure 4).

FIGURE 2. Coronal PET section shows multiple metabolically active left axillary lymph nodes.

Further mammographic and ultrasonographic work-up confirmed the abnormality (Figures 5 to 7). Planned mastectomy was deferred in favor of core needle biopsy of the suspected primary lesion. Poorly differentiated invasive ductal carcinoma was confirmed. The patient's

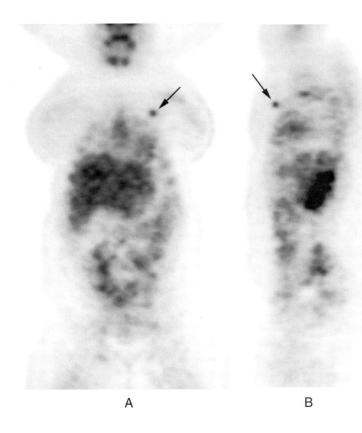

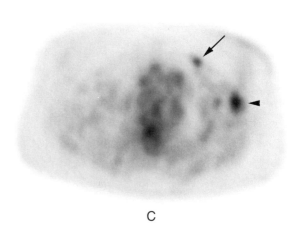

FIGURE 3. A more anterior coronal (**A**) and corresponding sagittal (**B**) and axial (**C**) sections show a separate hypermetabolic nodule in the left breast upper inner quadrant (*arrows*). The axial slice also visualizes one of the hypermetabolic axillary lymph nodes (*arrowhead*).

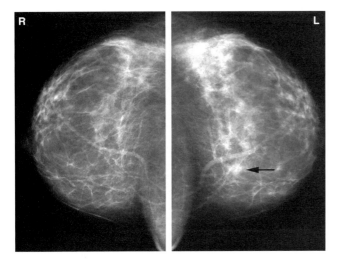

FIGURE 4. The patient's mammogram was re-reviewed with the PET information for correlation. On the craniocaudal views, a neodensity is visualized in the medial breast, new from the prior study (*arrow*). R, right; L, left.

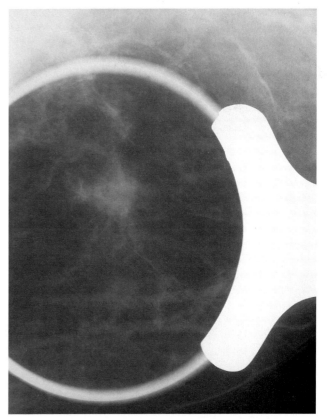

management was changed from mastectomy to lumpectomy. At pathology, a 1.5-cm poorly differentiated invasive ductal carcinoma was identified and 3 of 12 lymph nodes from axillary dissection were positive for malignancy. The largest lymph node measured 2.1 cm. Further therapy was undertaken with adjuvant chemotherapy and radiation.

FIGURE 5. Subsequently obtained spot compression view in craniocaudal projection shows suspicious features, with noncompressibility of the neodensity, irregular margins, and spiculation.

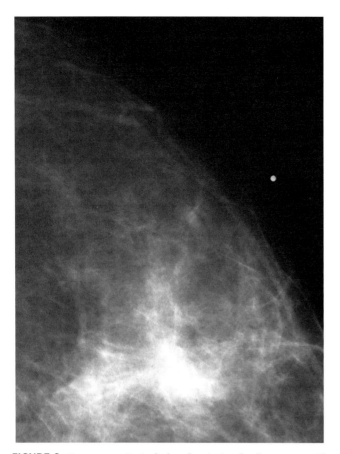

FIGURE 6. Spot compression in the lateral projection also shows a mass with spiculation and architectural distortion.

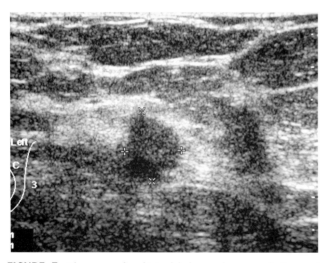

FIGURE 7. Ultrasonography obtained before performance of ultrasound-guided core biopsy shows suspicious ultrasonographic characteristics. Hypoechoic 1.1-cm solid mass (calipers) is taller than wide, with irregular margins and no capsule.

TEACHING POINTS

PET imaging was the initial study to locate this patient's breast carcinoma primary lesion. Overlooked initially on mammography, the addition of the PET information enabled the mammographic work-up to be redirected and the lesion successfully localized and sampled. The PET information also changed this patient's management. Until the lesion was confirmed on mammographic and ultrasonographic work-up, it was considered unable to be localized, and the patient was slated for mastectomy without consideration of breast conservation therapy. If the lesion had not been confirmed on the additional breast imaging work-up, enhanced breast MRI could have been considered as an appropriate next step in the imaging pursuit of this highly persuasive PET scan abnormality.

CASE 4 | Breast cancer restaging, normal post-lumpectomy and radiation breast findings

A 70-year-old woman with a history of stage IIA infiltrating ductal carcinoma of the right breast was referred for PET imaging and lumbar spine MRI. The patient was experiencing worsening low back pain, radiating from both groins to the feet. Bone metastases were thought unlikely owing to the generally favorable characteristics of the patient's tumor. A bone scan had shown degenerative activity in the lumbar spine. The PET scan was performed 1 year and 8 months after diagnosis and 14 months after radiation therapy concluded.

PET scan showed no evidence of recurrent breast cancer. Post-surgical and radiation therapy effects were noted in the right breast (Figures 1 and 2).

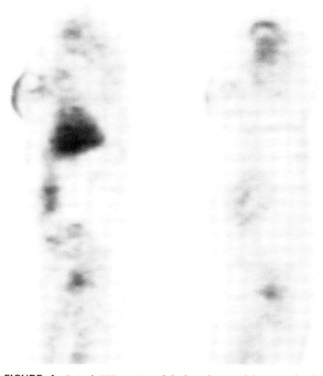

FIGURE 1. Sagittal PET sections (left through treated breast and right through opposite breast) show a normal appearance of the unaffected breast. In contrast, post-surgical changes are clearly evident on the post-lumpectomy side. A rim of mild metabolic activity outlines a photopenic defect, consistent with a postoperative seroma. There is marked asymmetry in the skin activity of the right breast compared with the untreated side, consistent with radiation therapy effects and analogous to the radiation-induced skin thickening seen on mammography.

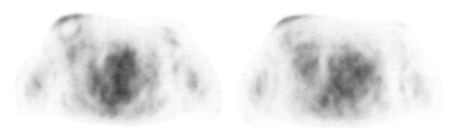

FIGURE 2. Axial PET sections through the breasts allow the two sides to be easily compared. No suspicious activity is seen on the treated side, and the findings are quite comparable to those typically seen in post-lumpectomy and radiation-treated breasts on mammography.

CASE 5 | *Post-surgical biopsy scar, post lumpectomy for infiltrating ductal carcinoma*

A 58-year-old woman with a history of node-negative invasive ductal carcinoma with aggressive features was referred for PET imaging for evaluation of elevated tumor markers. Her tumor was diagnosed about 22 months before as a 1.5-cm, poorly differentiated lesion and was treated with lumpectomy, four cycles of chemotherapy, and irradiation. Her CA19-9 was elevated, at 64 (normal <37). Imaging investigation for this was reportedly negative.

The PET scan showed a small focus of modest activity at the upper outer right breast level, in the region of the patient's prior surgery (Figure 1). A breast MRI was obtained for correlation (Figures 2 and 3). It showed a small spiculated focus at the surgical scar level, hypointense on all sequences and without abnormal enhancement. Physical examination noted thickness of the scar without a distinct palpable nodule. The patient had noted a slight puckering of the skin in the region. Because it was believed a local recurrence could not be excluded, a core needle biopsy was performed, followed a few weeks later by excisional biopsy. Both specimens showed similar findings, with a foreign-body giant cell reaction and fibrosis. Histologic appearance was consistent with the residua of a prior biopsy site.

TEACHING POINTS

Activity in a surgical scar may persist for variable lengths of time but usually resolves within months to upward of a year. It should be expected to be visualized for at least a month after surgery. Frequently, surgical scar activity is linear in configuration. Confounding features in this case are the focality of the activity and its presence so long after surgery (nearly 3 years). The MRI was probably overinterpreted as suspicious in this case in light of the PET scan findings. Both the PET scan and MRI features of this lesion are consistent with the final proven diagnosis of a surgical scar.

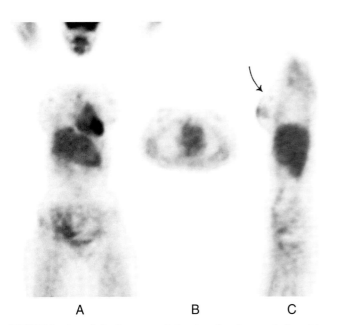

A   B   C

FIGURE 1. A small, focal, asymmetrical region of modest metabolic activity is seen on PET in the right upper outer quadrant, in the region of the patient's prior surgery nearly 3 years before. Coronal (**A**), transaxial (**B**), and sagittal (**C**) views are shown.

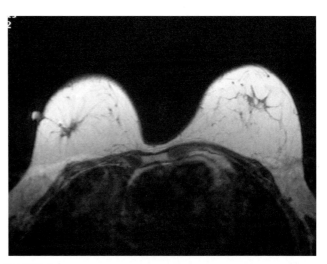

FIGURE 2. T1-weighted axial MR image of both breasts shows them to be predominantly fatty. A marker had been placed at the site of the patient's prior surgery. Subjacent to this is a spiculated hypointense focus.

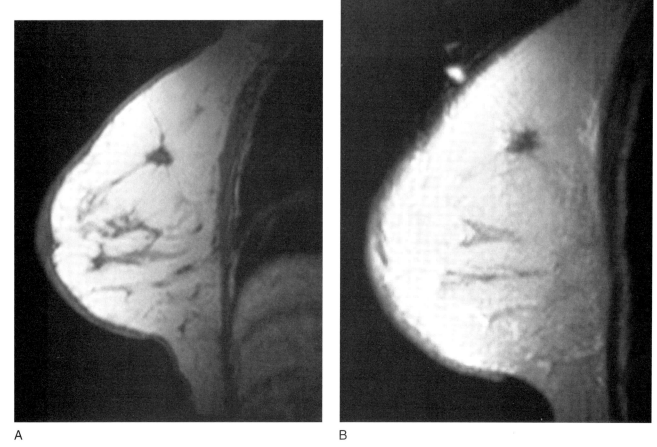

A   B

FIGURE 3. Sagittal T1-weighted (**A**) and T2-weighted (**B**) fast spin echo images of the right lateral breast show the spiculated focus, which is hypointense on both sequences and which did not enhance with contrast medium. MRI features are consistent with scar.

CASE 6 | *Recurrent inflammatory breast cancer*

A 52-year-old woman with recurrent inflammatory breast cancer was referred for PET imaging to aid in the restaging of her disease. She had originally been diagnosed with inflammatory breast cancer on the left 3 years before. She was initially treated with two cycles of paclitaxel (Taxol) and three cycles of docetaxel (Taxotere), after which she underwent a mastectomy with reconstruction. Her tumor histology was inflammatory breast carcinoma, stage III, with 7 of 10 positive lymph nodes. Microscopic margins were positive. Postoperatively she was treated with additional chemotherapy as well as chest wall and axilllary radiation. She was maintained on anastrozole (Arimidex), raloxifene (Evista), and local vaccine therapy. At the time of presentation for PET imaging, the patient had newly detected bilateral breast nodules. A biopsy confirmed right breast metastatic ductal carcinoma and left breast ductal carcinoma, with foci in the dermis and in breast fat. A PET scan was requested to assess the full extent of disease and identified multiple hypermetabolic foci in the right breast and at least three nodal foci in the right axilla (Figures 1 and 2). She subsequently underwent right mastectomy. Margins were negative, and 3 of 8 lymph nodes were positive. She was started on weekly docetaxel, on which she remained clinically stable.

TEACHING POINTS

At the time of referral for PET, this patient had an established diagnosis of locally recurrent disease. PET was requested as a whole-body staging examination to better direct therapy.

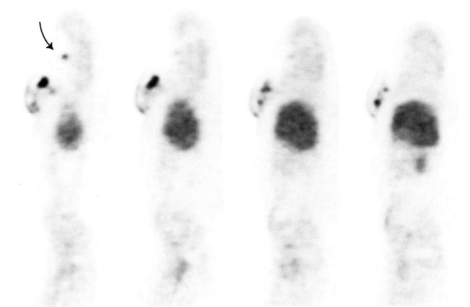

FIGURE 1. Sagittal PET images through the right breast show multiple discrete foci of hypermetabolic activity, consistent with multicentric disease. One metabolically active axillary lymph node is also depicted *(arrow)*.

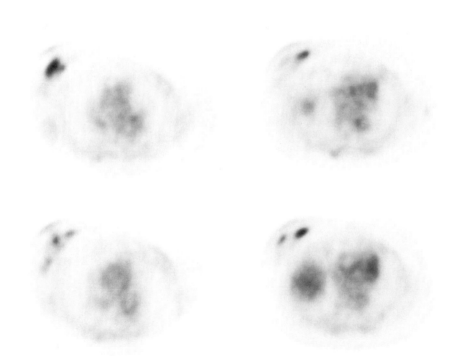

FIGURE 2. Axial PET images show the multiple metabolically active disease foci in the right breast.

CASE 7 | *Breast cancer restaging, neoadjuvantly treated infiltrating lobular carcinoma, with diffuse blastic bone metastases*

A 63-year-old woman was diagnosed with left breast cancer when she palpated a breast lump with nipple inversion. A 2-cm mass was confirmed on mammography in the upper outer quadrant. At the time of the initial oncologic evaluation, she had a large, palpable breast mass and palpable left axillary and supraclavicular adenopathy. She was evaluated for neoadjuvant therapy. A needle biopsy specimen was suggestive of infiltrating lobular carcinoma, with cell crush artifact. A bone scan showed no evidence of osseous metastatic disease (Figure 1). However, radiographs and spine MRI demonstrated diffuse blastic metastases (Figures 2 and 3). Small lung nodules were also noted on CT, suggesting lung metastases.

The patient was treated with neoadjuvant chemotherapy, with four cycles of doxorubicin/cyclophosphamide (Adriamycin/Cytoxan) and four cycles of taxane, with a marked decline in the size of the palpable breast mass and resolution of the axillary adenopathy. She then underwent PET scan before mastectomy. The patient's diffuse, confluent bony metastases were manifested only by a subtle, mottled, generalized increase in marrow activity (Figure 4). Localized left breast activity was seen at the level of the residual breast mass (Figures 5 and 6). Pathology from the mastectomy specimen showed a 1-cm residual infiltrating lobular carcinoma, moderately differentiated, with 17 of 17 lymph nodes positive.

TEACHING POINTS

This case serves to remind us of the myriad manifestations of bone metastases on different imaging modalities and to reinforce their complementary roles. That not all bone metastases are visible on bone scanning is well known, with visibility dependent on the lesion size

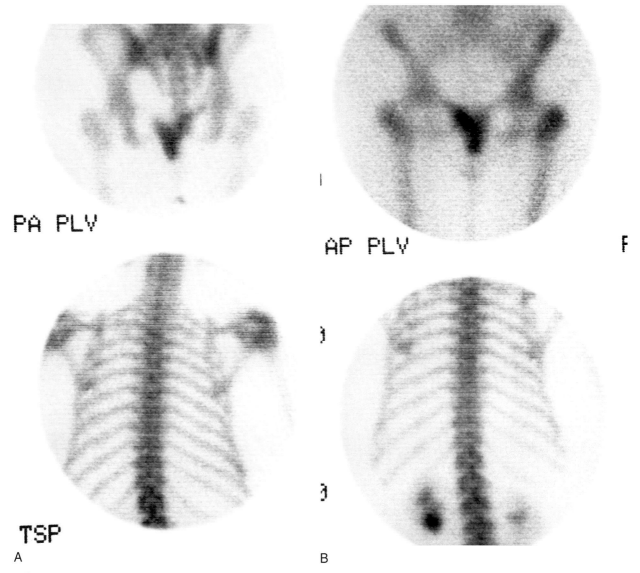

FIGURE 1. **A** and **B**, Posterior spine and anterior and posterior views of the pelvis from a bone scan show no evidence of osseous metastatic disease. Pelvic floor relaxation is noted from the bladder configuration and position. Kidneys are readily visualized, indicating this is not a superscan with the intensity poorly adjusted.

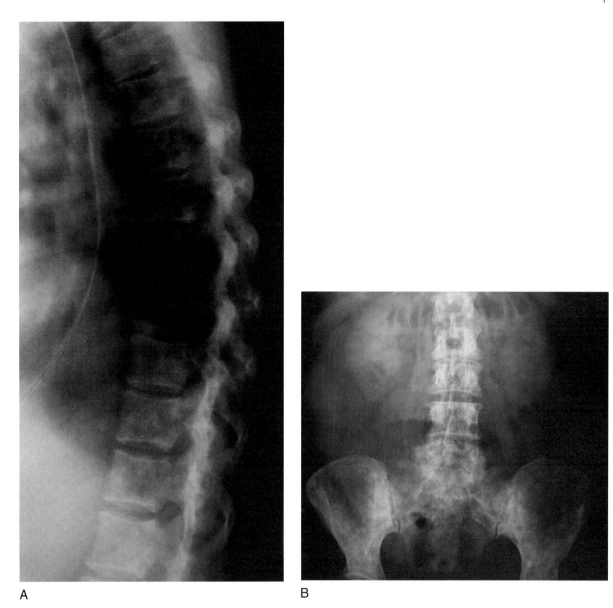

FIGURE 2. Radiographs (lateral thoracolumbar spine [**A**] and anteroposterior lumbar spine [**B**]) show obvious diffuse, blastic bone metastases.

and position, as well as the bone reaction elicited. In the case of breast cancer particularly, purely osteolytic metastases may be unappreciated on bone scan while osteoblastic lesions are generally readily visualized. However, here is a case in which the osteoblastic metastases are so extensive and confluent that they are obvious by x-ray and MRI but severely underestimated and overlooked by bone scintigraphy and subtle at best on PET. To some degree, our ability to identify a bone lesion depends on it contrasting to adjacent normal bone. Presumably, the extreme confluency of this osseous metastatic process contributed to the apparent normalcy of the skeletal findings on bone scan. Even on PET, the findings are subtle and may have been overlooked had the observer not been armed with the MRI information. On PET, this patient's diffuse blastic metastases manifested as an overall increase in bone marrow activity, with subtle slight increase in heterogeneity.

One useful practical clue to help in identifying these abnormalities is the ease of visualization of the sternum. The normal sternum is often difficult to discretely visualize, so the ease with which it is seen here is an important indication that the bone marrow is abnormal.

It is also interesting to note in this case that PET successfully demonstrated the patient's small (1 cm) residual infiltrating lobular carcinoma, after completion of chemotherapy and near-complete regression of the palpable mass clinically. One may speculate whether some of the unique features of this case may be related to the fact that this patient's primary tumor is infiltrating lobular carcinoma (ILC) rather than the more common infiltrating ductal carcinoma (IDC). In situ, IDC is more reliably demonstrable on PET imaging than ILC. On mammography, ILC can be notoriously difficult to recognize. It may present only as subtle architectural distortion, without a distinct mass.

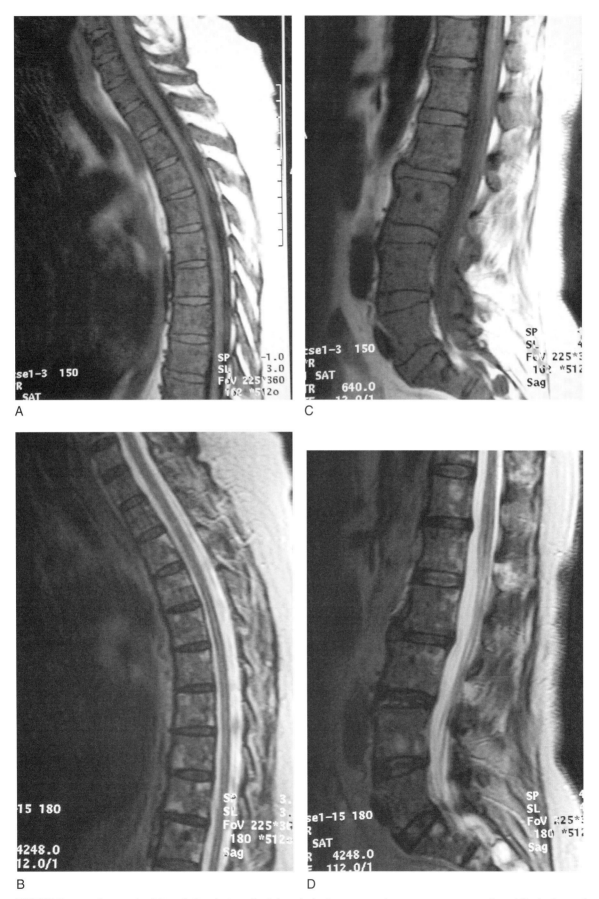

FIGURE 3. Sagittal T1-weighted (**A** and **C**) and T2-weighted (**B** and **D**) FSE sequences from a spine survey MRI show diffusely abnormal hypointense and heterogeneous bone marrow signal intensity, consistent with diffuse, confluent blastic metastases.

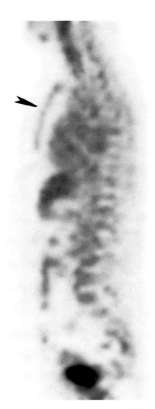

FIGURE 4. Sagittal view from PET scan shows subtle corresponding heterogeneously increased bone marrow activity, best appreciated by the ease of visualization of the sternum (*arrowhead*).

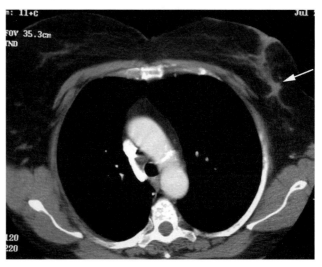

FIGURE 6. Enhanced chest CT image corresponding to the axial PET section (Figure 5C) shows the left breast cancer mass, with nipple retraction (*arrow*).

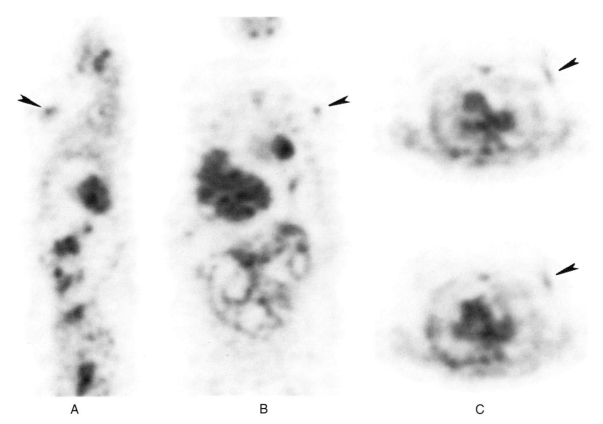

A   B   C

FIGURE 5. Sagittal (**A**), coronal (**B**), and axial (**C**) PET scan images through the left breast show focal activity in the lateral breast at the site of the known infiltrating lobular carcinoma (*arrowhead*).

CASE 8 | Breast cancer restaging, bone metastases

A 41-year-old woman with breast cancer and bone metastases was referred for PET imaging to assess her disease activity. The patient's right breast carcinoma was diagnosed 3 years before, with 15 positive lymph nodes. She was treated with mastectomy, lymph node dissection, chemotherapy, irradiation, and high-dose chemotherapy and stem cell transplantation. Seven months before PET imaging, bone scan showed evidence of metastases (Figure 1), confirmed radiographically (Figure 2). She was treated by irradiation to the right proximal femur and T10. PET scan identified multiple abnormalities, localizing to bone and consistent with metastases (Figure 3). Progression of osseous metastases was confirmed on a repeat bone scan 18 months later (Figure 4).

TEACHING POINTS

PET scanning can be useful in assessing the current activity of breast cancer metastases, particularly previously treated lesions. Bone metastases can be intrinsically lytic, sclerotic, or mixed, and sclerosis of a lesion can develop as a response to treatment. Bone scans may be confusing in assessing the status of breast metastases, because lytic foci may be underestimated and responding treated lesions may initially exhibit increased activity ("flare response").

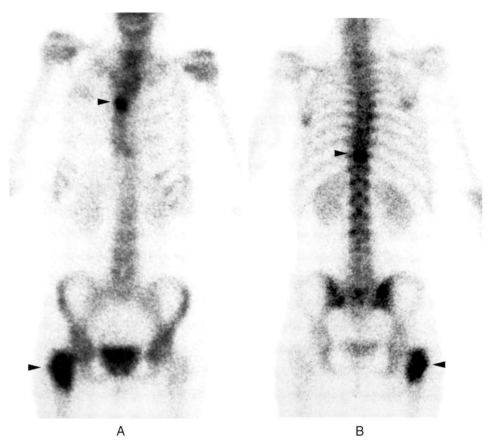

A   B

FIGURE 1. Anterior (**A**) and posterior (**B**) images from a whole-body bone scan show abnormally increased activity in the sternum, right proximal femur, and lower thoracic spine (*arrowheads*).

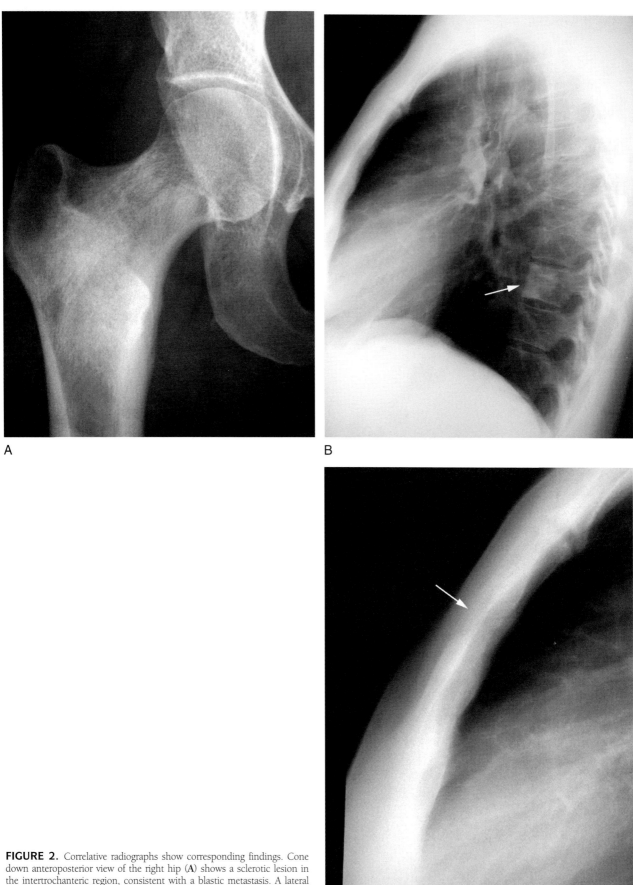

FIGURE 2. Correlative radiographs show corresponding findings. Cone down anteroposterior view of the right hip (**A**) shows a sclerotic lesion in the intertrochanteric region, consistent with a blastic metastasis. A lateral CXR (**B**) shows a sclerotic lower thoracic focus (*arrow*), and there is subtle lytic destruction of the sternum (**C**, *arrow*).

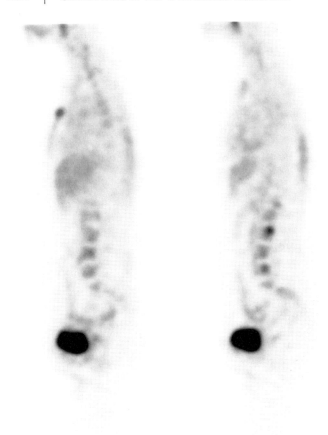

FIGURE 3. Two sagittal sections from the PET scan show hypermetabolic foci in the upper sternum and the lumbar spine, consistent with bone metastases. Lower thoracic bone marrow is not visualized, owing to radiation. Note increased activity of skin at irradiated levels.

BONE SCAN

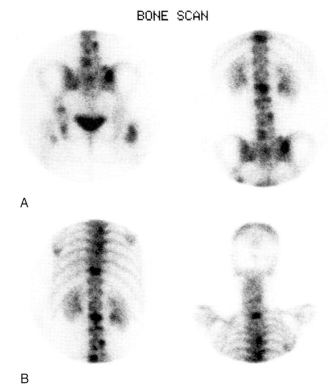

A

B

FIGURE 4. A and B, Subsequent bone scan (18 months later) shows progression to much more extensive osseous metastatic disease.

CASE 9 | *Breast cancer restaging, active bone metastases, treated liver metastases*

A 63-year-old woman with breast cancer, metastatic to bone and liver (Figures 1 to 3), was evaluated with PET when her previously declining serum tumor marker rebounded. Her diagnosis of breast cancer on the right was 3 years before and was treated with mastectomy. Three of 15 axillary lymph nodes were positive, and she underwent irradiation and chemotherapy. Subsequently, metastases were identified on bone scan when she was evaluated for fatigue and right groin pain (Figures 1 and 2). Development of liver metastases was confirmed by biopsy (Figure 3). About a year before PET scanning, the patient developed a pathologic femoral neck fracture, which was treated with femoral head replacement. At the time of PET scan evaluation, her tumor marker, which had been as high as 1000 the year before and had declined as low as 100 on weekly chemotherapy, rebounded to 150.

PET scan showed multiple foci of abnormal activity, all localizing to bone and correlating with persistent bone scan abnormalities (Figure 5). The liver showed no evidence of metastases, which correlated with the regressing findings on serial abdominal CTs (Figure 4). An additional PET finding was left upper extremity vascular activity, thought most likely to be phlebitis from the patient's weekly chemotherapy.

TEACHING POINTS

PET scan provided an alternative means to CT, bone scan, and serum tumor marker follow-up to assess the status of this patient's metastatic disease. At the time of PET scanning, the patient had been undergoing weekly chemotherapy for a year, with encouraging declines in her serum tumor marker and progressive regression by CT of her liver metastases. However, as is frequently the case, her liver lesions

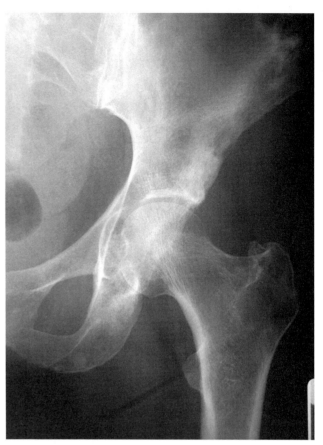

FIGURE 2. Cone down radiographic view of the left hip for correlation shows sclerotic metastases in the ilium and ischium, corresponding to bone scan findings.

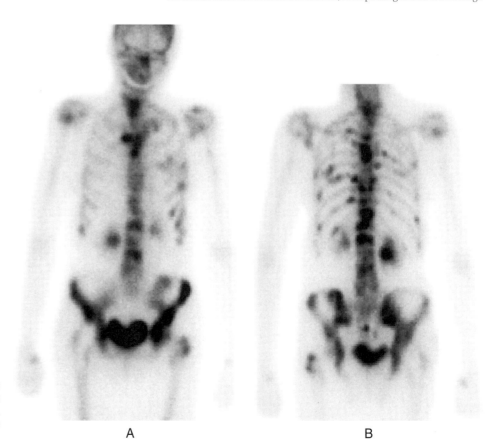

FIGURE 1. Anterior (**A**) and posterior (**B**) views from a bone scan, showing extensive metastases, especially involving the spine, pelvis, and ribs. Right femoral head has been replaced, owing to a pathologic fracture.

A   B

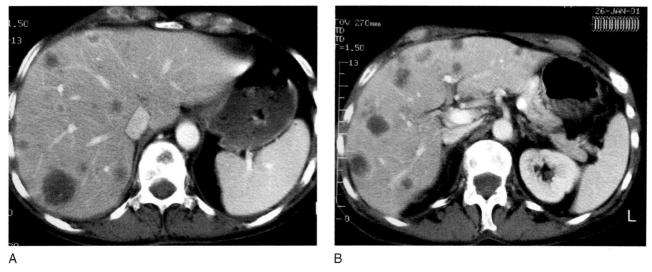

FIGURE 3. **A** and **B,** Enhanced abdominal CT images from 1 year before, showing multiple rim enhancing necrotic metastases. Three separate lesions were histologically sampled for confirmation of suspected metastases.

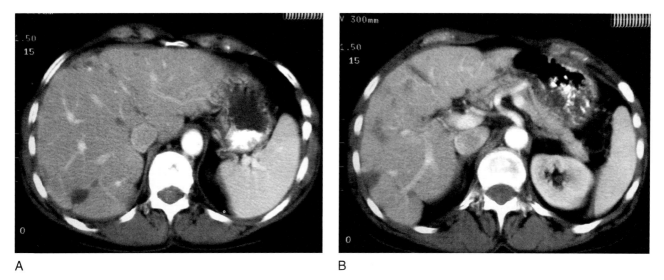

FIGURE 4. **A** and **B,** Counterpart enhanced abdominal CT images, 1 year later. The patient had been undergoing weekly chemotherapy. Findings of liver metastases are markedly improved. Some lesions have resolved; others have shrunk. Hypointense lesion residuals, with capsular retraction, at the site of some of the larger metastases, produce a "pseudo-cirrhosis" appearance of the liver.

regressed to a point, leaving the continuing question of whether the remaining findings are merely scar-like residua or active metastases. Her persistent bone scan abnormalities suggested that her bone metastases were not responding in keeping with the liver. PET provided an elegant means of addressing both questions in a whole-body modality and confirmed that her bony metastatic disease was active and even more extensive than demonstrated on bone scan. It also laid to rest the question of the significance of the residual liver CT findings.

Breast cancer bone metastases can be lytic, sclerotic, or mixed. In addition, initially lytic metastases can develop sclerosis as a treatment response, producing the "flare response" on bone scan. In general, bone scanning is most sensitive for identification of blastic metastases and may underestimate purely lytic disease. The converse is true of PET scanning, with PET being more sensitive to detection of lytic metastases than blastic. However, PET clearly can in some instances visualize blastic metastases, as demonstrated in this case.

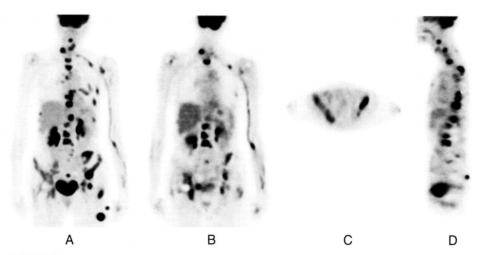

A   B   C   D

FIGURE 5. Coronally oriented projection image (**A**) and volume images in three planes (coronal, **B**; transaxial, **C**; and sagittal, **D**) show extensive PET scan abnormalities. Essentially all hypermetabolic abnormalities localize to bone. Correlation with the bone scan suggests even more active osseous metastatic foci than previously demonstrated. Foci apparently in the chest on the projection image prove on review to be in thoracic spine and ribs. The liver was normal in appearance on PET scan. Small active foci appearing to be on the liver surface in the projection image are in ribs. Coronal projection and volume images also visualize the left arm venous system, which is not normally seen. Phlebitis secondary to weekly chemotherapy was thought the most likely etiology.

CASE 10 | *Recurrent breast cancer, with extensive liver metastases*

A 68-year-old woman with a history of breast cancer was evaluated with bone scan and spine MRI when she developed back pain while lifting a box. Her breast cancer had been diagnosed the year before as a multifocal infiltrating ductal carcinoma, which was ultimately treated with a modified left radical mastectomy. Two of 26 lymph nodes demonstrated tumor. The patient declined chemotherapy and discontinued tamoxifen after 2 weeks.

Her bone scan showed intensely increased activity at the T11 level (Figure 1). A subsequent spine MRI showed findings of a pathologic compression fracture at this level, with complete replacement of the normal marrow (Figure 2). In addition, the scout view obtained on this study showed multiple hepatic lesions, indicating liver metastases (Figure 3). These were subsequently confirmed on CT (Figure 4). PET imaging showed corresponding findings, with the liver nearly replaced by hypermetabolic metastatic lesions (Figure 5). Radiation therapy was given to the lower thoracic spine for symptom palliation. Chemotherapy was also begun.

About 8 months later, the patient complained of dizziness, ataxia, and headache. MRI confirmed intracranial metastases, and the patient was treated with whole-brain radiotherapy.

TEACHING POINTS

When in the evaluation of a patient with cancer is PET scanning indicated? Arguably, in this patient, PET added only incremental information. In an era of limited resources, the request for a PET scan should be critically reviewed. The reader must be familiar with the tumor under investigation, the limitations and strengths of PET, and the potential impact on patient management of study results. The major strengths of PET include the potential for change in patient management, avoidance of noncurative, potentially morbid surgeries and invasive procedures, and the ability to accurately survey the entire body with one test (which may find disease before conventional imaging studies).

Although some may argue that the only measure of a test's value is an ultimate reduction in disease-specific mortality, most see tremendous benefit in improved patient management. PET has clearly demonstrated its ability to accurately stage disease, alter therapeutic decisions, and be cost effective.

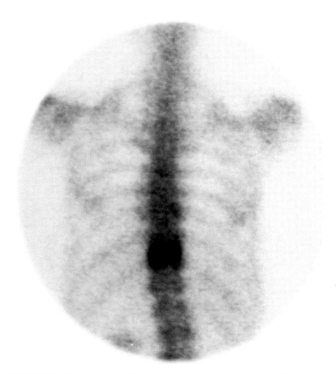

FIGURE 1. Posterior view of the thoracic spine from a whole-body bone scan shows intensely increased activity at the T11 level.

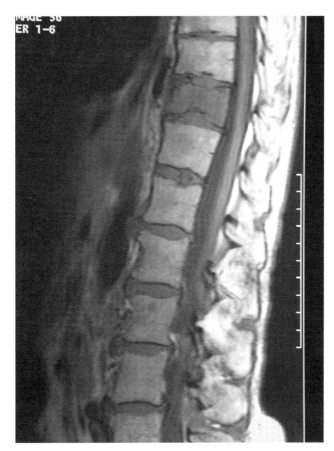

FIGURE 2. T1-weighted sagittal MR image shows the T11 vertebral body marrow signal to be replaced, and the centrum has lost height, consistent with a pathologic compression fracture. A small hypointense additional lesion is noted at L3, consistent with another bone metastasis.

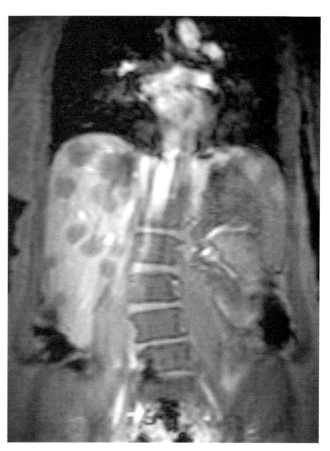

FIGURE 3. The coronal scout view from the spine MRI shows multiple focal liver lesions, consistent with metastases.

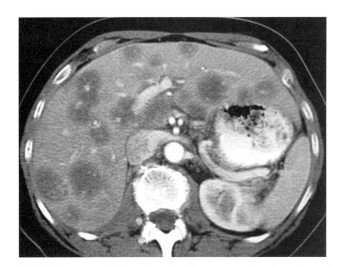

FIGURE 4. Innumerable hypodense liver lesions are confirmed on enhanced CT, consistent with metastases.

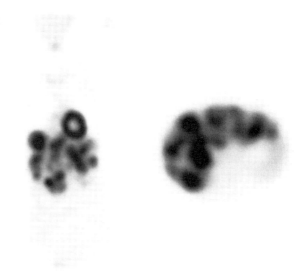

FIGURE 5. PET images in coronal and axial planes show the liver to be filled with hypermetabolic metastases.

CASE 11 | Breast cancer restaging, solitary liver metastasis

A 47-year-old woman with left breast carcinoma diagnosed 2 years before was treated with lumpectomy, one dose of doxorubicin (Adriamycin), radiation therapy, and 9 months of tamoxifen. She was referred for PET imaging based on suspicion of recurrence with a rising tumor marker level. PET imaging identified a solitary hypermetabolic lesion in the liver, consistent with a metastasis (Figure 1).

TEACHING POINTS

PET was utilized as a whole-body search method looking for recurrent disease and serves to direct subsequent imaging.

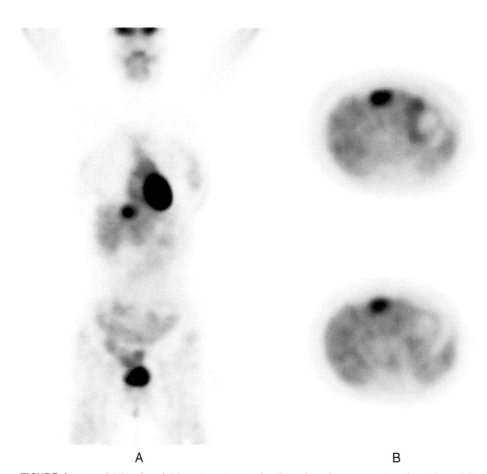

A   B

FIGURE 1. Coronal (**A**) and axial (**B**) PET scan images identify a solitary liver metastasis as the etiology of this patient's rising serum tumor marker. Low-level, post-surgical scar activity is noted in the left breast on the coronal view.

CASE 12 | Recurrent breast cancer, with chest wall and lung parenchymal disease

A 62-year-woman was evaluated with PET imaging when a right chest wall recurrence of breast cancer was confirmed by biopsy. She had originally been diagnosed with breast cancer 14 years before, with a right axillary presentation. After 18 months of chemotherapy, she underwent bilateral mastectomy and reconstruction. Two weeks before the PET scan, a palpable lump of the right chest wall was sampled and malignancy confirmed. The patient noted fullness in the supraclavicular and infraclavicular regions, suggesting adenopathy. Multiple foci of abnormal activity were confirmed on PET imaging in the right chest wall, axilla, and supraclavicular and infraclavicular regions (Figure 1). An additional probable lung nodule was noted in the posterior periphery of the right upper lobe (Figure 2). A chest CT was obtained subsequently and showed a corresponding irregularly marginated nodule (Figure 3). The appearance of the lung nodule suggested a small bronchogenic carcinoma, with breast cancer metastasis in the differential diagnosis. Underlying emphysema was evident of the lungs, and the patient was known to be a heavy smoker. Small right chest wall nodules corresponded to the PET scan findings (Figure 4). The patient was begun on chemotherapy. A repeat chest CT, 4 months later, suggested a possible slight increase in the size of the lung nodule. At that point,

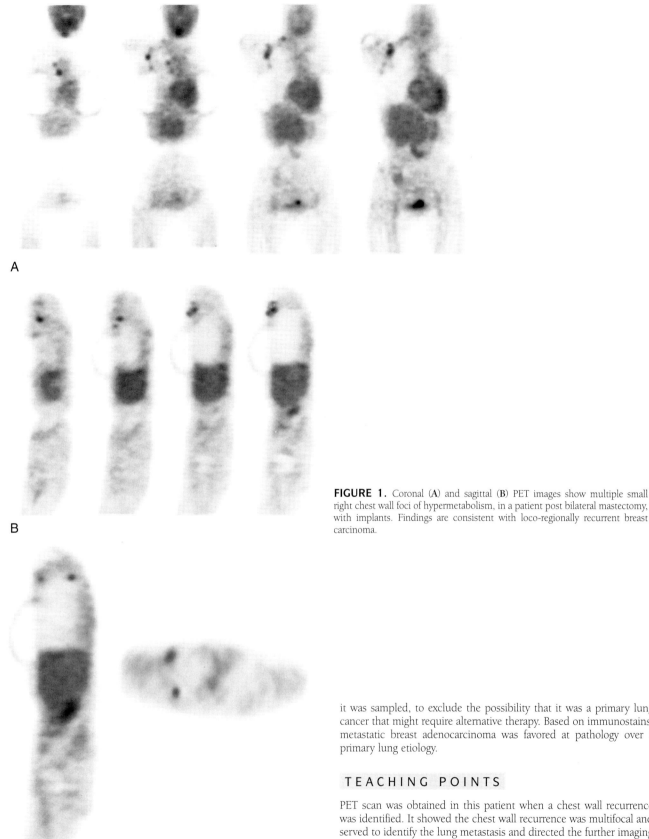

FIGURE 1. Coronal (**A**) and sagittal (**B**) PET images show multiple small right chest wall foci of hypermetabolism, in a patient post bilateral mastectomy, with implants. Findings are consistent with loco-regionally recurrent breast carcinoma.

FIGURE 2. Sagittal (**A**) and corresponding axial (**B**) PET images show an additional posterior right upper lobe lung hypermetabolic nodule, suggesting with the other findings a lung parenchymal metastasis.

it was sampled, to exclude the possibility that it was a primary lung cancer that might require alternative therapy. Based on immunostains, metastatic breast adenocarcinoma was favored at pathology over a primary lung etiology.

TEACHING POINTS

PET scan was obtained in this patient when a chest wall recurrence was identified. It showed the chest wall recurrence was multifocal and served to identify the lung metastasis and directed the further imaging restaging with CT. With knowledge of the PET scan information, the significance of the small right chest wall nodules can be fully appreciated. Without the PET data, an interpreter's attention is likely to be monopolized by the lungs and mediastinum, and the significance of the chest wall findings might well be overlooked (as it was in this case).

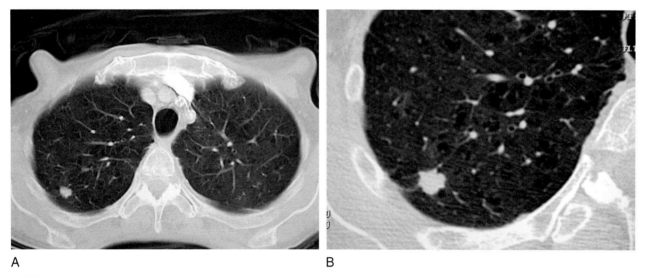

A   B

FIGURE 3. **A** and **B**, Chest CT lung windows confirm an irregularly marginated posterior RUL lung nodule. Lobular, irregular margins and background lung emphysema are best seen on the high-resolution detail view (**B**).

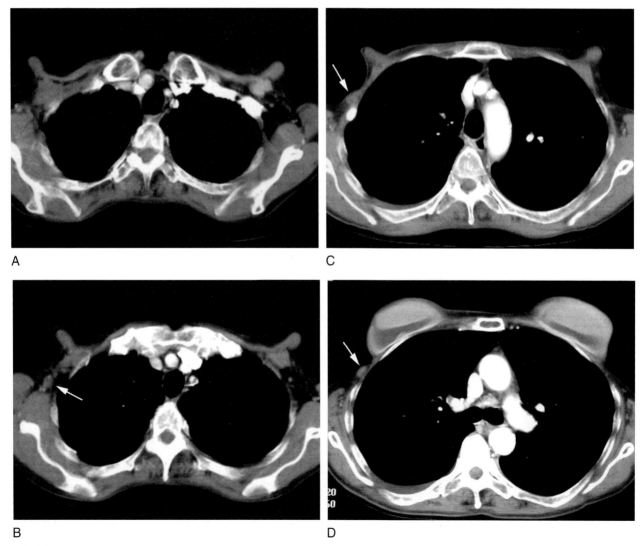

A   C

B   D

FIGURE 4. Enhanced chest CT images, from **A** to **D**, show asymmetrical right chest wall findings, above and lateral to the breast implant. These include multiple small (1 cm) nodules (*arrows*).

CASE 13 | Breast cancer restaging, axillary and chest wall involvement, and bone metastases

A 76-year-old woman with breast cancer bone metastases was referred for PET imaging for suspected recurrence. The patient was diagnosed with breast cancer 16 months before and underwent right mastectomy. Four of 12 lymph nodes were positive at the time of surgery. At the time of diagnosis and staging, her bone scan was negative. However, within 3 months, her bone scan changed and osseous metastases were suspected (Figure 1). Accordingly, she was treated postoperatively with chemotherapy and irradiation. Radiation therapy finished about a month before PET imaging, at which time chest wall recurrence was suspected based on a palpable parasternal lump. PET scan showed left axillary and chest wall hypermetabolic disease foci, as well as activity in rib metastases (Figure 2). PET scan findings were corroborated by findings on CXR and chest CT (Figures 3 to 5).

TEACHING POINT

Locally recurrent disease was suspected clinically in this patient at the time of PET imaging, based on a palpable parasternal nodule. PET scanning was able to confirm the local disease, including demonstrating disease in the axilla, where only mildly abnormal findings were depicted on CT. Rib and chest wall involvement are clearly demonstrated as well.

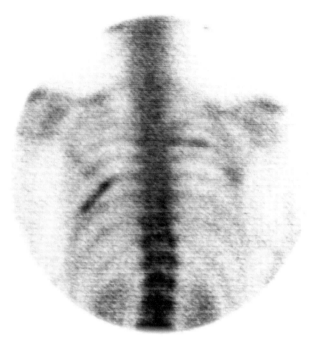

FIGURE 1. Posterior image of the thorax from a bone scan shows scintigraphic evidence of rib metastases, with long segments of abnormally increased activity in right sixth and left eighth ribs.

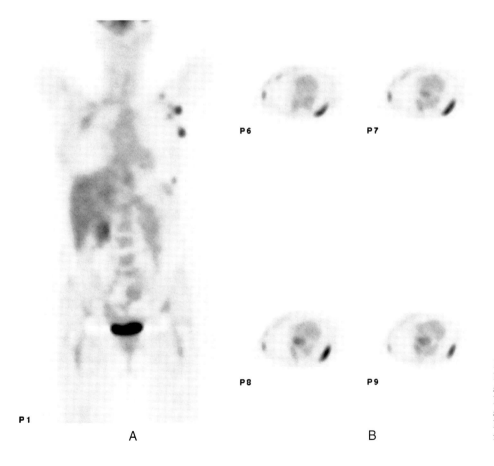

A

B

FIGURE 2. Coronal (**A**) and four axial (**B**) PET images show metabolically active left axillary and chest wall foci, consistent with locally recurrent disease. Axial sections show a long, curvilinear left posterior chest wall hypermetabolic focus, consistent with a rib metastasis, as suggested by bone scan.

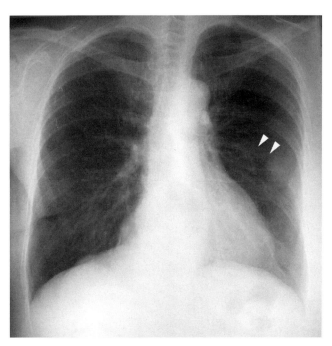

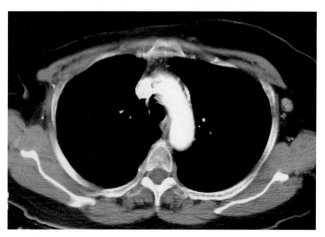

FIGURE 5. An additional chest CT section shows a round, minimally enlarged left axillary lymph node, corresponding to the PET scan.

FIGURE 3. Correlation was also made with this frontal CXR, showing indistinctness and lytic destruction of the left posterior eighth rib (*arrowheads*).

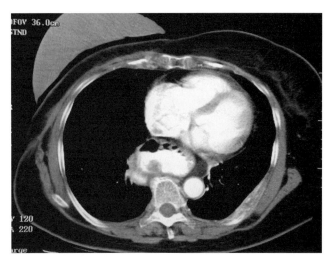

FIGURE 4. Chest CT section corresponding to the above shows lytic change and soft tissue replacement and expansion of the left posterior rib. The patient has undergone a right mastectomy and a prosthesis is in place. A large hiatal hernia is incidentally noted.

CASE 14 | *Breast cancer restaging, extensive local and nodal recurrence*

A 56-year-old woman presented with a 2-year history of breast cancer with multiple local recurrences. Her initial right lumpectomy 2 years before was for a 3-cm tumor. The margins were not clear, nor were they clear at reoperation 6 months later. Three months afterward, she underwent mastectomy with TRAM flap reconstruction. One involved axillary lymph node was noted. Radiation therapy was declined. The patient did undergo chemotherapy with paclitaxel (Taxol) for six cycles. Six months before presentation to a new oncologist and referral for PET scanning, a biopsy-proven TRAM flap suture line recurrence was confirmed. She chose to undergo alternative therapies in Mexico, including hyperthermia and ozone immunobooster, prior to presentation. Her physical examination identified 2- to 3-cm right axillary lymph nodes, right infraclavicular firmness, and a hard 2.5-cm mass in the midst of the reconstructed right breast. PET scan confirmed extensive disease involving the reconstructed right breast and chest wall, right axilla, and internal mammary and anterior mediastinal nodal stations (Figures 1 to 3). The patient declined additional chemotherapy and was referred for irradiation.

TEACHING POINTS

The patient presented with clinically advanced disease by physical examination. Just how extensive the process was became fully evident with PET scanning.

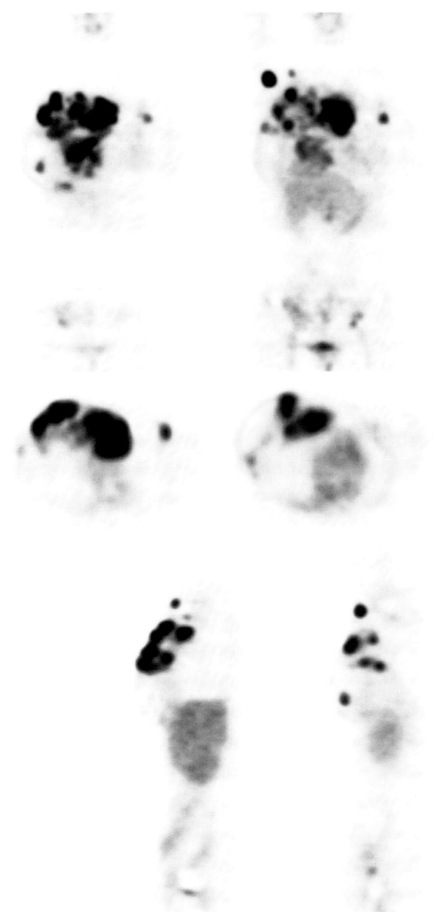

FIGURE 1. Two coronal PET images show advanced locally recurrent disease involving the reconstructed right breast, chest wall, axilla, and infraclavicular regions. A left breast focus of disease activity is also noted.

FIGURE 2. Axial PET sections allow more precise localization of the disease sites. The large midline hypermetabolic mass is within the chest and corresponds to prevascular anterior mediastinal adenopathy reported on an outside CT scan. The most extensive disease activity appears to be in the chest wall.

FIGURE 3. Two sagittal PET sections through the right breast show disease activity both within the reconstructed breast and axilla and extensively involving the skin.

CASE 15 | *Breast cancer restaging, local and nodal recurrences in axilla, supraclavicular neck, and mediastinum*

A 45-year-old woman with porphyria presented with a history of cancer of the left breast and was evaluated with PET for a clinically suspected recurrence. The diagnosis of breast cancer was made 9 months before by fine-needle aspiration of two adjacent palpable masses, although the patient was aware of a left breast mass for 2.5 years. Three months after diagnosis, following nutritional supplements only, the patient underwent surgical excision of the masses. No lymphadenectomy was performed.

At the time of referral for PET scan (7 months after surgical excision), the patient had found the week before a new palpable left breast mass, superolateral to the nipple, and noted progressive left axillary aching. PET scans showed focal intense left lateral breast activity at the site of the palpable lump, as well as multiple additional, presumably nodal, foci of activity (Figures 1 and 2). These abnormalities were noted in the left axilla and infraclavicular and supraclavicular regions, as well as in the subcarinal mediastinum and right hilus. Pulmonary parenchymal disease was also suggested.

TEACHING POINTS

PET scanning in this patient, with a history of porphyria and a holistic bent, allowed her new oncologist to noninvasively assess the

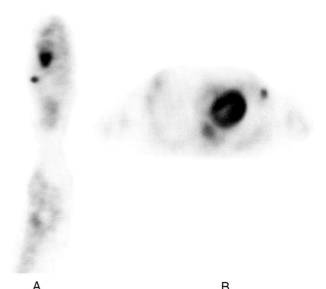

A   **B**

FIGURE 1. Sagittal (**A**) and axial (**B**) PET sections show an intense small focus of activity in the left lateral breast, at the site of the palpable local recurrence. In addition, the sagittal view also shows a larger hypermetabolic left axillary focus of metastatic disease.

full extent of her current disease activity after nonstandard therapy and management.

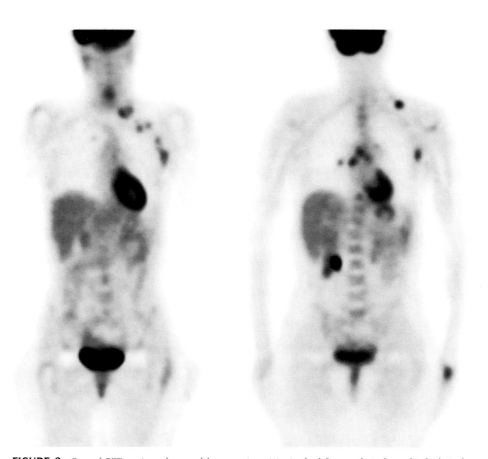

FIGURE 2. Coronal PET sections show nodal metastatic activity in the left supraclavicular and infraclavicular regions and in the left axilla. Nodal metastases are also identified in the subcarinal mediastinum and right hilus. A small, faint right upper lobe focus of pulmonary parenchymal activity suggests lung metastases as well.

CASE 16 | Breast cancer restaging for mediastinal, neck, and supraclavicular nodal recurrences

A 43-year-old woman with recurrent breast cancer was evaluated with PET for a persistent palpable left supraclavicular abnormality 1 year after finishing chemotherapy for left neck nodal disease.

The patient was first diagnosed with a 1-cm left breast infiltrating ductal carcinoma at age 32 and treated with mastectomy. Fifteen lymph nodes were negative. Two and a half years before PET scanning, left neck nodal recurrence was found and treated with 6 months of chemotherapy. Six months later, she again developed a recurrent left neck lump and was treated with an additional eight cycles of chemotherapy, which finished 1 year before. At the time of PET evaluation, she had a persistent hard, fixed palpable left supraclavicular nodule. MRI showed only a normal size (1 cm) left supraclavicular lymph node at that level (Figure 1).

PET scan confirmed a small left supraclavicular hypermetabolic nodule at the level in question (Figure 2). A trial of hormonal therapy yielded no clinical response, so 3 months later, the node was surgically excised and proven to be metastatic breast cancer. She was restarted on chemotherapy and had completed four cycles when she was re-evaluated with neck and chest MRI and PET scan. Unfortunately, these studies showed interval progression, with new prevascular mediastinal and bilateral neck and supraclavicular foci of activity on PET, which correlated with MRI masses (Figures 3 to 6).

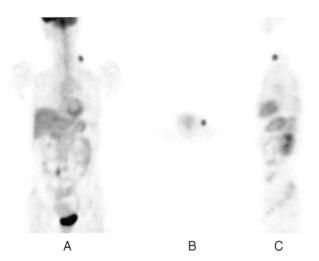

A   B   C

FIGURE 2. PET scan images show a small hypermetabolic nodule of activity at the left supraclavicular level, corresponding precisely to the normal size lymph node in question on MRI. This was subsequently excised and proven to be metastatic breast cancer. Coronal (**A**), transaxial (**B**), and sagittal (**C**) views are depicted.

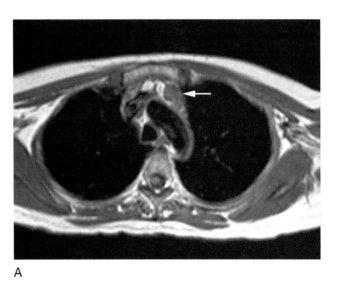

A

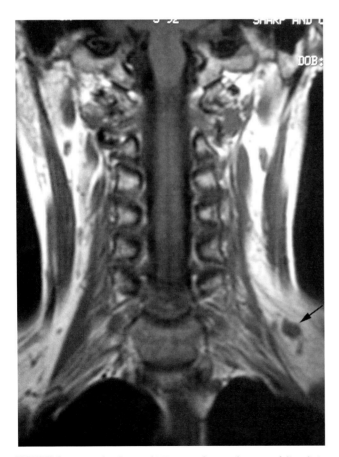

FIGURE 1. T1-weighted coronal MR image shows only a normal (1 cm) size left supraclavicular lymph node (*arrow*) and was the only MR finding relevant to the persistent palpable abnormality in this region.

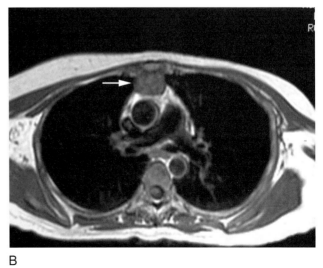

B

FIGURE 3. **A** and **B**, T1-weighted axial MR images through the superior mediastinum show two prevascular soft tissue masses (*arrows*).

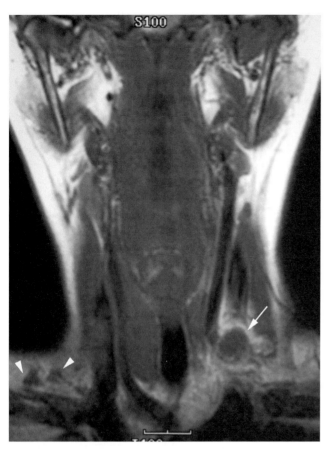

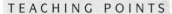

FIGURE 4. T1-weighted coronal MR image through anterior neck shows a round, new left supraclavicular nodule *(arrow)*. Smaller soft tissue nodules are noted in the right supraclavicular fat *(arrowheads)*.

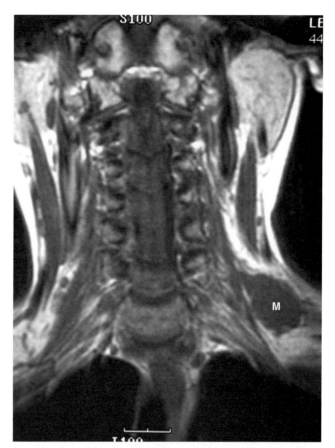

A

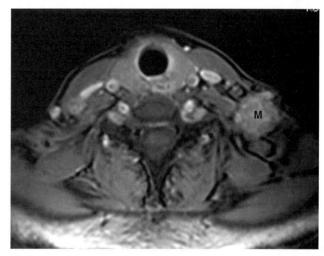

B

TEACHING POINTS

At the time of this patient's initial PET scan, she had had a protracted course with left neck recurrent disease and was left with a palpably suspicious hard and fixed left neck lump. The corresponding MRI showed only a normal size lymph node. This discordance was bridged with the addition of PET imaging, which showed this node to be intensely hypermetabolic. Metastatic breast cancer was subsequently confirmed at this site by surgical excision. PET also confirmed the progressive findings demonstrated subsequently on imaging follow-up.

FIGURE 5. T1-weighted coronal (**A**) and enhanced, fat-saturated FMPSPGR (gradient echo) (**B**) axial sequences show a new, lobular mass (M) in the left posterior triangle.

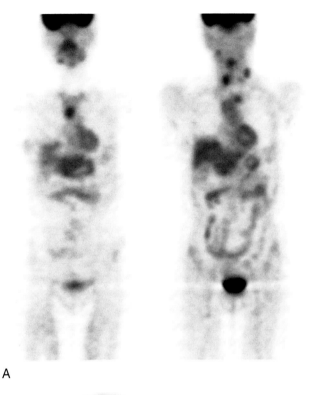

A

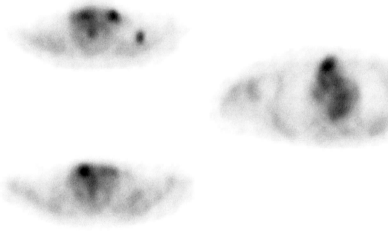

B

FIGURE 6. Corresponding coronal (**A**) and axial (**B**) PET scan images show some of the multiple new foci of activity in the anterior mediastinum and neck, corresponding to the MRI findings.

CASE 17 | *Breast cancer restaging, hilar nodal involvement, progression to liver and bone metastases*

A 68-year-old woman presented with breast cancer. The patient's initial diagnosis of node-positive disease had been made 15 years before, at which time she was treated with mastectomy, 6 months of chemotherapy, and tamoxifen. Three years before PET scan referral, metastatic brachial plexus involvement had been confirmed by exploratory surgery and treated with radiation. The patient did well for 1 year before developing worsening upper extremity symptoms. Additional chemotherapy was given, which concluded 5 months before PET scan was requested for restaging (Figure 1). Outside MRI of the brachial plexus reportedly was inconclusive. PET did not show

evidence of disease activity at the brachial plexus but did identify right hilar nodal activity. Subsequent CT did not identify pathologic findings at this level.

The patient returned 10 months later for repeat PET scan, with worsened symptoms in the hand and arm. PET scan showed progressive disease, with development of liver and bone metastases (Figures 2 and 3).

TEACHING POINTS

The brachial plexus is a difficult anatomic region to image, particularly when the region has been previously treated. This patient's persistent and progressive upper extremity symptoms drove her imaging evaluation. PET is an important adjunct to anatomic modes of imaging of the brachial plexus, because it generally is less affected by surgical or other

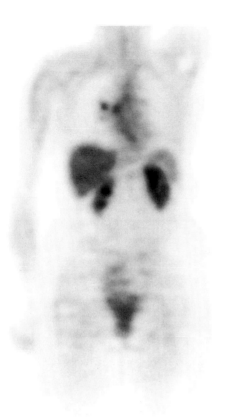

FIGURE 1. Coronal PET image shows small, discrete, presumably nodal foci of activity in the right hilus. No other suspicious finding was noted. The right brachial plexus shows no findings to particularly indicate disease activity at this level.

FIGURE 2. Follow-up PET scan, 10 months later. The right hilar activity persists. New hypermetabolic disease sites are now visualized within the liver, consistent with metastases. Increased activity is seen at the right thoracic inlet level.

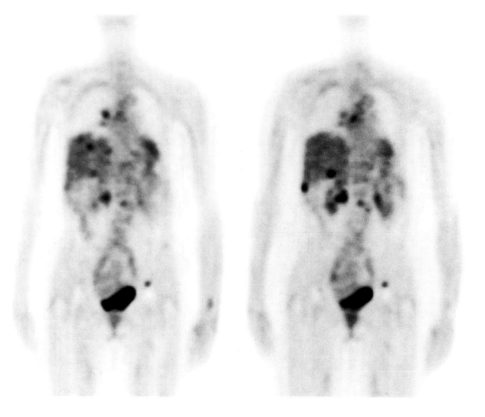

FIGURE 3. Additional coronal PET images from the follow-up study show more liver lesions, as well as other sites of activity, including in the right hilus and subcarinal region. A new metastatic focus is also seen at the left acetabular level.

treatment interventions and can identify disease before tumor nodules or masses are pathologically enlarged. Of course, size limitations apply here as elsewhere with PET; and if a process is infiltrative or subcentimeter in size, it may not be identified.

In this case, the initial PET scan showed evidence of disease only at the right hilar level. However, because no pathologically enlarged lymph nodes were found on a subsequent CT, these were observed, with no additional diagnostic procedures or therapy. The follow-up PET study 10 months later showed disease progression, both in the mediastinum and hilus, as well as new disease in the liver and bone.

CASE 18 | Restaging, thoracic (nodal and pulmonary parenchymal) metastases

A 37-year-old woman with infiltrating ductal breast carcinoma metastatic to the thorax was referred for PET imaging to assess disease activity. She had initially been diagnosed about 3 and a half years before when she palpated a right breast mass soon after delivering a child. Pathology showed the tumor to be 4 × 3 × 2.5 cm, with a completely excised extensive intraductal component and negative margins. Histologically, the tumor displayed poor differentiation, with a high mitotic rate and marked nuclear pleomorphism. Axillary node dissection revealed tumor in 1 of 18 lymph nodes. Adjuvant chemotherapy with four cycles of doxorubicin (Adriamycin) and cyclophosphamide (Cytoxan), followed by four cycles of paclitaxel (Taxol), was completed 2 years before. Relapse was diagnosed about a year and a half before in the mediastinum and lungs and confirmed by percutaneous lung biopsy. This was treated with a variety of chemotherapeutic regimens, which were altered when CT showed progression in response. The most recent CT had shown stability to slight decrease in one nodule. PET scanning was requested to assess the disease activity and extent. It showed precise concordance with the chest CT findings, with subcarinal and right hilar nodal foci of activity and multiple metabolically active pulmonary nodules (Figures 1 to 7).

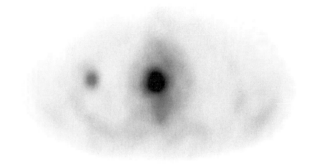

FIGURE 2. Axial PET image through the mediastinum shows hypermetabolism of a subcarinal nodal mass, as well as in a right lower lobe nodule.

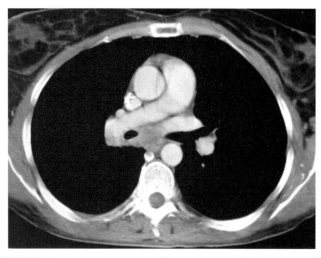

FIGURE 3. Corresponding enhanced chest CT image shows the enlarged subcarinal nodal mass.

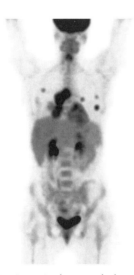

FIGURE 1. Projection image in the coronal plane shows hypermetabolic disease activity in the subcarinal mediastinum and right hilus, with bilateral lower lobe hypermetabolic metastatic lung nodules.

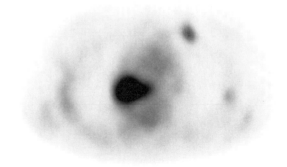

FIGURE 4. A more inferior axial PET section shows a hypermetabolic right hilar nodal mass, as well as two metabolically active left lower lung nodules.

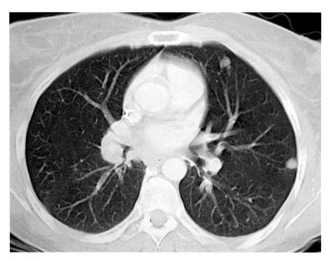

FIGURE 5. Corresponding chest CT lung window at the same level shows the right hilar enlargement and the 1-cm metastatic left lung nodules.

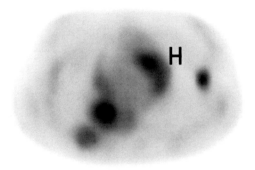

FIGURE 6. A more inferior axial PET image, through the heart (H), shows increased metabolic activity of two adjacent, larger right lower lobe lung masses, as well as an additional left lower lobe metastatic nodule.

TEACHING POINTS

PET was utilized in this case as an alternative to anatomic imaging in the assessment of disease response to chemotherapy. It clearly demonstrates all the patient's measurable disease to be metabolically active and viable tumor. The longitudinal follow-up of measurable lesions on CT can be difficult at times, requiring bidimensional measurements and comparison. At times, it may be hard to say by measurements alone whether there has been a response, owing to differences in sectioning, slice thickness, and depth of respiration.

There are emerging data that standardized uptake value (SUV) measurements may be of value in serial assessment of response to therapy. With careful attention to imaging variables (including injected dose, plasma glucose level, reproducible uptake phase, timing of study after therapy, and use of attenuation corrected images), changes in SUVs may prove to be a very accurate method to evaluate treatment changes.

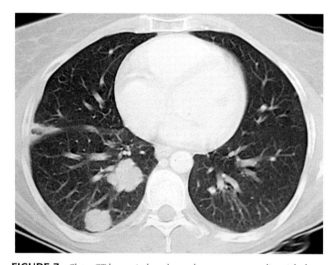

FIGURE 7. Chest CT lung window shows the two corresponding right lower lobe metastatic pulmonary parenchymal masses.

CASE 19 | *Breast cancer restaging, assessment of chemotherapy efficacy, mediastinal and bone metastases*

A 54-year-old woman with a 15-year history of breast cancer and bone metastases presented for PET scan assessment of her disease status. Her initial diagnosis of right breast cancer was treated with lumpectomy and irradiation. Local recurrence 4 years later was treated with bilateral mastectomy with reconstruction and chemotherapy. Bone metastases developed 4 years later and were treated with tamoxifen,

oophorectomy, and chemotherapy, which induced remission. About 8 months before the current evaluation, a rising carcinoembryonic antigen (CEA) level prompted re-investigation. Bone scan showed new evidence of metastases, for which the patient was started on anastrozole (Arimidex) and pamidronate (Aredia). However, the CEA level continued to rise and the patient was switched to exemestane (Aromasin). A repeat bone scan reportedly was stable. The patient was referred at this point to assess her disease activity.

PET scan identified multiple hypermetabolic foci, consistent with metastases (Figure 1). These localized both to bone and to mediastinum. She was treated with two courses of docetaxel (Taxotere),

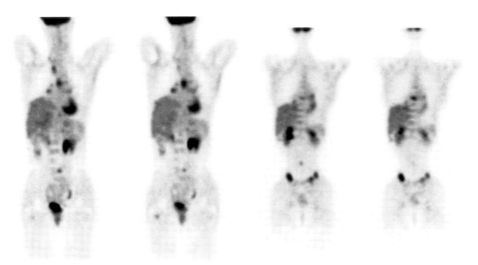

FIGURE 1. Coronal PET sections show multiple hypermetabolic disease sites. In the chest, activity is noted in nodal regions of the mediastinum, including the right paratracheal, subcarinal, and right hilar levels. The most posterior section *(right)* shows a thoracic focus localizing to spine. Most other identifiable foci localize to bone, such as in the lumbar spine, ilia bilaterally, and right proximal femur.

with a decline in her CEA level; and the PET scan was repeated (Figure 2). The follow-up study showed marked interval improvement, with osseous sites of activity smaller and less intense in activity compared with the prior study, indicating a favorable response. Similarly, the mediastinal nodal disease activity showed near-complete regression.

TEACHING POINTS

PET imaging provided a whole-body method of assessing this patient's disease status, a helpful capability in a patient with such a long and complex history of multiple recurrences and therapies. It also provided an objective means of assessing the success of a new therapeutic approach.

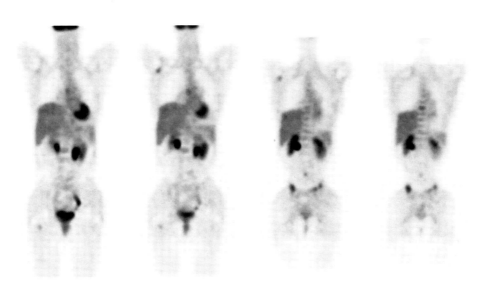

FIGURE 2. Comparable coronal PET sections from a repeat study, 2 months later after two courses of docetaxel (Taxotere), show a favorable response. Improvement is particularly notable in the mediastinum. Even osseous disease sites, including midthoracic and lumbar spine levels, and iliac pelvic bones, appear both smaller and decreased in activity.

Miscellaneous Tumors

PET has been shown to be of value in many tumors that are less common or routinely evaluated by other methods. In some cases (e.g., thyroid cancer), PET is especially useful in a particular subset of patients—those with an elevated thyroglobulin level and negative iodine-131 whole-body scan. In other cases, such as sarcoma, tumor grade plays a major role in predicting the efficacy of PET. For ovarian, cervical, and testicular cancers, PET has proven quite valuable as a "problem-solving" tool, often dramatically influencing patient management. Evidence is accumulating that PET may play an important role in the management of multiple myeloma.

There are a number of examples presented in this chapter (e.g., thymoma, transitional cell carcinoma, prostate, endometrial, and nonmelanoma skin malignancies) without accompanying introductory text. This is primarily because of the relatively small number of such cases documented in the literature. One noteworthy exception is prostate cancer, where data indicate a marginal role for FDG-PET because of low sensitivity. However, newer, non–FDG-based radiopharmaceuticals have shown promise in this common malignancy.

Relatively poor sensitivity for low metabolic rate cancers (e.g., prostate, neuroendocrine, and bronchoalveolar lung cancer) and tumors whose evaluation is hampered by physiologic activity (i.e., those of bladder and heart) has stimulated research into alternate radiopharmaceuticals and procedural modifications.

This chapter reviews the use of FDG-PET in patients with these "miscellaneous" tumors, with emphasis on the unique information provided by PET.

THYROID CANCER

There are approximately 17,000 cases of thyroid carcinoma diagnosed each year in the United States. Most patients present with a solitary nodule. The vast majority are differentiated tumors: 50% to 80% papillary and 10% to 20% follicular.

Although the outlook is generally favorable, negative prognostic factors include age at diagnosis, gender, tumor stage, and history of rapid growth. The low mortality rate of thyroid cancer is attributable to effective surgery, the subsequent use of radioactive iodine, and sensitive methods available for patient follow-up.[1] Surveillance is performed with a combination of serum thyroglobulin (Tg) measurement and imaging. Tg does not provide localization information and the test may be falsely negative in the presence of antithyroglobulin antibodies. Imaging is therefore of crucial importance. The preferred study remains the iodine-131 whole-body survey, supplemented by ultrasonography, and occasionally CT or MRI.

The less differentiated types of thyroid cancer account for a high percentage of the fatal cases. These tumors typically are unable to concentrate radioactive iodine (RAI). Additionally, nearly one fourth of patients with differentiated thyroid cancer with recurrent or metastatic disease are incapable of concentrating RAI.[2] Options for care include attempts to localize disease with other imaging modalities or treating empirically with high doses of radiolabeled iodine. The latter approach may result in reduction of Tg level, as well as identification of metastatic sites on post-therapy scans. However, evidence that this treatment provides important benefit is debatable.[3] Ultrasonography and MRI may be helpful in imaging the neck in thyroid cancer follow-up but offer only regional evaluation. Radiopharmaceuticals such as thallium, sestamibi, and tetrofosmin are relatively sensitive but are limited by lesion size and physiologic accumulation, especially below the diaphragm.

There appears to be an inverse relationship between ^{131}I uptake and FDG uptake.[1,4-6] Those tumors with little or no iodine-concentrating ability (e.g., less well-differentiated, Hürthle cell, anaplastic, medullary) typically demonstrate FDG uptake. This allows PET to image these suspected recurrences/metastases accurately and to significantly impact patient management.

Many studies have been published on the use of FDG-PET in patients with elevated Tg and negative ^{131}I scans, with sensitivities ranging from 68% to 100%.[6-11]

There is some evidence that the higher the Tg level, the more likely PET is to be positive.[1,12] Although patients have been studied under both thyroid-stimulating hormone stimulated and suppressed conditions, the current recommendation is to perform PET while the patient remains on thyroid hormone suppression. PET may be able to select patients who can benefit from curative surgery.

As with PET scanning in general, false-positive studies may occur in inflammatory sites. False-negative results are possible with lesions below the level of resolution for PET imaging (i.e., ≈1 cm), including minimal disease in cervical lymph nodes.[1] When surgical excision is planned based on a positive FDG-PET study, it is recommended that confirmatory anatomic imaging with CT or MRI be performed.

REFERENCES

1. Wang W, Macapinlac H, Larson SM, et al: [18-F]-2-fluoro-2-deoxy-D-glucose positron emission tomography localizes residual thyroid cancer in patients with negative diagnostic I-131 whole body scans and elevated serum thyroglobulin levels. J Clin Endocrinol Metab 1999;84:2291-2302.
2. Alnafisi NS, Driedger AA, Coates G, et al: FDG-PET of recurrent or metastatic I-131 negative papillary thyroid carcinoma. J Nucl Med 2000;41:1010-1015.
3. McDougall IR: I-131 Treatment of I-131 negative whole body scan and positive thyroglobulin in differentiated thyroid carcinoma: What is being treated? Thyroid 1997;7:669-672.
4. McDougall IR, Davidson J, Segall GM: Positron emission tomography of the thyroid, with an emphasis on thyroid cancer. Nucl Med Commun 2001;22:485-492.
5. Shiga T, Tsukamoto E, Nakada K, et al: Comparison of 18F-FDG, I-131 Na, and 201Tl in diagnosis of recurrent or metastatic thyroid carcinoma. J Nucl Med 2001;42:414-419.
6. Muller SP, Georges R, Brandt-Mainz K, et al: The role of FDG-PET and 201Tl imaging as a preoperative diagnostic tool in recurrent Hürthle cell carcinoma of the thyroid. J Nucl Med 2000;41:306P.
7. Diehl MS, Risse JH, Brandt-Mainz K, et al: 18F fluorodeoxyglucose positron emission tomography in medullary thyroid cancer: results of a multicentre study. J Nucl Med 2001;42:132.
8. Moog F, Linke R, Manthey N, et al: Influence of thyroid-stimulating hormone levels on uptake of FDG in recurrent and metastatic differentiated thyroid carcinoma. J Nucl Med 2000;41:1989-1995.
9. Macapinlac HA: Clinical usefulness of FDG PET in differentiated thyroid cancer. J Nucl Med 2001;42:77-78.
10. June-Key G, So Y, Lee JS, et al: Value of FDG PET in papillary thyroid carcinoma with negative I-131 whole-body scan. J Nucl Med 1999;40:986-992.
11. Grunwald F, Kalicke T, Feine U, et al: Fluorine-18 fluorodeoxyglucose positron emission tomography in thyroid cancer: results of a multicentre study. Eur J Nucl Med 1999;26:1547-1552.
12. Schluter B, Bohuslavizki KH, Beyer W, et al: Impact of FDG PET on patients with differentiated thyroid cancer who present with elevated thyroglobulin and negative I-131 scan. J Nucl Med 2001;42:71-76.

CASE 1 | Recurrent thyroid carcinoma, lungs and neck

A 62-year-old man with papillary thyroid carcinoma was reevaluated for increasing thyroglobulin. His ^{131}I whole-body scan was negative. The patient had undergone thyroidectomy 5 years previously, followed by postoperative ^{131}I therapy (200 mCi). He had been treated for recurrences with two additional 200-mCi doses of ^{131}I at 8 months and 4 years after initial therapy. At the time of the most recent ^{131}I whole-body scan, the patient's serum Tg level had risen to 753 ng/mL from less than 2 eight months earlier. PET scanning was performed to evaluate for suspected recurrence after the ^{131}I whole-body scan was negative (Figure 1).

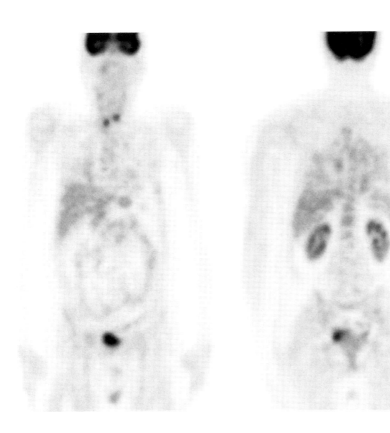

FIGURE 1. Two coronal PET scan images (right more posterior than left) show two discrete hypermetabolic foci in the low anterior neck. There also is diffuse low-level lung activity, more easily seen on the posterior image.

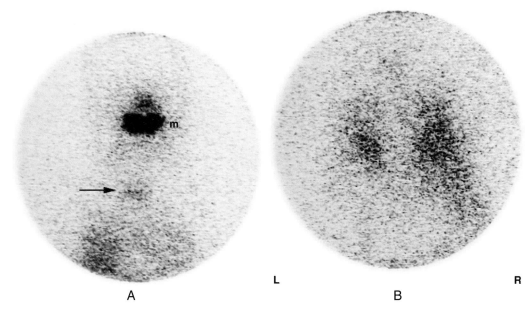

FIGURE 2. [131]I whole-body scan (anterior head and neck [**A**] and posterior chest [**B**] shown), 10 days after treatment with 206 mCi ^{131}I, shows corresponding sites of ^{131}I activity in the lungs, right greater than left, and in the low anterior neck (*arrow*). R, right; L, left; m, mouth (oropharyngeal activity).

It confirmed recurrent thyroid carcinoma with discrete hypermetabolic foci in the low anterior neck and thoracic inlet. In addition, diffuse low-level pulmonary parenchymal activity was noted (right greater than left), suggesting recurrent lung metastases. The patient was thought to have recurrent thyroid carcinoma that had dedifferentiated and no longer incorporated iodine. Because of the limited treatment options, he was re-treated with another 206 mCi of [131]I. Imaging 10 days later showed ^{131}I accumulation in distributions corresponding to the PET scan, including the superior mediastinum and lower neck, as well as the lungs (right greater than left) (Figure 2).

TEACHING POINTS

A rising serum Tg value strongly suggests recurrence of thyroid carcinoma. PET can be useful in the evaluation for recurrent thyroid cancer if the ^{131}I whole-body scan does not identify an abnormality. In this case, PET confirmed recurrent disease not identified by ^{131}I scanning. Imaging after administration of the treatment dose of ^{131}I proved that the patient's malignancy was still able to incorporate iodine. It is well recognized that higher doses of ^{131}I will demonstrate more thyroid carcinoma than smaller diagnostic doses.

The question could be raised: why not treat this patient empirically with ^{131}I, based on the suspicion of recurrence raised by the rising thyroglobulin? The answer is that PET demonstration of recurrent disease can guide therapy, depending on the number and location of recurrent disease sites. An isolated recurrence identified by PET in this scenario may preferentially be treated by surgery, rather than [131]I (see Case 2).

CASE 2 | *Recurrent thyroid carcinoma, isolated neck lymph node*

A 46-year-old woman with papillary thyroid carcinoma with lymph node involvement was treated with surgery and ^{131}I ablation with 153 mCi. A year later, she underwent an ^{131}I whole-body scan, which was negative (Figure 1). A PET scan was obtained, because her Tg level was elevated

to 70 ng/mL. PET scanning identified a solitary focus of increased activity in the left lower anterior neck, suggesting a pathologic lymph node (Figure 2). MRI was recommended for correlation, which confirmed a single, sub-centimeter lymph node at the same level (Figures 3 to 5). The patient underwent surgery, which confirmed a single lymph node with metastatic papillary thyroid cancer. The patient has shown no evidence of disease in 1.5 years of follow-up, with normal Tg levels and two subsequent negative ^{131}I whole-body scans.

TEACHING POINTS

[131]I whole-body scans remain the mainstay for follow-up evaluation of patients with the most common histologies of thyroid carcinoma (papillary and follicular). PET scan is an important modality to evaluate a subset of these patients: those with elevated Tg levels (and therefore high suspicion of residual or recurrent disease) with negative ^{131}I scans. In these patients, PET may be able to identify metastatic disease not revealed by low dose (usually 3 mCi) [131]I whole-body scans. In this particular patient, PET identified a solitary lymph node, enabling the

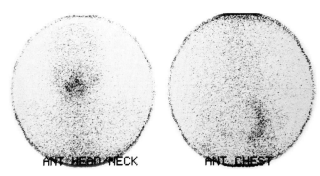

FIGURE 1. Anterior views from an ^{131}I whole-body scan show physiologic activity in the oropharynx and the stomach but no pathologic site of ^{131}I accumulation to explain the patient's elevated thyroglobulin level.

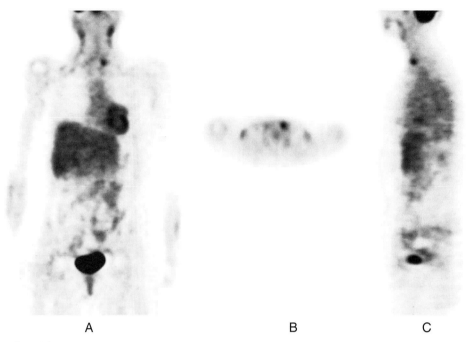

FIGURE 2. PET scan images in all three planes (coronal, **A**; transaxial, **B**; and sagittal, **C**) show a solitary, small focus of intensely increased activity in the left low anterior neck, suggesting a metastatic lymph node. Symmetrical neck muscular activity is also displayed on the coronal view.

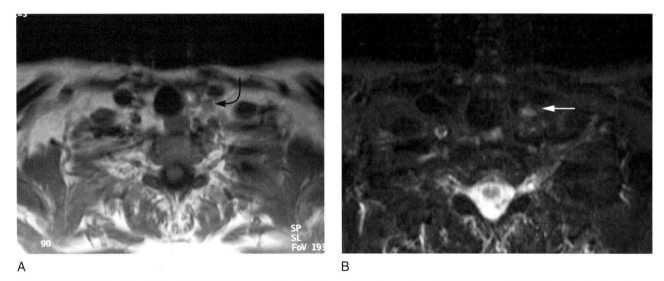

FIGURE 3. Axial T1-weighted (**A**) and STIR (**B**) MR images of the neck show a sub-centimeter (normal) sized left supraclavicular lymph node (*arrows*).

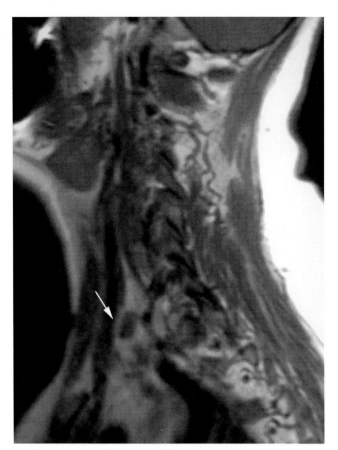

FIGURE 4. Normal-sized lymph node is seen in the sagittal plane with T1 weighting (*arrow*).

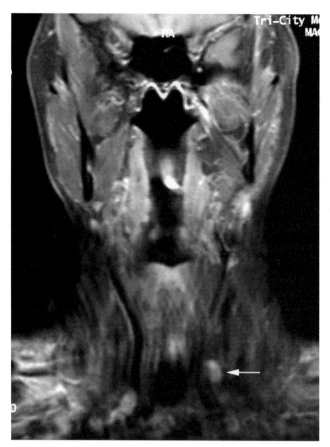

FIGURE 5. The lymph node in question enhances on a coronal, fat-saturated, enhanced T1-weighted MR image (*arrow*).

patient to be treated surgically, rather than be re-treated with ^{131}I. The PET scan findings also directed and limited the subsequent imaging evaluation to the area of interest and enabled more importance to be attached to the finding of a normal-sized lymph node than would be possible based on imaging alone.

CASE 3 | *Recurrent thyroid carcinoma to neck, low metabolic rate*

A 51-year-old woman with recurrent papillary thyroid carcinoma was referred for PET imaging for restaging. Her history dated back 3 years when she underwent thyroidectomy and neck dissection for a 4.5-cm papillary carcinoma diffusely involving both lobes, with capsular invasion, local soft tissue and skeletal muscle metastases, with 17 of 20 lymph nodes positive. She had been treated on three separate occasions with a total of 400 mCi ^{131}I and had most recently received 150 mCi 9 months before. At that time, her 2-mCi ^{131}I whole-body scan was negative but her Tg level was rising.

Before undergoing PET scan evaluation, a left neck node had been palpated and confirmed on ultrasound (Figure 1) and MRI (Figure 2). Biopsy confirmed metastatic papillary thyroid carcinoma. PET scan showed only very modest metabolic activity at this left neck level (Figure 3). This was interpreted as being caused by a low metabolic rate tumor. Metastatic papillary thyroid cancer was confirmed on subsequent surgical excision.

TEACHING POINTS

Thyroid carcinomas vary in histology, aggressiveness, and metabolic rate. This papillary thyroid cancer, although locally aggressive, proved to be relatively low in metabolic rate, as evidenced by the modest activity displayed here by a proven recurrence. This metastasis is more impressive on morphologic than metabolic grounds.

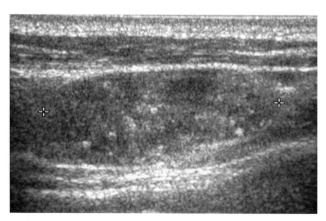

FIGURE 1. Longitudinal left neck ultrasound image shows an ovoid, smoothly marginated heterogeneous mass, delineated by cursors.

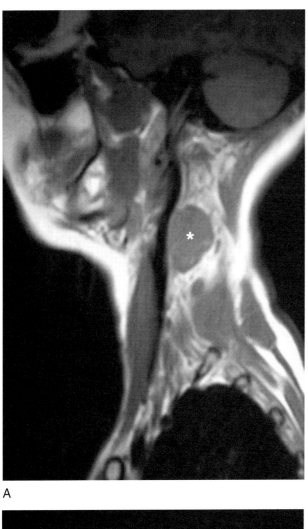

A

FIGURE 2. MR images (T1-weighted sagittal [**A**], T1-weighted axial [**B**], fat-saturated T2-weighted fast spin echo axial [**C**], fast inversion recovery coronal [**D**], and enhanced T1-weighted coronal [**E**] sequences) from neck soft tissue study show a lobular, ovoid, sharply marginated left posterior triangle nodal mass (*asterisks*). T1-weighted axial sequence (**B**) shows the mass is deep to the sternocleidomastoid muscle, and palpable, as evidenced by the presence of a skin marker.

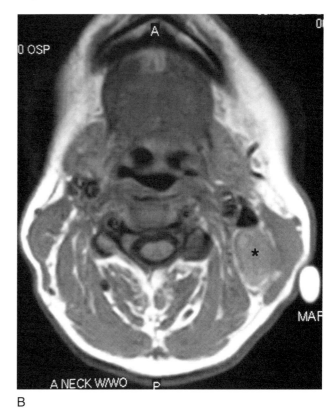

B

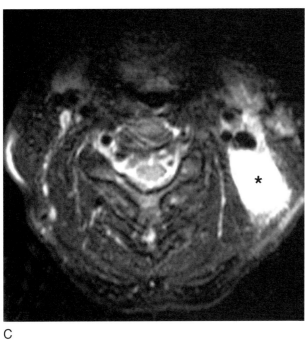

C

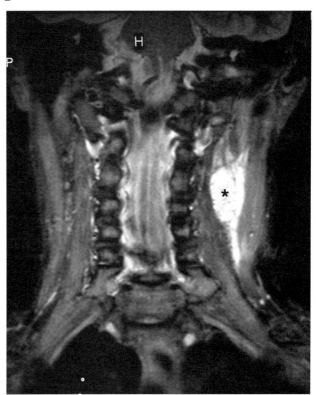

D

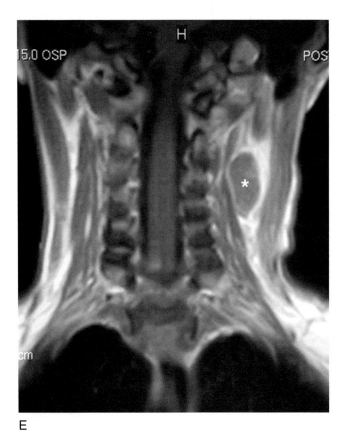

E

FIGURE 2 (cont'd).

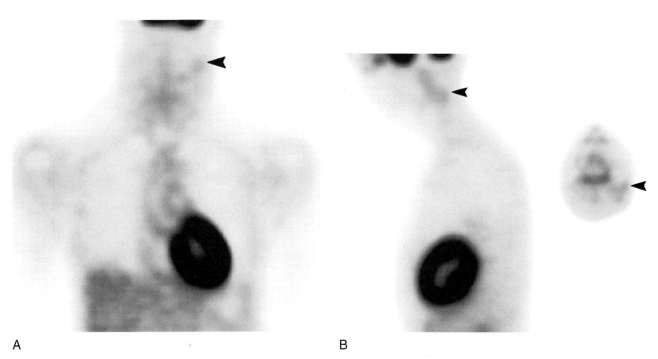

A

B

FIGURE 3. A and B, PET scan images show subtle asymmetry, with only modest activity at the level in question, presumed due to a low tumor metabolic rate (*arrowheads*).

CASE 4 | *Pitfall: Suspected recurrent thyroid carcinoma to mediastinum, false positive (thymus)*

A 25-year-old woman underwent surgery for papillary thyroid carcinoma, with 13 positive paratracheal lymph nodes. Tumor reportedly breached the gland capsule, involving the trachea. About 6 weeks after surgery, the patient was treated with 267 mCi of [131]I. The post-therapy ^{131}I scan showed uptake in an anterior mediastinal mass and cervical lymph nodes. A diagnostic 3-mCi ^{131}I scan obtained 7 months after surgery was negative. Concurrent with this, the stimulated Tg increased from 6 to 35 ng/mL. PET scanning was performed a month later and showed anterior mediastinal activity, thought suggestive of metastatic papillary thyroid carcinoma (Figure 1). MRI was recommended for correlation. An MRI at another facility identified a 5 × 5 × 2-cm mass surrounding the aortic arch, superior vena cava, and right innominate artery. A median sternotomy was performed to remove the mass, to which the patient's shortness of breath was attributed. The mass proved to be benign thymus. Subsequent evaluations for persistent Tg elevation were also negative, including neck node biopsy. The patient was treated with a second course of [131]I.

TEACHING POINT

This case proved to be a false positive for suspected persistent thyroid carcinoma, with anterior mediastinal activity identified in a young patient, which was proven to be benign thymus. Presumably, involvement of the thymus by thyroid carcinoma was not overlooked at histologic evaluation, because the patient's Tg level remained elevated after thymectomy. Uptake of FDG in normal thymus must be considered in the scintigraphic differential diagnosis whenever anterior mediastinal activity is identified on a PET scan in a young oncology patient. However, this does not allow exclusion of involvement of the thymus by the neoplasm. Conversely, development of new anterior mediastinal activity in thymic rebound can be seen on PET, particularly after recovery from chemotherapy, such as for lymphoma (see Case 16 in Chapter 4).

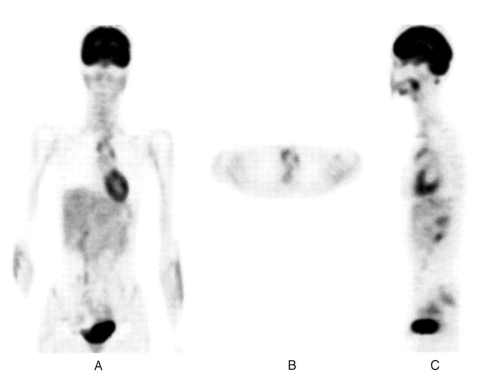

A   B   C

FIGURE 1. PET images show modest intensity anterior mediastinal activity, clearly increased over normal mediastinal uptake. No imaging studies were available for correlation at the time, so MRI was recommended. Identification of activity within the anterior mediastinum in a young person could be within thymus or in prevascular lymph nodes. The mediastinal activity does display a linear, paired configuration suggesting thymus. Given the previous demonstration of ^{131}I uptake in the mediastinum, identification of thymic uptake does not allow differentiation between activity in a normal thymus versus activity within a thymus involved with thyroid carcinoma. Coronal (**A**), transaxial (**B**), and sagittal (**C**) views are shown.

GENITOURINARY MALIGNANCIES

Renal Carcinoma

Renal cancer represents approximately 3% of cancers in adults, with a male:female ratio of 2:1. As with most cancers, the probability of cure is related to tumor stage and degree of dissemination at diagnosis. The overall 5-year survival is approximately 40%, but patients with advanced disease have a 0% to 20% 5-year survival.[1] An important subgroup is those with a solitary metastasis. Their 5-year survival approaches 50%.

Typically, patients with renal cell carcinoma (RCC) are evaluated with CT. Some patients are initially diagnosed by ultrasound, and some may benefit from MRI. The first report of the use of PET in humans with RCC was by Wahl and colleagues in 1991.[2] Their pilot study of five patients showed FDG uptake in all primary as well as metastatic sites. Subsequent reports have confirmed the efficacy of PET for RCC in selected patients. There appears to be no real advantage for PET versus CT in the primary tumor diagnosis.

PET may be useful in the detection of metastases, assessment of response to therapy, and determination of the nature of renal masses.[3] The sensitivity of PET for detection of metastatic RCC appears to correlate with tumor aggressiveness.[4] Although Miyauchi and associates looked only at primary RCC, they found that those that were well visualized had a higher grade and higher expression of GLUT-1 transporters and tended to be larger than poorly visualized tumors.[5] Of note, only 6 of 11 patients had a positive PET study in their series. Even though the total number of patients reported who have been evaluated for recurrence or metastases is relatively small, preliminary data suggest that PET alters therapeutic management and may be of value in assessing renal bed recurrence.[1]

Data on evaluating response to therapy are preliminary but do indicate a potential role for PET.[6] The investigation of the nature of renal masses may include PET in the problem case if other imaging tests and/or tissue sampling are inconclusive. Although one series showed PET to be useful for indeterminate renal cysts,[7] false-positive PET scans have been reported in angiomyolipoma, pericytoma, and pheochromocytoma.[8]

Summarily, early studies with PET in RCC are encouraging. The overall accuracy is in the range of 80%,[9] and PET may currently be viewed as a diagnostic aid in difficult cases, with special emphasis on metastatic assessment.

REFERENCES

1. Ramdave S, Thomas GW, Berlangieri SU, et al: Clinical role of F-18 fluorodeoxyglucose positron emission tomography for detection and management of renal cell carcinoma, J Urol 2001;166:825-830.
2. Wahl RL, Harney J, Hutchins G, et al: Imaging of renal cancer using positron emission tomography with 2-deoxy-2-(F18)-fluoro D-glucose: pilot animal and human studies. J Urol 1991;146:1470-1474.
3. Gambhir SS, Czernin J, Schwimmer J, et al: A tabulated summary of the FDG PET literature. J Nucl Med 2001;42:56S-57S.
4. Lang O, Brouwers AH, Mergenthaler HG, et al: Value of whole-body 18F-FDG-PET in metastatic renal cell carcinoma-correlation with tumor aggressiveness? J Nucl Med 2000;41:117P.
5. Miyauchi RS, Brown HB, Grossman K, et al: Correlation between visualization of primary renal cancer by FDG-PET and histopathological findings. J Nucl Med 1996;37:64P.
6. Hoh CK, Seltzer MA, Franklin J, et al: Positron emission tomography in urological oncology. J Urol 1998;159:347-356.
7. Goldberg MA, Mayo-Smith WW, Papanicolaou N, et al: FDG PET characterization of renal masses: preliminary experience. Clin Radiol 1997;52:510-515.
8. Bachor R, Kotzerke J, Gottfried HW, et al: Positron emission tomography in diagnosis of renal cell carcinoma. Urologe A 1996;35:146-150.
9. Safali A, Hoh CK, Seltzer MA, et al: The usefulness of 18F deoxy-glucose PET imaging for staging of renal cell cancer. J Nucl Med 2000;41:117P.

CASE 5 | *In situ primary tumor, presenting as pleural metastases*

A 68-year-old man presented with the sudden onset of right flank pain. On CXR, there was a large right pleural effusion, nearly opacifying the hemithorax (Figure 1). CT of the chest showed pleural nodularity and thickening within the large right pleural effusion, highly suggestive of a malignant etiology (Figure 2). The abdomen showed a 5.5-cm heterogeneous right renal mass, consistent with RCC (Figure 3). Thoracentesis of the pleural fluid showed lymphocytosis but did not identify malignancy on cytology. The clinical picture was that of an RCC metastatic to pleura. The patient underwent a right kidney core biopsy, confirming RCC. PET scan was obtained to clarify the nature of the pleural disease, in the absence of firm confirmation of its suspected malignant nature. PET scan showed multiple hypermetabolic foci along the periphery of the right hemithorax, correlating with the pleural disease and confirming the malignant nature of the pleural findings (Figure 4). The right lower pole RCC mass itself was essentially

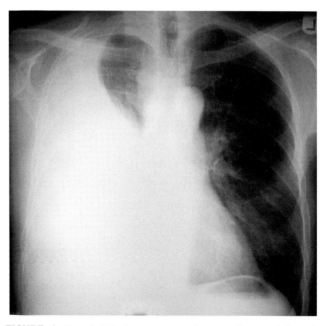

FIGURE 1. Frontal CXR shows near complete opacification of the right hemithorax from a huge right pleural effusion.

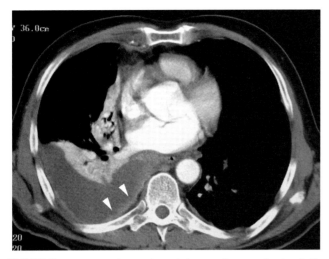

FIGURE 2. Contrast medium–enhanced chest CT shows a right pleural effusion, accompanied by nodular thickening and enhancement of the pleura *(arrowheads)*, indicating the effusion is malignant. The right lower lobe is atelectatic.

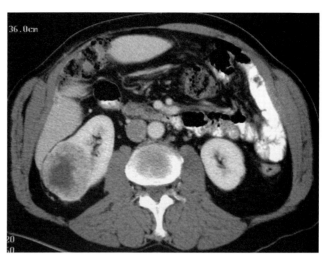

FIGURE 3. Enhanced CT image through the kidneys shows a heterogeneously enhancing right renal mass. Central hypodensity suggests necrosis. Appearance is quite typical of a renal cell carcinoma. Stranding of perirenal fat is seen along the posterolateral aspect of the mass.

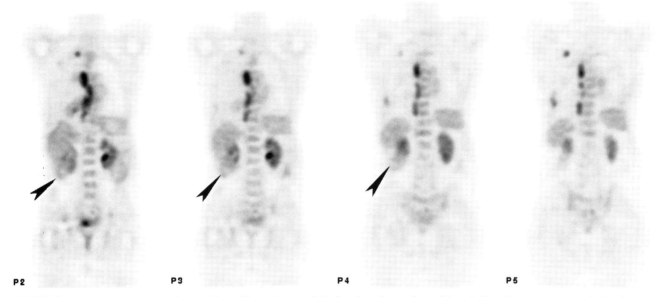

P2   P3   P4   P5

FIGURE 4. Coronal PET scan images show nodular and linear hypermetabolic foci along the periphery of the right hemithorax, consistent with pleural metastases. The right lower pole renal cell carcinoma is visualized with more difficulty, with the periphery isointense to renal parenchyma and central photopenia where CT had shown necrosis *(arrowheads)*. The primary tumor is not frankly hypermetabolic compared with background renal activity.

isointense with the renal parenchyma, with central photopenia where CT showed necrosis. The patient was initially hesitant to institute systemic interleukin therapy, because he was relatively asymptomatic at presentation and instead sought alternative therapy. Three months after the first PET scan, another PET study was obtained, which showed clear interval progression of the pleural metastases (Figure 5). The patient then began interleukin therapy but only received one dose before again electing alternative therapy. He died 3 months later.

TEACHING POINTS

This case illustrates well some of the peculiarities and limitations of the use of PET in RCC. There are a number of RCC varieties, which vary in their aggressiveness and, by extension, their metabolic activity. Identification of RCC primary lesions on PET is dependent on their size, location within the kidney, and intrinsic metabolic activity level of the tumor. These factors, balanced against the expected background

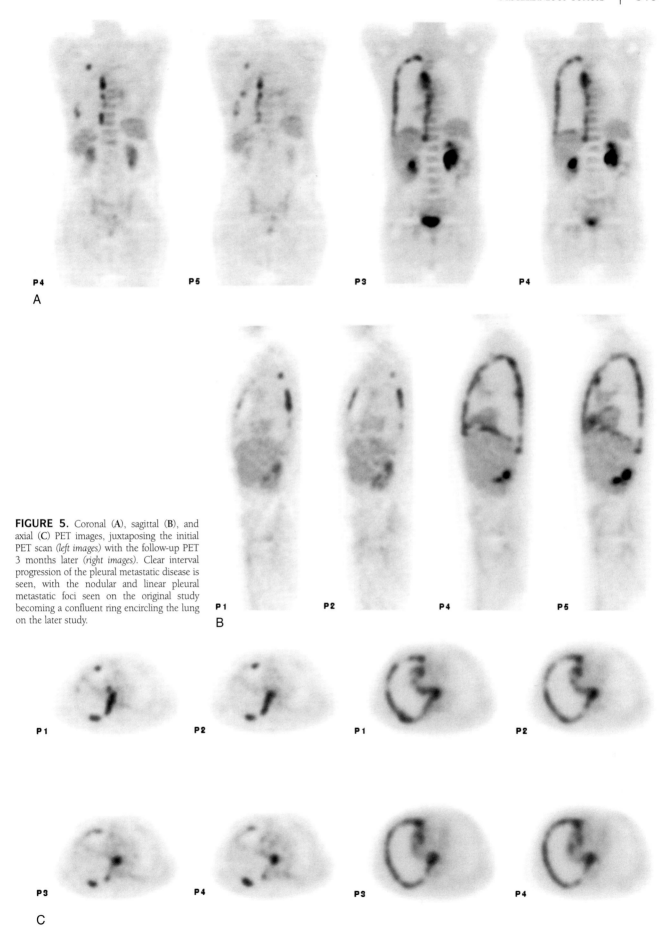

FIGURE 5. Coronal (**A**), sagittal (**B**), and axial (**C**) PET images, juxtaposing the initial PET scan (*left images*) with the follow-up PET 3 months later (*right images*). Clear interval progression of the pleural metastatic disease is seen, with the nodular and linear pleural metastatic foci seen on the original study becoming a confluent ring encircling the lung on the later study.

activity level of the native kidney, determine whether a renal mass can even be visualized on PET. Although the normal renal parenchyma is only modest in its FGD accumulation, the intensity and variable amount of collecting system activity are contentious factors. For these reasons, the use of PET to aid in the differential diagnosis of indeterminate renal masses is fraught with difficulty. In this case, although the primary tumor is relatively sizeable and in a favorable location, it was comparatively difficult to visualize on PET and might well have been overlooked prospectively without foreknowledge of its location by imaging.

CASE 6 | Sarcomatoid renal cell carcinoma, with retroperitoneal metastases

A 53-year-old woman with squamous cell anal-vaginal septal carcinoma had been treated with abdominoperineal resection and radiation therapy. An enlarged left supraclavicular node was identified 15 years later. Biopsy was interpreted as metastatic squamous cell carcinoma. This was initially regarded as a late metastasis from the patient's prior primary tumor. CT restaging showed bilateral renal abnormalities, with a chronically obstructed appearance of the right and bilateral, solid, indeterminate renal masses (Figure 1). Two pathologically enlarged retroperitoneal lymph nodes were also noted (Figure 2). Subsequent PET scan showed hypermetabolic activity at the nodal sites (Figure 3). No renal abnormality was recognized on PET scan (Figure 4). The patient refused treatment, opting instead to self-treat with immunotherapy and nutritional supplements. Approximately a year later, she developed abdominal pain and weakness and, on CT, marked interval growth was seen of the right renal mass (Figure 5). She underwent right nephrectomy, adrenalectomy, and lymph node dissection. Pathology showed sarcomatoid renal cell cancer. Review of the prior year's supraclavicular node pathology in conjunction with this result was reinterpreted as consistent with metastatic RCC.

TEACHING POINT

There are inherent limitations in evaluating the kidneys with PET, secondary to the expected intense activity of the intrarenal collecting system from excreted FDG. The renal parenchyma itself displays modest activity on FDG PET. Depending on the size and location (central vs. exophytic), renal masses may or may not be seen on PET scans.

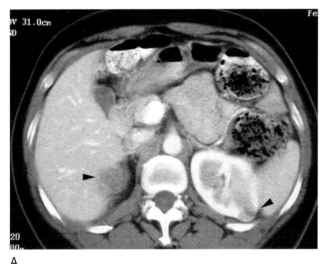

A

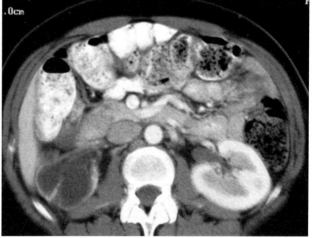

C

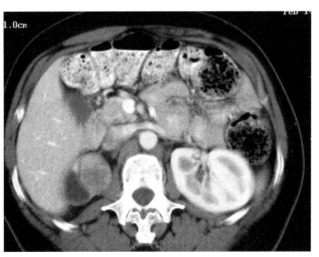

B

FIGURE 1. A to C, Three sections through the kidneys from an enhanced abdominal CT show bilateral solid indeterminate renal masses, at the right upper pole and posterior left upper pole levels (arrowheads). No normal right kidney is seen, with the remaining kidney consisting of a dilated collecting system with a thin rim of atrophic cortical tissue.

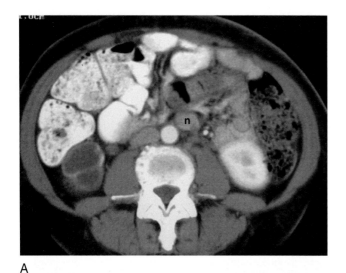

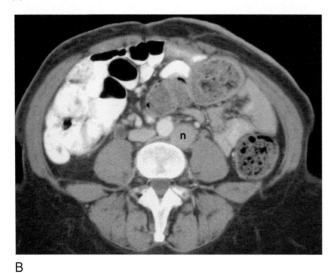

FIGURE 2. **A** and **B**, Enhanced abdominal CT sections through the mid-abdomen show two left para-aortic enlarged lymph nodes (n). Chronic right renal obstruction is again noted, with cortical atrophy, and hydroureteronephrosis.

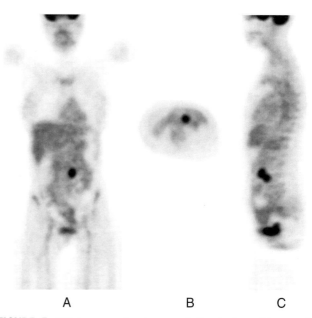

FIGURE 3. PET images confirm hypermetabolism in the nodal retroperitoneal findings (two foci are best demonstrated on the sagittal section). Coronal (**A**), transaxial (**B**), and sagittal (**C**) views are shown.

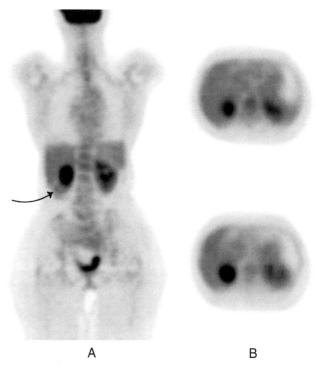

FIGURE 4. Coronal (**A**) and two axial (**B**) PET sections through the kidneys show intense hypermetabolic activity at the right renal level, thought initially to represent the hydronephrotic, chronically obstructed right kidney. In retrospect, the activity corresponds to the solid, indeterminate right upper pole mass on CT, with the lower intensity activity noted on the coronal section below this the only possible correlate for the hydronephrotic sac of the remaining kidney (*arrow*).

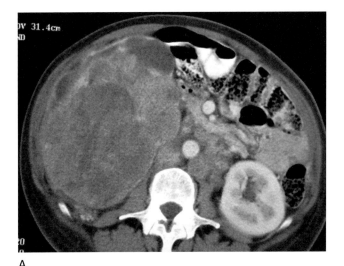

A

B

FIGURE 5. A and B, Ten months later, after alternative therapies only, the right kidney mass and adenopathy have dramatically progressed. Subsequent excision of the right kidney confirmed sarcomatoid renal cell carcinoma.

Accordingly, it may be difficult to sufficiently visualize an indeterminate renal mass to assess its metabolic activity. To add to these difficulties, RCCs vary in their metabolic activity rates. Administration of furosemide (Lasix) can promote diuresis of intrarenal collecting system activity and may aid in improving visualization of renal masses. For patient comfort, bladder catheterization will likely be required if furosemide is given.

This case demonstrates some additional pitfalls. The solid, indeterminate left renal mass is small, minimally exophytic, and not visualized. The right kidney is chronically obstructed. The intense right renal fossa activity seen on PET was misinterpreted initially as representing the dilated collecting system, filled with excreted FDG. In retrospect, this seems unlikely given the extreme cortical atrophy present here; there is essentially not enough normally functioning renal tissue left to produce the volume of urine it would take to result in this PET appearance. Presumably, the right renal fossa activity corresponds to the heterogeneous, solid right upper pole mass, which was proven subsequently to be a sarcomatoid RCC.

CASE 7 | *In situ primary tumor, with inferior vena cava tumor extension*

A 69-year-old man was ill for several months, with abdominal pain, nausea, anorexia, weight loss, rib pain, microscopic hematuria, anemia, and leg swelling. CT identified a 10-cm right renal mass (Figures 1 to 3). RCC was presumed, and tumor thrombus invaded the renal vein and inferior vena cava. This was confirmed by MRI (Figure 4). PET scan was requested to assess metastatic status. The right kidney was dominated by the metabolically active mass. Linear hypermetabolic activity extended cephalad from the kidney along the course of the inferior vena cava, consistent with metabolically active tumor thrombus and venous invasion (Figure 5). The advanced disease and patient's debility precluded aggressive treatments, and he died in a skilled nursing facility 1 month later.

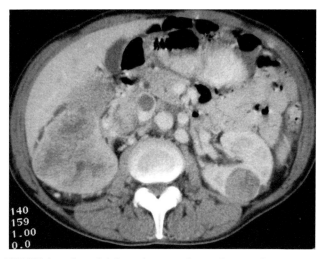

FIGURE 1. Enhanced abdominal CT scan shows a dominant, heterogeneous mass replacing the right kidney. Anterior, extrarenal extension is noted. Similar-appearing tumor thrombus distends the right renal vein. Thrombus (probably bland) is seen in the inferior vena cava at this level. A smaller, heterogeneously enhancing mass, suggestive of a second renal cell carcinoma, is seen in the left posterior kidney.

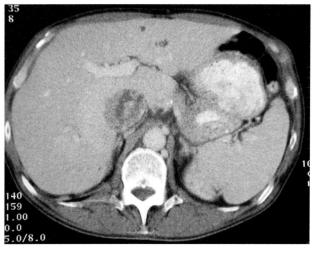

FIGURE 2. A more cephalad section shows heterogeneously enhancing tumor thrombus distending the intrahepatic inferior vena cava.

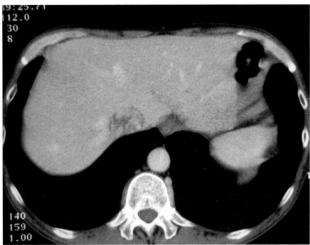

FIGURE 3. A higher section, at the level of the hepatic venous confluence with the inferior vena cava, showing the most cephalad extent of the tumor thrombus.

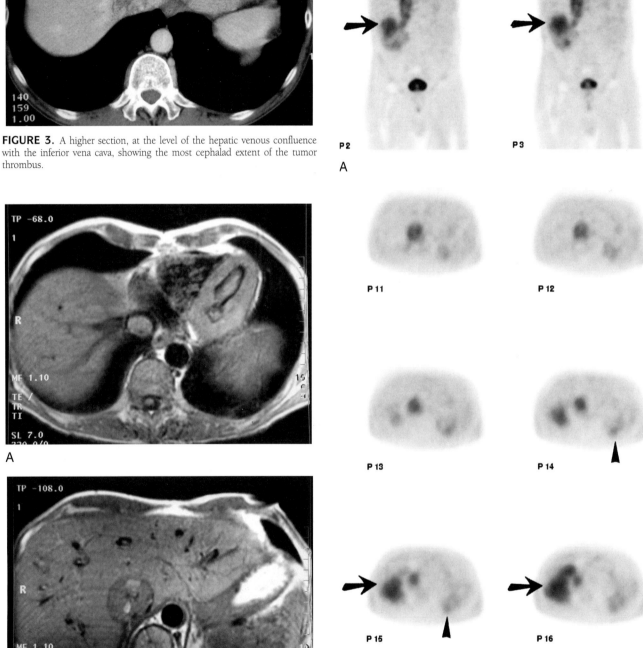

A

B

FIGURE 4. A and B, T1-weighted axial MR sections show comparable findings, with tumor thrombus invading the intrahepatic inferior vena cava.

FIGURE 5. Coronal (A) and axial (B) PET images show the metabolically active right RCC (*arrows*). Linear intraluminal activity of similar intensity extends cephalad from the primary tumor and outlines the inferior vena cava to the level of the right atrium, confirming the CT impression of venous invasion by tumor thrombus. The suspected left second RCC is only modest in metabolic activity, although increased enough over background renal parenchymal activity to be identifiable (*arrowhead*). Symmetrical, normal variant neck muscular activity (versus activated brown fat) is incidentally noted.

TEACHING POINT

Other cases have illustrated how variable in metabolic activity primary RCCs can be. This large, aggressive and advanced stage lesion could be readily visualized on PET, as could the venous invasion by tumor thrombus. However, the second left-sided lesion illustrates the difficulties of applying PET to the evaluation of smaller indeterminate renal masses, particularly those that are entirely intrarenal.

CASE 8 | *Renal cell carcinoma, lung metastasis*

A 58-year-old man developed a LUL lung nodule on CXR, 5 months after undergoing a right nephrectomy for a 10-cm clear cell renal carcinoma. Chest CT confirmed the noncalcified LUL nodule to be abutting the pleura (Figures 1 and 2). CT-guided biopsy returned only atypical cells. PET scan showed the nodule to be hypermetabolic and consistent with tumor (Figure 3). One month later, the patient underwent left upper lobectomy, with chest wall resection and reconstruction,

as well as hilar and mediastinal lymphadenectomy. At pathology, the mass measured 5 × 4.5 × 3.5 cm and was a clear cell carcinoma, consistent with metastasis from renal carcinoma. No metastases were identified in six intraparenchymal or six hilar lymph nodes. Extension to, but not through, the visceral pleura was noted, and margins were negative. Within a month after surgery, the patient developed profound fatigue and anorexia, as well as weight loss, and a CXR 3 months after surgery showed multiple new pulmonary metastases. The patient died 3 months later, 10 months after the first pulmonary metastasis was identified.

TEACHING POINT

RCC can vary in the virulence and time course of recurrences. Some patients with relatively indolent disease fare well with surgical resection of isolated metastases. This patient's metastasis proved to be aggressive and rapidly progressive, as suggested by the discrepancy between the apparent size of the LUL metastasis on chest CT and PET, performed only 2 months apart. The lesion was growing rapidly, as confirmed by the surgical pathology results identifying a much larger mass than seen on CT.

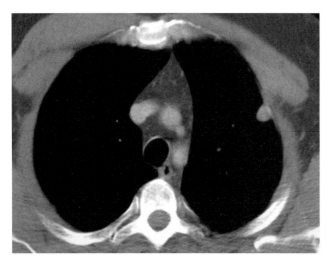

FIGURE 1. Unenhanced chest CT (mediastinal window) shows a noncalcified LUL nodule, abutting the pleura, which is focally thickened.

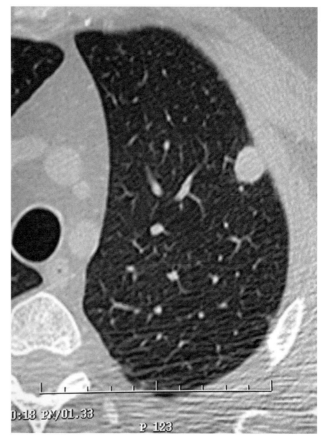

FIGURE 2. High-resolution lung window image shows slight margin irregularity of the nodule.

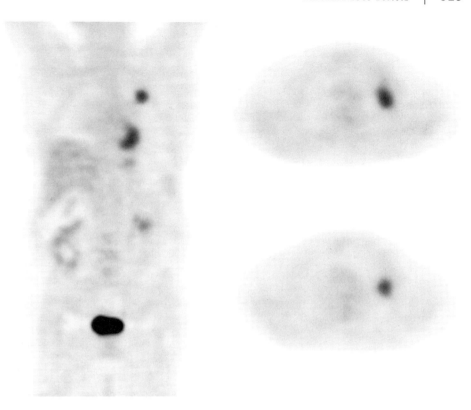

FIGURE 3. PET scan confirms the nodule is hypermetabolic, therefore malignant. Interval growth is suggested by correlation with the CT, performed approximately 2 months before the PET scan. No other lesions are found.

CASE 9 | *Recurrent renal cell carcinoma, hilar and vertebral metastases*

A 70-year-old man, 3.5 years post left nephrectomy for renal cell carcinoma, was evaluated for back pain and found by CT to have lytic change at the L1 vertebral body. This was sampled, and malignancy consistent with renal cell metastasis was identified. He was also noted to have an enlarged right hilus on CXR (Figure 1). CT evaluation for this was inconclusive, being compromised by the inability to administer contrast agent owing to allergy. He was referred for PET scan for further evaluation. PET showed abnormally increased activity at both the

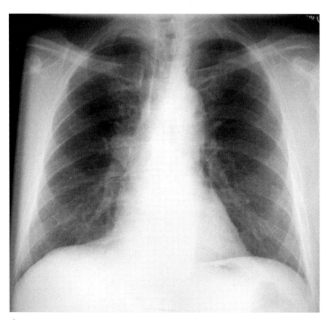

A

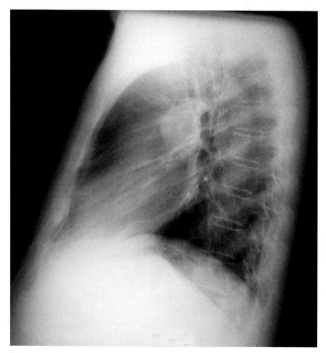

B

FIGURE 1. Posteroanterior (**A**) and lateral (**B**) CXR views show an enlarged, dense right hilus, suggestive of a mass or adenopathy.

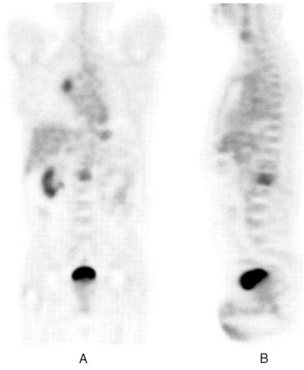

A   B

FIGURE 2. Coronal (**A**) and sagittal (**B**) PET images show increased uptake at the right hilus, corresponding to the CXR finding. The L1 vertebral body is also abnormally hypermetabolic and was known by biopsy to be replaced by metastatic RCC. The left kidney is surgically absent.

right hilus and the L1 vertebral body, consistent with metastases (Figure 2).

TEACHING POINTS

PET can be useful in the evaluation of RCC, particularly for remote metastases. The variable metabolic rate of renal carcinomas and the relatively high normal activity level of kidneys on FDG-PET limit PET's utility in the assessment of renal masses suspected to be RCCs. Larger renal masses may be adequately visualized on PET, but smaller masses may not be identifiable against the background renal parenchymal activity and intense activity of excreted FDG in the collecting systems. However, away from the renal fossa, these limitations do not hinder PET's utility in the evaluation of suspected metastatic RCC.

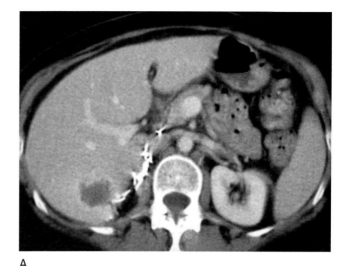

A

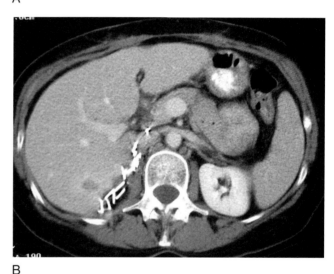

B

FIGURE 1. **A,** Enhanced abdominal CT image shows multiple surgical clips in the right retroperitoneum from prior right nephrectomy. A low-density, necrotic-appearing mass with rim enhancement in the posterior segment of the right lobe of the liver had grown from the prior study 4 months before. **B,** This comparison study, obtained 1 month after resection of right RCC that focally invaded the liver, showed findings at this level that were thought to be postresection changes.

CASE 10 | *Locally recurrent clear cell renal cell carcinoma, with lung metastases*

A 54-year-old woman was referred for PET evaluation of recurrent disease 6 months after right nephrectomy for clear cell RCC. At the time of surgery, tumor extension into the liver was surgically excised. CT follow-up showed evidence of local recurrence in the surgical bed, as well as new tiny lung nodules, suggesting pulmonary metastases (Figures 1 and 4). At the time of PET imaging, the patient had completed a postoperative 3-month course of autologous lymphocyte infusion therapy. PET scan confirmed the CT abnormalities were metabolically active and

consistent with local recurrence of RCC and pulmonary metastases (Figures 2, 3, and 5).

TEACHING POINTS

This case illustrates two different forms of recurrent RCC, with local recurrence at the surgical bed level and tiny hematogenous lung metastases. PET can be a useful adjunct to anatomic imaging when a local recurrence is suspected in the renal fossa, particularly if extensive postoperative changes render the imaging evaluation difficult. This case also depicts detectable metabolic activity in remarkably small lung nodules (on the order of 5 to 6 mm), at the lower limit of PET resolution.

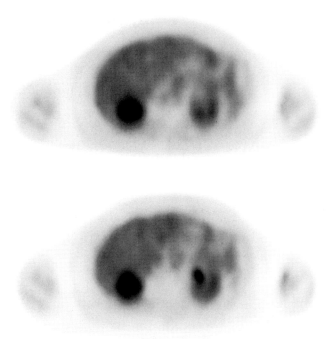

FIGURE 2. Axial PET images at the level of the kidneys show intense hypermetabolic activity at the right posterior liver level, corresponding to the growing CT abnormality and consistent with locally recurrent RCC.

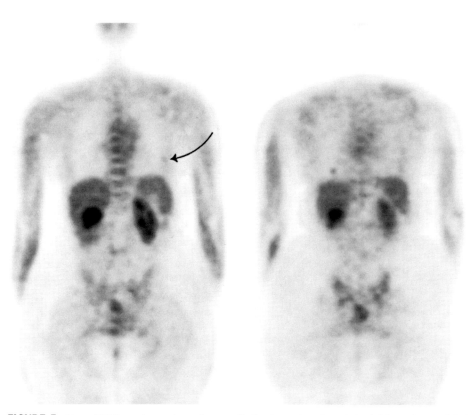

FIGURE 3. Coronal PET scan image shows the same finding in another plane. A tiny left lower lung nodule is barely discernible (*arrow*). The more posterior coronal section (*right*) shows a small, metabolically active right posterior basal lower lobe nodule.

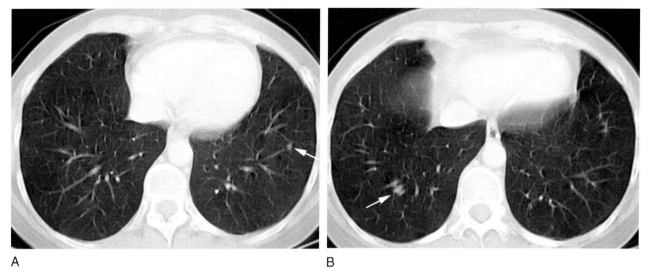

A   B

FIGURE 4. Corresponding chest CT lung windows show tiny, sub-centimeter lung nodules (*arrows*), new from a prior study. The constellation of findings is consistent with lung metastases.

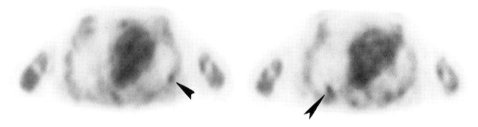

FIGURE 5. Corresponding axial PET sections showing tiny metabolically active foci in the LLL and RLL, at the levels of the largest of the new tiny lung nodules (*arrowheads*).

Testicular Cancer

Germ cell tumors (GCT) are rare, but testicular cancer is the most common malignancy in men aged 15 to 35.[1] The two main types, seminoma and teratoma (nonseminoma), are highly curable (>90%). As with other tumors, potential roles for PET include primary diagnosis, follow-up, characterization of a post-therapy mass, and use in patients with elevated tumor markers.

Data are scant on primary diagnosis/initial staging. The few published studies document a good positive predictive value for identifying metastases.[2-4] However, sensitivity and negative predictive value are suboptimal, owing to the inability of PET to find sub-centimeter retroperitoneal lymph node disease.[2,3]

The use of PET for restaging, including those patients with elevated serum tumor markers (i.e., α-fetoprotein, β-hCG) and negative conventional studies, shows promise.[5] Although PET may be helpful for restaging, caution must be exercised because of the potential for false-positive results in patients with inflammatory lesions.[6,7] With respect to elevated tumor markers, the data are also preliminary. Once again, the positive predictive value is relatively high but the negative predictive value may be as low as 50%.[8,9]

A perplexing dilemma in management of testicular cancer is the residual mass after therapy. Some authors have shown benefit from PET in the evaluation of post-therapy residual masses in seminoma.[1,10,11]

Both visual assessment and quantitative standardized uptake value measurements have been able to separate viable tumor from either scar/necrosis or mature teratoma. However, a prospective study reached the opposite conclusion, seeing no apparent benefit for PET in the evaluation of post-therapy masses.[12]

Monitoring response to treatment is based on PET's ability to demonstrate reduction in FDG accumulation in previously positive regions. To be of value, this must also predict a durable or long-term remission. It may be important to delay PET imaging for some weeks after completion of therapy to avoid false-positive scans due to activated white blood cell response.[6] The few studies published that have addressed monitoring have shown encouraging results but are less than fully convincing because of the small number of patients reported.

As with many tumors currently under investigation, the role of PET in GCT is not conclusively established. The term *problem-solving tool* appropriately applies, with PET of great benefit in selected patients.

REFERENCES

1. Sugawara Y, Zasadry KR, Grossman HB, et al: Germ cell tumor: differentiation of viable tumor, mature teratoma, and necrotic tissue with FDG PET and kinetic modeling. Radiology 1999;211:249-256.

2. Hain SF, O'Doherty MJ, Timothy AR, et al: Fluorodeoxyglucose PET in the initial staging of germ cell tumours. Eur J Nucl Med 2000;27:590-594.

3. Cremerius U, Wildberger JE, Borchers H, et al: Does positron emission tomography using 18-fluoro-2-deoxyglucose improve clinical staging of testicular cancer?—results of a study in 50 patients. Urology 1999;54:900-904.

4. Albers P, Bender H, Yilmaz H, et al: Positron emission tomography in the clinical staging of patients with stage I and II testicular germ cell tumors. Urology 1999;53:808-811.

5. Hain SF, O'Doherty MJ, Huddart RA, et al: The value of FDG-PET in recurrent testicular carcinoma. J Nucl Med 1999;40:105P.

6. Cremerius U, Effert PJ, Adam G, et al: FDG PET for detection and therapy control of metastatic germ cell tumor. J Nucl Med 1998;39:815-822.

7. Nuutinen JM, Leskinen S, Elomaa I, et al: Detection of residual tumours in post-chemotherapy testicular cancer by FDG-PET. Eur J Cancer 1997;33:1234-1241.

8. Maszelin P, Lumbroso J, Theodore C, et al: Fluorodeoxyglucose (FDG) positron emission tomography (PET) in testicular germ cell tumors in adults: preliminary French clinical evaluation, development of the technique and its clinical applications. Prog Urol 2000;10:1190-1199.

9. Hain SF, O'Doherty MJ, Timothy AR, et al: Fluorodeoxyglucose positron emission tomography in the evaluation of germ cell tumours at relapse. Br J Cancer 2000;83:863-869.

10. DeSantis M, Bokemeyer C, Becherer A. et al: Predictive impact of 2-18-fluro-2-deoxy-D-glucose positron emission tomography for residual post-chemotherapy masses in patients with bulky seminoma. J Clin Oncol 2001;19:3740-3744.

11. Muller-Mattheis V, Reinhardt M, Gerharz CD, et al: Positron emission tomography with [18F]-2-fluoro-2-deoxy-D-glucose (18 FDG-PET) in diagnosis of retroperitoneal lymph node metastases of testicular tumors. Urologe A 1998;37:609-620.

12. Ganjoo KN, Chan RJ, Sharma M, et al: Positron emission tomography scans in the evaluation of post-chemotherapy residual masses in patients with seminoma. J Clin Oncol 1999;17:3457-3460.

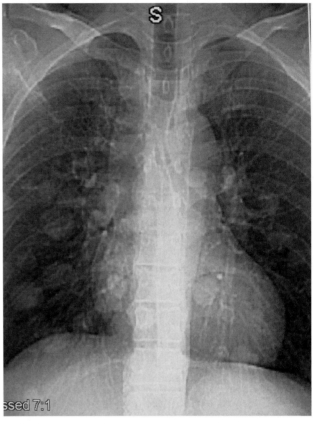

FIGURE 1. Multiple lung nodules are seen bilaterally on frontal CXR, consistent with metastases.

CASE 11 | *Widely metastatic testicular carcinoma, response to chemotherapy*

A 37-year-old man was diagnosed with a nonseminomatous GCT at orchiectomy. His initial staging studies showed metastatic disease. On CXR, multiple pulmonary parenchymal nodules were seen (Figure 1). Abdominal CT showed suspicious liver lesions, as well as retrocrural and retroperitoneal adenopathy and left adrenal infiltration (Figure 2). PET imaging confirmed multiple hypermetabolic disease foci in the chest and abdomen (Figure 3). He was treated with high-dose chemotherapy, followed by stem cell transplantation. Follow-up PET scan, 2.5 months after his first study, showed resolution of all disease findings (Figure 4).

TEACHING POINTS

PET has shown value in testicular carcinoma in staging and monitoring response to therapy. The assessment of a primary lesion remains the province of physical examination, ultrasonography, MRI, and histologic evaluation.

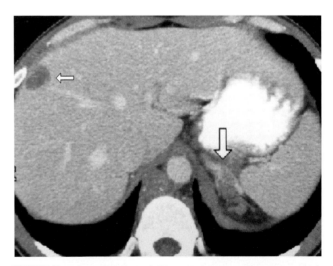

FIGURE 2. Enhanced abdominal CT image shows an indeterminate peripheral liver lesion (*small arrow*), as well as low-density retrocrural adenopathy and infiltration of the left adrenal gland (*large arrow*).

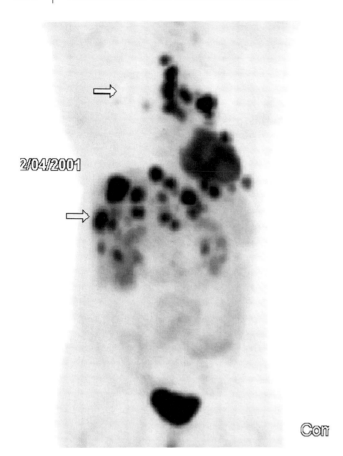

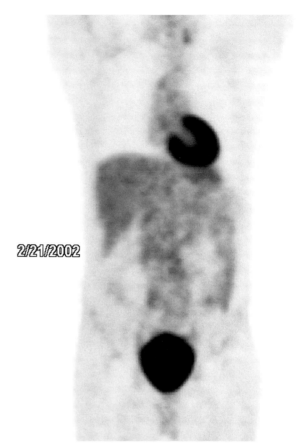

FIGURE 3. Coronal PET image shows innumerable pathologic foci of hypermetabolism in the chest and abdomen (*arrows*), consistent with extensive metastases.

FIGURE 4. Repeat PET scan, 2.5 months later, after high-dose chemotherapy and stem cell transplant, has normalized.

CASE 12 | *Suspected recurrence, disseminated sarcoidosis*

A 44-year-old man with a history of retroperitoneal seminoma developed evidence of splenic lesions, as well as a mass at the splenic hilus. The patient had a history of seminoma 2 years previously that was treated with retroperitoneal dissection. No testicular site was identified. The patient was treated with chemotherapy when a recurrence was identified a year after initial diagnosis. A "sarcoid-like" reaction was noted on analysis of nodal material. When CT surveillance showed splenic parenchymal and hilar mass lesions, the patient was referred for PET scan for further evaluation. At this time, the patient clinically was well. PET imaging showed innumerable foci of hypermetabolic activity, including in nodal regions (mediastinum, supraclavicular, retroperitoneal, and pelvic), viscera (especially spleen), bone (spine, pelvis, and left femur), and left pleura (Figures 1 to 3). Findings were regarded with suspicion for metastatic testicular carcinoma. Sarcoid was considered in the differential diagnosis but was thought less likely. The patient underwent removal of inguinal nodes. These showed noncaseating granulomas and no evidence of malignancy.

TEACHING POINTS

Active granulomatous processes, such as sarcoid, can be positive on PET scanning and can closely mimic neoplastic processes, especially metastatic disease and lymphoma. As always, PET provides an excellent whole-body map of the distribution and extent of metabolically active diseases but does not differentiate among neoplastic and active inflammatory and granulomatous processes. PET may help identify more readily accessible sites to guide biopsy, but tissue is required to confirm specific diagnoses.

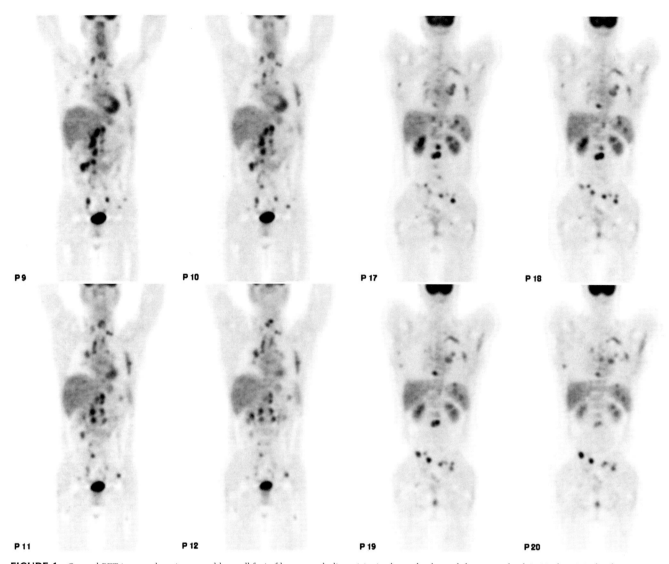

FIGURE 1. Coronal PET images show innumerable small foci of hypermetabolic activity in the neck, chest, abdomen, and pelvis. Neck activity localizes to supraclavicular regions bilaterally. Chest activity is consistent with mediastinal and hilar nodal activity, with more linear left hemithoracic activity indicative of pleural disease. In the abdomen and pelvis, hypermetabolic nodal activity follows retroperitoneal and iliac chains, and small active foci are seen within the spleen. Multiple osseous foci are also seen, including in the spine, pelvis, and left proximal femur.

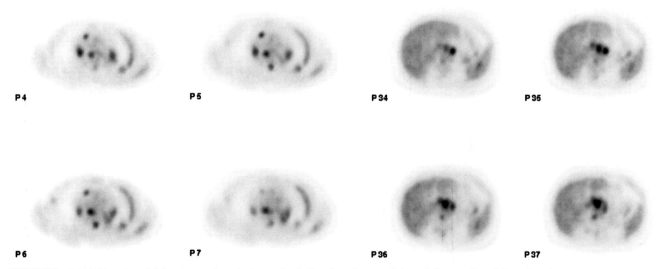

FIGURE 2. Axial PET sections (left four images through chest and right four through upper abdomen) show small, nodal-type foci of activity in the mediastinum, hila, and retroperitoneum. The left hemithoracic curvilinear activity is consistent with pleural involvement.

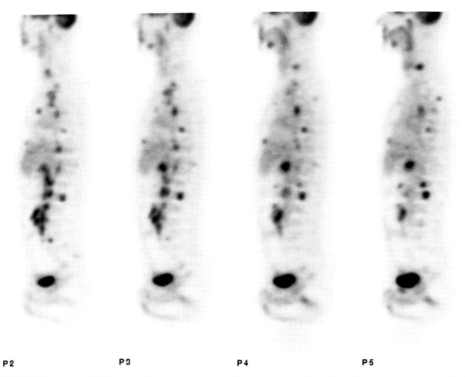

P2   P3   P4   P5

FIGURE 3. Sagittal PET sections better show the prespinal retroperitoneal nodal activity, as well as osseous foci within the thoracic and lumbar vertebrae.

Other Genitourinary Malignancies
TRANSITIONAL CELL CARCINOMA

CASE 13 | *In situ primary transitional cell carcinoma*

An 84-year-old woman developed persistent pain in the LLQ and flank. Her past medical history included a remote history four decades before of cancer of the left breast treated by mastectomy and a history of LUL lung cancer, treated surgically 6 years previously. A local recurrence of the lung cancer to the left paraspinal region 18 months before had been irradiated (Figure 1). A PET scan was obtained because of left flank pain, and interpreted as essentially negative (Figure 2). She returned 6 months later, with persistent complaints of left flank and abdominal pain. Repeat PET scan showed a left hemipelvic focus of pathologic hypermetabolic activity, progressive from the prior study (Figure 3). The smaller focus on the prior study was erroneously presumed to be focal left ureteral activity. Correlation with CT showed corresponding findings of a left distal ureteral level soft tissue mass obstructing the left kidney (Figures 4 and 5). This proved to be transitional cell carcinoma (TCC), a third primary tumor in this patient.

TEACHING POINTS

TCC is potentially identifiable on PET imaging, as this case illustrates, but PET is clearly not the usual preferred modality for initial evaluation. Although TCC masses are FDG avid and hypermetabolic, the usual small size of the tumors and identical intensity to excreted FDG within

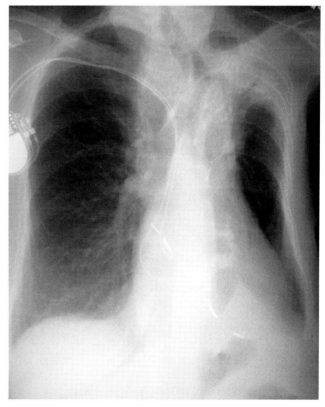

FIGURE 1. Frontal CXR shows opacified and contracted left lung apex from prior surgery and radiation therapy.

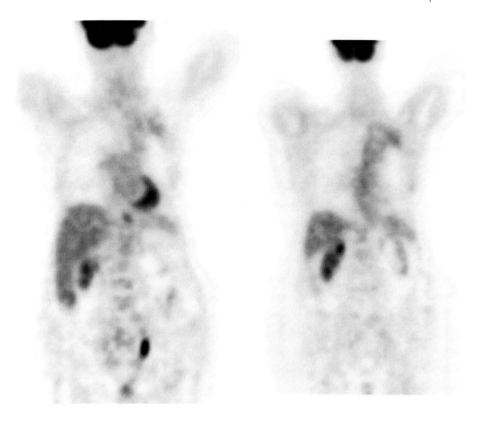

FIGURE 2. Initial PET study. Coronal image on left shows an oblong focus of activity in the left hemipelvis, along the course of the left distal ureter. One clue to its pathologic nature is provided by the asymmetry of the kidneys on the more posterior section on the right. Activity is seen within the intrarenal collecting system on the right, whereas the PET equivalent of a "negative pyelogram" (due to a distended, unopacified collecting system) is present on the left. An additional clue is that there is little excreted FDG in the bladder. Both images show a left hemithoracic apical cap of low level activity, secondary to prior radiation therapy.

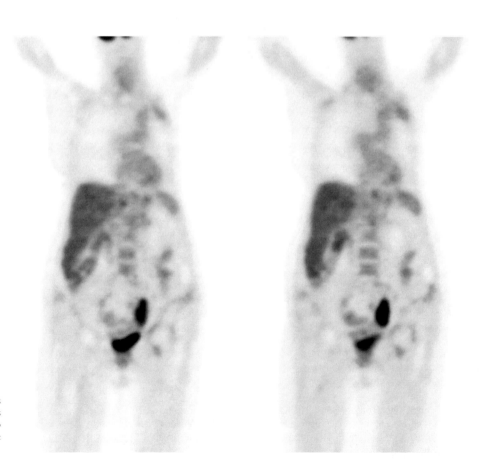

FIGURE 3. Repeat PET scan, 6 months later. The left hemipelvic focus of activity is larger and more mass-like, now clearly too bulky to be mistaken for excreted FDG in the distal ureter.

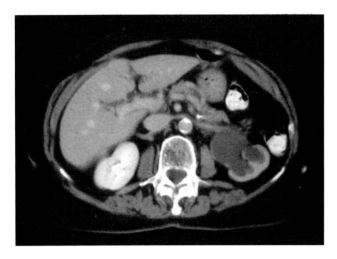

FIGURE 4. Enhanced CT through the kidneys shows chronic left hydronephrosis, with cortical thinning.

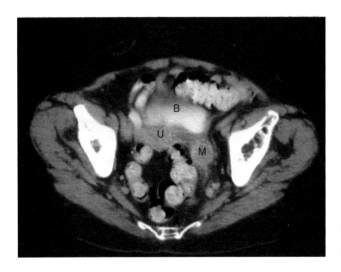

FIGURE 5. Pelvic CT shows a round, soft tissue density mass at the left distal ureteral level, just above the ureterovesical junction level. Above this level, the dilated ureter was traceable to the mass. M, mass; U, uterus; B, bladder.

the collecting system precludes the routine use of PET imaging in the evaluation of TCC in all but the most unusual of cases. The urothelium is better assessed for masses indirectly by traditional radiography with collecting system opacification (intravenous urography, retrograde pyelography) or by direct visual inspection, such as cystoscopy. In the unusual situation where PET is indicated and TCC is in the differential diagnosis, the examination technique can be modified by the addition of bladder catheterization and/or lavage and diuretics can be administered. When TCC is suspected remote from the collecting systems (e.g., in retroperitoneal lymph nodes), PET imaging may be complementary to CT.

This case also illustrates a pitfall in interpretation. The significance of this distal ureteral activity was not initially recognized. The activity was assumed to be a focus of excreted FDG in the ureter. The clues that may have enabled its recognition are subtle but evident in retrospect.

The activity itself is along the course of the ureter, with the same elongated orientation. One could argue that the caliber of the activity is greater than usually seen with excreted FDG in a normal ureter. Another observation that could have been made is the paucity of urine in the bladder itself; excreted FDG activity in the ureters should be accompanied by visualization of the bladder itself. The final critical observation is the asymmetry of the kidneys; there is no excreted FDG in the intrarenal collecting system on the left, although there is on the right. In fact, there is the PET equivalent of the intravenous urographic "negative pyelogram" sign on the left, with photopenia in place of the distended and obstructed collecting system.

This case again underscores the value of correlating PET with anatomic imaging studies, which may help avoid such an interpretative pitfall.

CASE 14 | *Widely metastatic transitional cell carcinoma*

A 67-year-old man was evaluated with PET imaging for staging of recently diagnosed TCC. Two months before he underwent left nephroureterectomy and cystectomy for TCC. Preoperative CT raised a question of abnormal pelvic lymph nodes. The patient's past medical history included a prior prostatectomy for prostate carcinoma over 6 years before, with radiation therapy 1 year after diagnosis for recurrence.

PET imaging showed extensive metastatic disease, to both bone and soft tissue, including the liver and left renal fossa (Figure 1).

The findings were thought most likely to be metastases from advanced TCC.

TEACHING POINTS

PET imaging in this patient identified much more advanced metastatic disease than suspected based on preoperative and surgical staging. The presumptive diagnosis is widely metastatic TCC. This is based on probabilities, because the only other malignancy history in this patient is of prostate carcinoma, which most commonly is PET negative unless dedifferentiated (compare with Case 15).

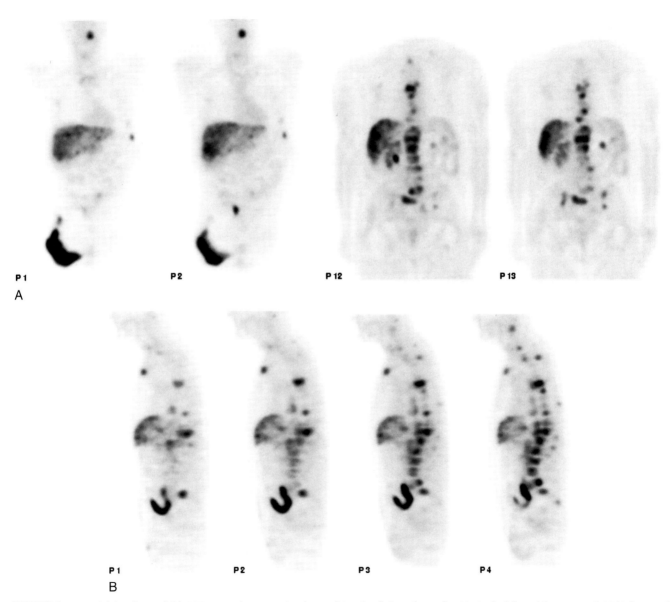

FIGURE 1. Coronal (**A**) and sagittal (**B**) PET images show extensive abnormalities. A soft tissue focus of activity in the left renal fossa is noted. Multiple sites of increased bone activity are noted, consistent with osseous metastases. Particularly confluent involvement is seen in the lumbar spine, with involvement also at cervical and thoracic levels and of the sternum and pelvis. The liver is also abnormal, with multiple foci of abnormal activity noted, particularly in the right lobe. The most anterior coronal sections show excreted activity in the right-sided ileostomy bag.

PROSTATE CANCER

CASE 15 | *Widely metastatic prostate cancer, dedifferentiated*

A 56-year-old man presented with a pathologic fracture and epidural mass at T4, with impending spinal cord compression. He underwent T3 and T4 laminectomy, with fusion from T1 through T6. Pathology confirmed adenocarcinoma, possibly of prostatic origin. However, the primary origin was not clearly established. The patient's past medical history was remarkable only for prostate carcinoma (Gleason score of 9), treated about 2 years before with retropubic prostatectomy. Reportedly, there was extracapsular extension at surgery, but negative lymph nodes. The prostate-specific antigen (PSA) test at that time was 2.2. A bone scan performed after the prostate surgery apparently showed no bone metastases.

PET scan was obtained 1 month after the patient's spinal surgery. PET showed innumerable hypermetabolic foci, consistent with extensive metastatic disease (Figure 1). Most of the sites localized to bone. The largest single focus was at the T4 level of the known pathologic fracture and cord encroaching mass. Lower intensity posterior soft tissue activity is seen above and below this level, related to the recent surgery.

TEACHING POINTS

This is a case of presumed prostate carcinoma metastatic to bone. The patient's only known malignancy history was of prostate carcinoma. Spinal decompression material identified adenocarcinoma, possibly of prostate origin.

In general, PET imaging is of limited utility with prostate carcinoma. Most prostate carcinomas are slow-growing, low metabolic rate tumors. However, tumors that become undifferentiated and thereby aggressive may be visualized on PET imaging, as is presumed to have occurred in this case.

BENIGN ADRENAL HEMANGIOENDOTHELIOMA

CASE 16 | *Benign adrenal hemangioendothelioma*

A 77-year-old man presented with depressed appetite and weight loss of 40 pounds over 8 to 9 months. Past medical history was significant for drinking five alcoholic beverages per day. His work-up included CT, which showed innumerable tiny hypodense liver lesions, on the order of 5 mm and less. A heterogeneously enhancing left adrenal mass and gastric wall thickening were also noted (Figure 1). Upper endoscopic biopsy of the stomach showed chronic active gastritis and *Helicobacter pylori* but no evidence of malignancy. PET scan was requested for suspicion of metastatic disease, based on the liver lesions and the adrenal mass. The liver was unremarkable on PET, but the small size of the lesions may have been limiting. Given the history of significant alcohol intake, nodular steatosis was favored to explain the liver findings. The adrenal gland displayed moderate metabolic activity and was regarded as suggestive of malignancy (Figure 2). It was sampled, and a vascular neoplasm was identified, classified as an epithelioid hemangioendothelioma, a benign lesion of unpredictable biologic behavior.

TEACHING POINTS

This represents an unusual adrenal mass histology. This vascular neoplasm is not clearly malignant. Its appearance on PET is intermediate in activity between the two extremes seen with the two most common adrenal masses, namely, benign adenomas and adrenal metastases. Benign adenomas generally are inactive and not visualized on PET, whereas adrenal metastases are usually intensely hypermetabolic, greater than the moderate activity level noted here.

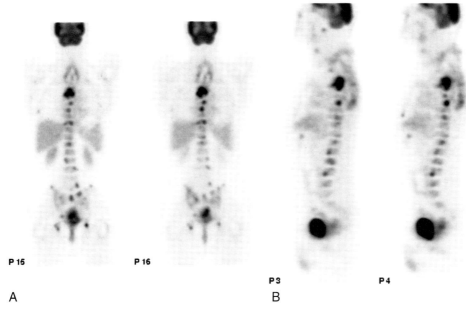

P 15   P 16

A   B

P3   P4

FIGURE 1. Coronal (**A**) and sagittal (**B**) PET images show a large hypermetabolic focus at T4, at the site of the known pathologic fracture and threatened cord compression. Multiple smaller foci of vertebral activity are seen, and foci of activity are also noted in other osseous sites, including the pelvis, ribs, and sternum. Note the lower intensity posterior soft tissue activity at upper thoracic levels, from decompression and spinal fusion surgery the month prior.

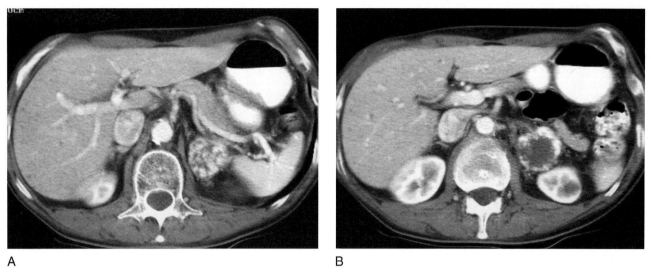

A   B

FIGURE 1. **A** and **B,** Adjacent enhanced abdominal CT sections show innumerable tiny hypodense foci in the liver. There is also a left adrenal gland mass of distinctly unusual appearance. Intense, heterogeneous and peripheral enhancement is noted of the adrenal mass, suggesting a vascular lesion. Central hypodensity is seen, which usually suggests necrosis.

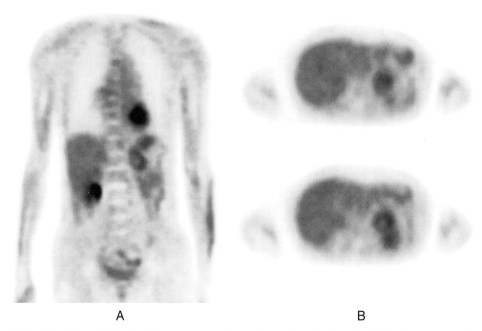

A   B

FIGURE 2. Coronal (**A**) and axial (**B**) PET images show no liver lesions. The tiny size of the lesions seen on CT is below the threshold for reliable visualization on PET. The adrenal mass is moderate in metabolic activity level and centrally photopenic.

GYNECOLOGIC MALIGNANCIES

The value of PET for gynecologic malignancies is less well established than for most other tumors. In part, this is because there is a relative paucity of firm data. However, in selected women with ovarian and cervical cancer, PET offers valuable additional information.

Ovarian Cancer

Annually, more than 25,000 new cases of ovarian cancer are diagnosed. Approximately 14,500 deaths occur each year, making it the fifth leading cause of death from cancer in women.[1] Because a significant percentage of patients develop metastases within a year of surgical resection, typical management includes second-look laparotomy. Additional methods for follow-up include imaging with ultrasound, CT, or MRI and measurement of serum CA-125. Because all of these modalities, including laparotomy, have limitations, FDG-PET has been evaluated for its potential in detecting recurrence. Most studies are small but report good sensitivity (range: 83% to 100%) and specificity (range: 67% to 100%) for the identification of macroscopic disease.[2-5] FDG-PET, like other imaging modalities, is of no value for micrometastases. At present, the role of PET seems to be for problem solving and as a complementary test in the patient with suspected recurrence. This is also true for cervical cancer.[6]

There are data that support the use of PET in managing patients with recurrent ovarian carcinoma to identify that subset of patients who could avoid second-look surgeries (i.e., FDG-PET negative). This may also result in significant cost savings.[1] Thus far, clinical evidence of PET efficacy for the evaluation of ovarian masses, preoperative staging, or monitoring response to therapy is preliminary.

REFERENCES

1. Smith GT, Hubner KF, McDonald T, et al: Cost analysis of FDG PET for managing patients with ovarian cancer. Clin Pos Imag 1999;2:63-70.
2. Yen RF, Sun SS, Shen YY, et al: Whole body positron emission tomography with 18F-fluoro-2-deoxyglucose for the detection of recurrent ovarian cancer. Anticancer Res 2001;21:3691-3694.
3. Zimny M, Siggelkow W, Schroder W, et al: 2-[fluorine-18]- fluoro-2-deoxy-D-glucose positron emission tomography in the diagnosis of recurrent ovarian cancer. Gynecol Oncol 2001;2:310-315.
4. Nakamoto Y, Saga T, Ishimore T, et al: Clinical value of positron emission tomography with FDG for recurrent ovarian cancer. AJR Am J Roentgenol 2001;176:1449-1454.
5. Kubik-Huch RA, Dorffler W, von Schulthess GK, et al: Value of (18F)-FDG positron emission tomography, computed tomography, and magnetic resonance imaging in diagnosing primary and recurrent ovarian carcinoma. Eur Radiol 2000;10:761-767.
6. Grigsby PW, Dehdashti F, Siegel BA: FDG-PET evaluation of carcinoma of the cervix. Clin Pos Imag 1999;2:105-109.

CASE 17 | Recurrent ovarian carcinoma, response to chemotherapy

A 57-year-old woman was referred for PET evaluation of recurrent ovarian carcinoma. Her diagnosis was made 1 year before at surgery, at which she underwent total abdominal hysterectomy, bilateral salpingo-oophorectomy, omentectomy, partial cystectomy, and cecectomy. She was treated with chemotherapy for 1 year with paclitaxel (Taxol) and carboplatin. Her CA-125, 1200 U/mL at diagnosis, had declined to unmeasurable, but at the time of referral for PET scanning, it had rebounded to 58 U/ml. Imaging evaluation with CXR and abdominal and pelvic CT scans reportedly was negative.

PET scan showed multiple hypermetabolic disease sites in the abdomen and pelvis, consistent with ovarian carcinoma (Figure 1). Foci localized to peritoneal surfaces, particularly on the liver surface and in the right flank. The patient sought a second opinion subsequent to this study and underwent three courses of topotecan before being reevaluated with PET. This study (not shown) showed a similar disease distribution, with mild worsening.

The patient then underwent a debulking surgery, at which time cholecystectomy, splenectomy, and partial colectomy of both the ascending and descending colon was performed. Chemotherapy was reinstituted, including intraperitoneal cisplatin. PET scanning was performed 1 year later for reevaluation (Figure 2). The serosal surface implants previously noted overlying the liver and in the right flank were no longer evident, consistent with the interval debulking. However, multiple new, small, scattered foci of activity were now identifiable within the abdomen and pelvis.

TEACHING POINTS

PET scanning can be useful in the imaging evaluation of patients with ovarian carcinoma. Patients with demonstrable disease by PET potentially could be spared "second look" laparotomies, and PET provides a noninvasive complement to CT for assessing chemotherapy responses. However, caution must be exercised, because ovarian carcinoma that manifests as peritoneal carcinomatosis and/or omental cake, with only tiny tumor deposits studding peritoneal surfaces, may be severely underestimated on PET, as on CT.

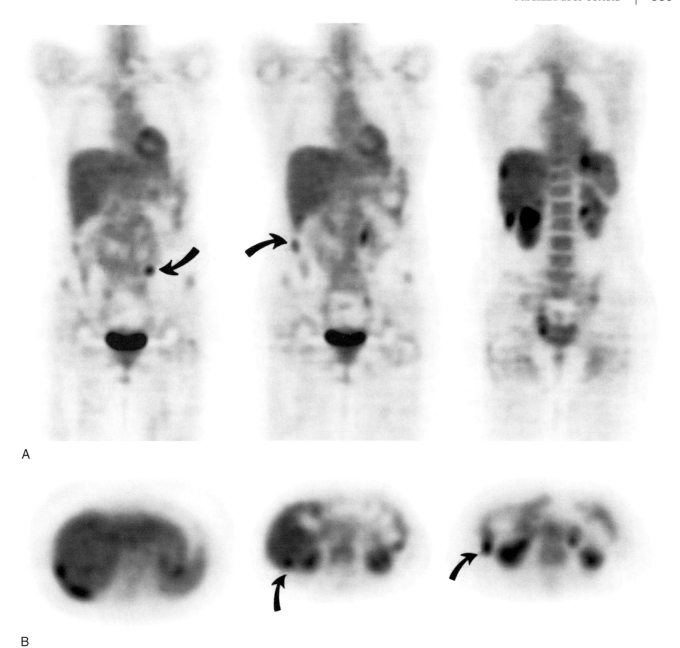

FIGURE 1. Coronal (**A**) and axial (**B**) PET images show foci of hypermetabolic activity localizing to serosal surfaces, typical of ovarian carcinoma. The perihepatic sites are on the liver surface, not within the liver parenchyma. There also are foci in juxtasplenic and right flank locations (*arrows*).

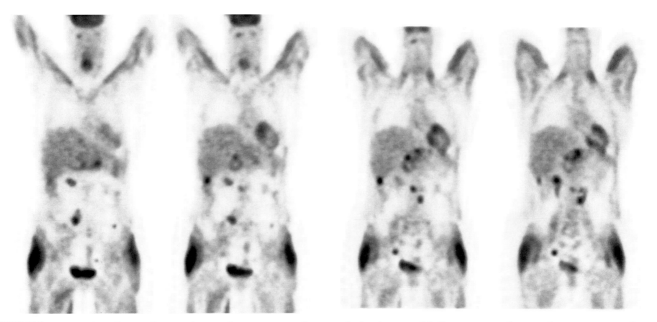

FIGURE 2. One year later, foci noted previously are no longer apparent. The patient had undergone a debulking surgery in the interval. However, scattered new disease sites are evident.

CASE 18 | *Recurrent ovarian carcinoma, with parathyroid adenoma*

A 70-year-old woman was referred for PET scanning for suspicion of recurrent ovarian carcinoma, based on a recent increase in her CA-125. She had been treated for ovarian carcinoma 7 years before, with surgery and chemotherapy. The patient was asymptomatic but was hypercalcemic. PET imaging identified two pathologic sites of presumed recurrent ovarian carcinoma, one in the LUQ and another in the LLQ (Figures 1 and 2). An additional site of hypermetabolism was noted in the left low anterior neck (Figure 3). The patient had been previously evaluated for hyperparathyroidism by sestamibi parathyroid scintigraphy (Figure 4), and ultrasonography (Figure 5), with findings consistent with a left parathyroid adenoma.

TEACHING POINTS

Recurrent ovarian carcinoma was suspected in this patient based on an elevated CA-125 level. PET imaging provides an excellent whole-body capability in the imaging evaluation of such patients. The major limitation of PET scanning in the evaluation of ovarian carcinoma is lesion size. Small tumor nodules of 1 cm and less in size may be readily overlooked on CT, and lesions of this size may not be visualized on PET either. Carcinomatosis, with tiny tumor foci studding peritoneal surfaces, is an ovarian carcinoma disease pattern that may be severely underestimated on both CT and PET.

Hypermetabolic activity can be seen in both benign and malignant thyroid nodules and in parathyroid adenomas. If a focus of activity is identified on PET in the thyroid region, this suggests imaging correlation be performed to identify a corresponding nodule. In this case, there was already strong clinical suspicion of hyperparathyroidism, with an imaging work-up identifying a presumed parathyroid adenoma already having been completed.

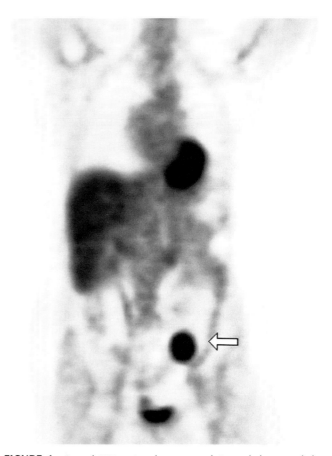

FIGURE 1. Coronal PET section shows a round, intensely hypermetabolic left lower quadrant focus, consistent with a site of recurrent ovarian carcinoma *(arrow)*.

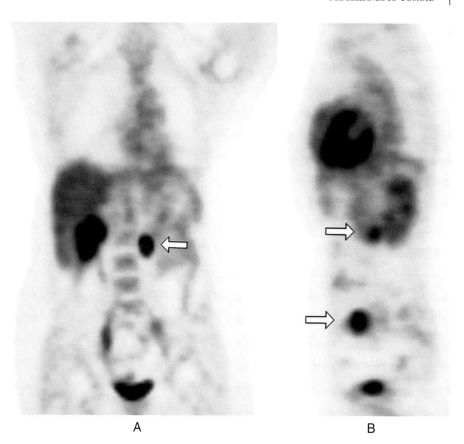

FIGURE 2. Coronal (**A**) and sagittal (**B**) PET images show a second intra-abdominal site of pathologic activity in the LUQ. On the coronal view, the focus (*arrow*) might be mistaken for renal pelvic activity, analogous to the hydronephrotic right renal collecting system activity seen on the same image. However, correlation with the sagittal plane clearly demonstrates this focus to be anterior and separate from the lower pole of the left kidney (*arrow*). The LLQ disease site is well shown in this plane as well (*arrow*).

A

B

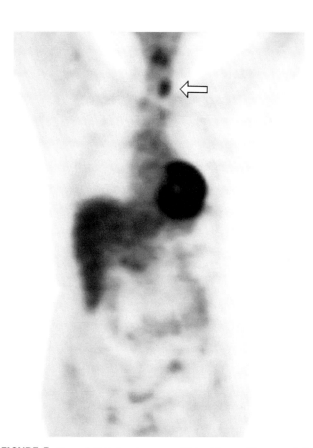

FIGURE 3. Coronal PET slice shows an additional focus of hypermetabolic activity in the left inferior neck (*arrow*).

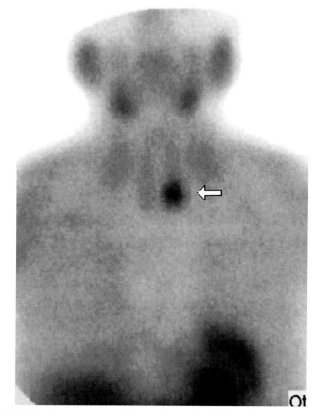

FIGURE 4. Correlation with this patient's additional studies shows a corresponding lesion (*arrow*), consistent with an adenoma, on a parathyroid sestamibi study performed for suspected hyperparathyroidism.

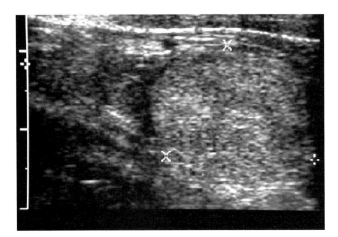

FIGURE 5. Neck ultrasonography also identifies a corresponding homogeneous nodule (cursors).

Cervical Cancer

Spread of carcinoma of the cervix is by local extension or by lymphatic spread to the pelvic, para-aortic, and supraclavicular lymph nodes. Subsequently, metastases may occur to lung, bone, brain, and liver. Conventional imaging modalities are limited in their ability to assess lymph node metastases. PET has been shown to be of value because of a high avidity for FDG documented in cervical cancer.[1,2] Studies comparing PET versus CT or MRI for the evaluation of lymph node involvement have documented a clear advantage for PET, with sensitivities in the range of 57% to 100% and specificities of 92% to 100%.[1,3-7] The lower sensitivity values tend to be in the para-aortic nodes.

Excreted FDG within the bladder may be problematic, and some centers have found the use of post-void images, bladder irrigation, and diuretic administration to be of value. Although PET has been shown to be highly accurate for lymph node metastasis and demonstrates high negative predictive value, it cannot replace anatomic imaging studies, which are necessary for treatment planning.

REFERENCES

1. Rose PG, Adler LP, Rodriguez M. et al: Positron emission tomography for evaluating para-aortic nodal metastasis in locally advanced cervical cancer before surgical staging: a surgicopathologic study. J Clin Oncol 1999;17:41-45.
2. Sugawara Y, Eisbruch A, Kosuda S, et al: Evaluation of FDG PET in patients with cervical cancer. J Nucl Med 1999;40:1125-1131.
3. Sun SS, Chen TC, Yen RF, et al: Value of whole body 18F-fluoro-2-deoxyglucose positron emission tomography in the evaluation of recurrent cervical cancer. Anticancer Res 2001;21:2957-2961.
4. Park DH, Kim KH, Park SY, et al: Diagnosis of recurrent uterine cervical cancer: computed tomography versus positron emission tomography. Korean J Radiol 2000;1:51-55.
5. Grigsby PW, Siegel BA, Dehdashti F: Lymph node staging by positron emission tomography in patients with carcinoma of the cervix. J Clin Oncol 2001;19:3745-3749.
6. Reinhardt MJ, Ehritt-Braun C, Vogelgesang D, et al: Metastatic lymph nodes in patients with cervical cancer: detection with MR imaging and FDG PET. Radiology 2001;218:776-782.
7. Narayan K, Hicks RJ, Jobling T, et al: A comparison of MRI and PET scanning in surgically staged loco-regionally advanced cervical cancer: potential impact on treatment. Int J Gynecol Cancer 2001;11:263-271.

CASE 19 | Advanced cervical carcinoma, initial staging

A 44-year-old woman was referred for PET for staging of newly diagnosed squamous cell carcinoma (SCC) of the cervix. Retroperitoneal nodal metastases were suspected based on MRI. She presented with heavy menses and iron-deficiency anemia, with weight loss of 100 pounds over 1 year (from 350 to 250 pounds) without dieting. Her Papanicolaou smear had been negative 1.5 years before.

Pelvic MRI showed the uterus to be enlarged and lobular, with many hypointense fibroids (Figure 1). The cervical carcinoma mass was accompanied by adenopathy, measuring up to 2 cm at the left para-aortic lower retroperitoneal level (Figure 2). The patient was referred for CT-guided biopsy of the retroperitoneal lymph node to confirm the impression of advanced disease. Because of her size and the necessary approach, this would have required use of a 17-cm needle. At this point, PET scanning was considered as an alternative to biopsy. It showed the in situ cervical carcinoma mass to be intensely hypermetabolic (Figure 3). The enlarged myomatous uterus was comparatively low in metabolic activity. The nature of bilateral juxtauterine masses, previously thought to be exophytic fibroids, became clearer. Their intense hypermetabolism suggested they represented pathologically

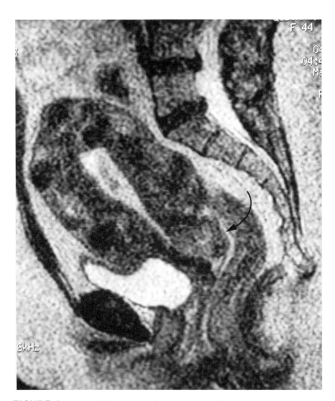

FIGURE 1. Sagittal T2-weighted fast spin echo MR image through the midline of the pelvis shows the enlarged myomatous uterus, with multiple hypointense fibroids. The signal of the cervical carcinoma mass contrasts to the normal stromal hypointensity of the cervix (arrow).

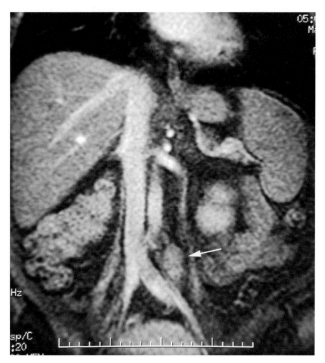

FIGURE 2. Coronal-enhanced SPGR MR section shows a 2-cm, enlarged left para-aortic lymph node, at the level of the aortic bifurcation.

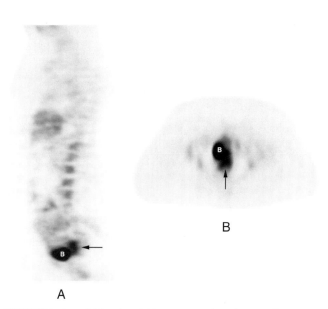

A

B

FIGURE 3. Sagittal (**A**) and axial (**B**) PET images show the cervical carcinoma mass (*arrow*) posterior to the urinary bladder (B) to be hypermetabolic. The enlarged uterus is of relatively low metabolic activity. Marrow activity of the visualized lumbar spine is abnormally increased and was attributed to the patient's anemia and marrow hyperplasia.

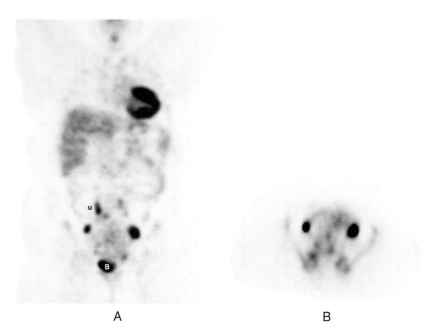

FIGURE 4. Coronal (**A**) and axial (**B**) PET sections show the enlarged, myomatous uterus to be low in metabolic activity. Intensely hypermetabolic masses, left larger than right, flank the uterus. A segment of the right ureter (u) is included on the coronal slice. B, bladder.

A

B

enlarged pelvic nodes (Figures 4 and 5). The left para-aortic lower retroperitoneal lymph node in question was also hypermetabolic, providing presumptive confirmation of involvement (Figures 6 and 7).

TEACHING POINTS

This case broaches many topics for discussion. No special patient preparation was utilized here because the nature of the retroperitoneal lymph node was the primary question in this case and the diagnosis of

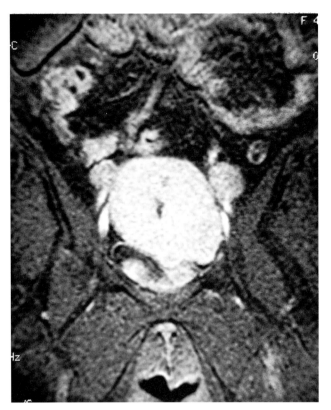

FIGURE 5. Enhanced SPGR coronal MR section through the uterus at a corresponding level shows bilateral enhancing "ears" projecting off both sides of the uterus. These represent pathologically enlarged pelvic lymph nodes.

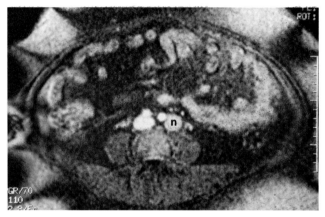

FIGURE 7. Corresponding axial SPGR image showing the enlarged left para-aortic node (n) at the aortic bifurcation level.

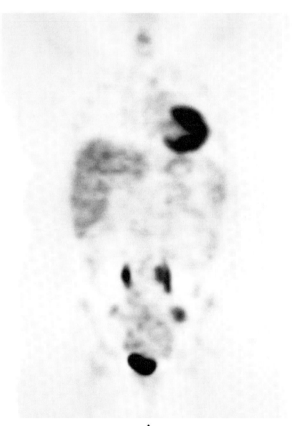

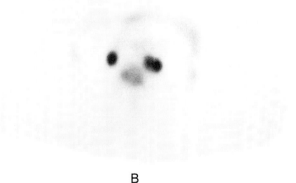

FIGURE 6. Coronal (**A**) and axial (**B**) PET images through the distal ureters and adjacent left para-aortic node, producing a double intensity on the left. The node is medial to the ureter. Activity is also seen in an enlarged left pelvic node on the coronal image.

A

B

cervical carcinoma was already established. There is no difficulty distinguishing between activity in the bladder anteriorly and the SCC mass posteriorly. If the patient had not been able to empty the bladder well, this potentially could have been more of an issue. Protocols for PET imaging of gynecologic and pelvic malignancies at some centers include maneuvers to minimize bladder activity, such as Foley catheter placement and administration of furosemide. Because catheterization rarely results in complete absence of activity in the bladder, the potential exists for confusion arising from a less firm identification of the partially collapsed and visualized bladder. One could argue that the presence of the bladder, as long as it is not overly distended, serves a useful landmark in localization.

Another interesting facet of this case is the low activity level of the diffusely myomatous uterus. Normal uterine and fibroid activity can occasionally and unpredictably be relatively intense. If that had occurred in this case, it could have made recognition of the activity of the cervical SCC more difficult. The low uterine and fibroid activity in this case allowed more ready recognition of the significance of the bilateral juxtauterine activity. Not previously identified as pathologic and probably assumed to be exophytic fibroids on imaging, it seems unlikely that bilateral fibroids would be hypermetabolic when the numerous other fibroids in the uterus are not. Although that possibility exists, it seems much more likely that these foci represent pathologically enlarged, metastatic pelvic nodes. It also cannot be entirely excluded that these represent bilateral adnexal masses, secondary to ovarian metastases.

Finally, PET provided a "metabolic biopsy" alternative for evaluation of the para-aortic lymph node in this patient, in whom actual biopsy would have been technically difficult.

CASE 20 | Widely metastatic cervical carcinoma (brain, porta hepatis, supraclavicular, and presacral nodes)

A 36-year-old woman presented with acute development of vaginal bleeding and was found to have stage IIB poorly differentiated SCC of the cervix. She was treated with primary external beam radiation, with cisplatin (Platinol) chemotherapy. About 2 months after diagnosis, on the day the patient was admitted to begin intracavitary irradiation, she developed seizures and right-sided weakness. Brain CT showed a 3-cm left parietal lesion with edema and midline shift. Brain MRI confirmed the lesion to be solitary and consistent with a neoplasm. Pathology from a CT-guided biopsy returned a diagnosis of metastatic poorly differentiated carcinoma, consistent with a cervical primary tumor. Further metastatic work-up with chest, abdomen, and pelvis CT showed no additional evidence of disease. The patient underwent a left parieto-occipital craniotomy with gross total removal of the tumor, followed by whole-brain irradiation. The tumor bed was further treated with gamma knife radiation therapy.

About 5 months later, left supraclavicular adenopathy was found on a routine follow-up examination. Physical examination also suggested a presacral abnormality. CT of the chest, abdomen, and pelvis was obtained to restage her disease and identified nodal metastatic disease in the porta hepatis (Figure 4). Repeat brain MRI and PET scan were requested to complete her restaging. The brain MRI showed interval growth, with central necrosis, of the left parietal mass, with an

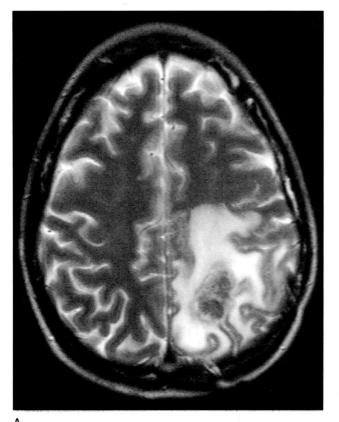 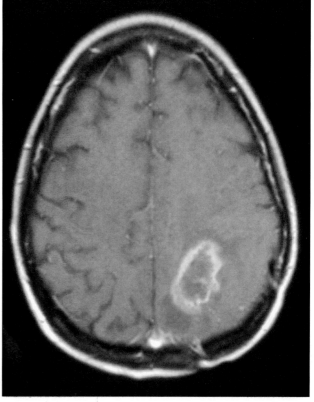

A B

FIGURE 1. T$_2$ fast spin echo (**A**) and enhanced T1-weighted (**B**) axial MR images show a ring-enhancing left parietal metastasis, with accompanying edema and mass effect with sulcal effacement. There was clear interval progression from a prior examination 4 months before.

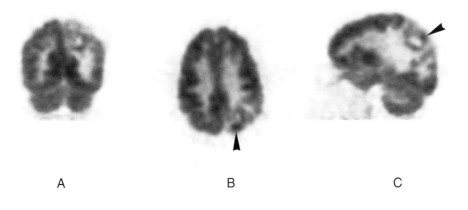

A   B   C

FIGURE 2. Brain PET images show generalized hypometabolism of the left parietal lobe, attributable to the edema. Within this is seen a ring lesion, centrally hypometabolic, with a metabolically active surrounding rim. Most of the rim is comparable to brain cortical activity in intensity, but there is a more discrete nodule of hypermetabolic activity noted at the posterosuperior margin of the lesion, consistent with tumor *(arrowheads)*. Coronal (**A**), transaxial (**B**), and sagittal (**C**) views are shown.

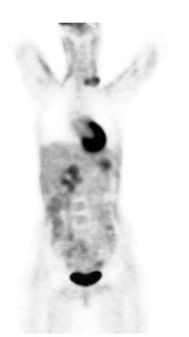

accompanying marked increase in edema (Figure 1). The PET scan showed multiple abnormalities, consistent with multifocal metastatic disease (Figures 3 and 5). Abnormal activity was noted at the site of the palpable left supraclavicular adenopathy, in the liver hilus corresponding to adenopathy on CT, and in the left presacral region. This latter focus showed necrosis and corresponded to a juxtacolonic mass on CT, not previously recognized (Figure 6). A dedicated brain PET study was also performed, which showed the lesion to be hypometabolic centrally, surrounded by a rim of metabolic activity, which was pathologically increased at the posterosuperior margin of the lesion (Figure 2). The patient died 3 months later.

TEACHING POINTS

Lymphatic spread of cervical cancer progresses via internal iliac, external iliac, or presacral chains, all routes leading to the common iliac nodes and more proximally. Cervical cancers have a high avidity for FDG. PET has been shown to be extremely accurate in identifying para-aortic nodal disease, as well as distant metastases. Comparative studies with CT suggest an advantage for FDG-PET in sensitivity and perhaps specificity.

FIGURE 3. Coronal PET image shows activity at the site of the palpable supraclavicular adenopathy. Right subhepatic activity correlates with porta hepatis adenopathy on CT. LUQ activity is normal stomach.

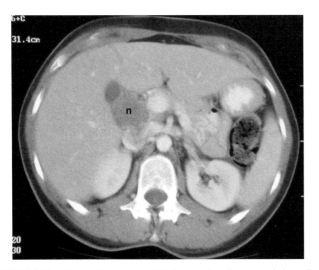

FIGURE 4. Enhanced abdominal CT shows a low-density, pathologically enlarged porta hepatis lymph node (n), corresponding with RUQ findings on PET.

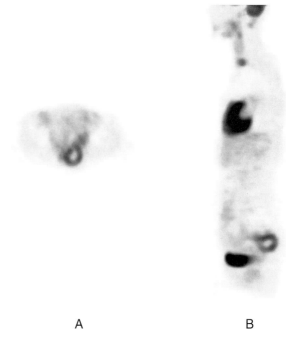

A   B

FIGURE 5. Axial (**A**) and sagittal (**B**) PET images show a ring of left presacral activity, consistent with a necrotic metastasis. Review of a concurrent CT confirmed a juxtacolonic mass at this level, not previously recognized.

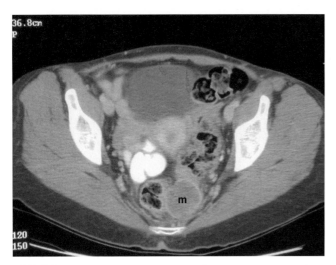

FIGURE 6. Enhanced pelvis CT shows a low-density, necrotic, presacral, juxtacolonic mass (m), corresponding to the PET abnormality.

Endometrial Carcinoma

CASE 21 | *Uterine corpus carcinoma, with vaginal metastasis*

A 55-year-old woman presented with postmenopausal vaginal spotting. Physical examination identified a 1.5-cm lower vaginal mass, near the urethral meatus. Biopsy showed nonkeratinizing carcinoma. A concurrent uterine biopsy showed a similar histology. Pelvic MRI evaluation reported marked thickening of the endometrium. A staging laparotomy with para-aortic and pelvic lymphadenectomy, cystoscopy, and examination under anesthesia was performed. Eighteen lymph nodes were examined and showed no evidence of nodal metastases. PET scan was requested before initiation of preoperative radiation therapy to the pelvis. The PET scan showed intense uterine corpus activity, as well as focal hypermetabolism at the level of the lower vaginal metastasis (Figures 1 and 2). No evidence of distant metastatic disease was seen.

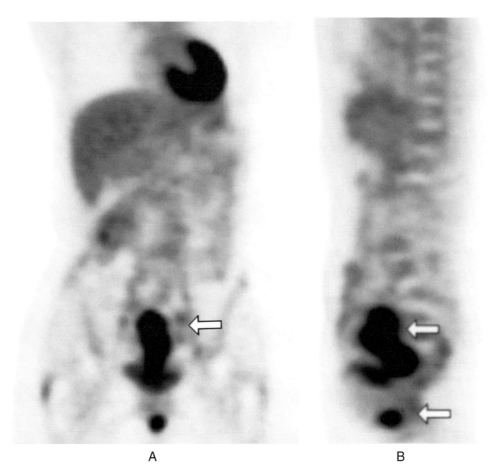

A   B

FIGURE 1. Coronal (**A**) and sagittal (**B**) PET images show intense hypermetabolism in the uterine corpus and at the level of the vaginal metastasis, above and below activity of excreted FDG in the urinary bladder.

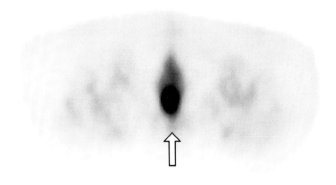

FIGURE 2. Axial PET section shows the focally hypermetabolic uptake at the lower vaginal level.

TEACHING POINTS

Although endometrial carcinoma is the most common gynecologic malignancy, the imaging utility of PET in endometrial carcinoma has been less well studied than for cervical and ovarian carcinomas. Endometrial carcinoma can be visualized on FDG PET imaging, as demonstrated here, and can be a cause for focal uterine uptake on PET. Note should be made that uterine corpus uptake can uncommonly be seen as a benign variant in menstruating females and that fibroids can display activity, ranging from negligible to intense.

In preparing for PET imaging of a patient with a known or suspected pelvic malignancy, it may be prudent to consider maneuvers to minimize excreted FDG activity in the urinary bladder. Some centers elect to place a Foley catheter in the bladder and to encourage diuresis with hydration and furosemide (Lasix). Other sites prefer to keep the examination as noninvasive as possible and "read around" urinary bladder activity. At a minimum, the patient should void immediately before scanning and, if the pelvis is the area of greatest interest, scanning should commence there. As demonstrated in this case, often the presence of urinary bladder activity poses no great interpretive difficulty.

SOFT TISSUE SARCOMAS

Experience with PET and soft tissue sarcomas is relatively small but quite encouraging. These tumors may arise essentially anywhere in the body and can reach massive size. They may invade locally or metastasize distantly, often to the lungs. Traditional evaluation relies on plain radiographs, CT, and MRI. Important issues include differentiation of benign from malignant, estimation of histologic grade of malignancy, selection of biopsy site, search for metastases, assessment of recurrent lesions after therapy, and monitoring treatment response.

Differential Diagnosis: Benign Versus Malignant

Although high-grade soft tissue sarcomas are reliably identified by FDG-PET, low-grade malignancies cannot be differentiated from benign lesions owing to low FDG uptake.[1-3]

Histologic Grading of Malignancy

As with most tumors, the higher the grade, the greater the FDG uptake. Histologic grade is determined on the basis of cellularity,

nuclear atypia, mitotic activity, and necrosis.[4] Histology may be subject to sampling bias and interpretive disagreement. PET has shown there is a strong correlation between glucose metabolic rate and tumor malignancy grade in soft tissue sarcoma.[3-9] This can be assessed visually (qualitatively) or semi-quantitatively with standardized uptake values; however, these values may not be able to reliably separate benign from malignant masses, as noted earlier.[6]

Selection of Biopsy Site

Clearly, MRI remains the imaging modality of choice in the initial evaluation of a soft tissue mass. However, even MRI may have significant difficulty in localizing the most appropriate site for biopsy. PET can direct the specialist to the most metabolically active region, increasing the likelihood of definitive tissue sampling.

Search for Metastases

Similar to the investigation of other tumor types, PET allows for whole-body evaluation with a single study. Although local recurrence may be better depicted with MR, and pulmonary metastases are more sensitively detected with CT, the entire body is most accurately surveyed with FDG-PET. Numerous studies have confirmed PET's ability to identify more lesions than other imaging studies.[1,4,10]

Assessment of Recurrent Lesions after Therapy

Many patients are evaluated for recurrent masses at the site of an earlier resection (some having received radiation therapy). CT and MR studies may be indeterminate for separating benign, post-treatment changes from malignant recurrence. PET has proven extremely valuable in this scenario. With the usual caveats vis-à-vis inflammatory or early postirradiation uptake, high FDG activity typically suggests recurrence of soft tissue sarcomas and absence of uptake indicates post-therapy changes.[2,11-12]

Monitoring Treatment Response

As with many other tumors and their various treatments, the use of PET to monitor response to therapy is under active investigation in soft tissue sarcomas. Preliminary results are encouraging in both the neoadjuvant and post-treatment settings.[13] Generally, absence of FDG uptake suggests a favorable response to treatment, whereas high uptake predicts treatment failure and may direct a change in therapeutic management.

REFERENCES

1. Lucas JD, O'Doherty MJ, Cronin BF, et al: Prospective evaluation of soft tissue masses and sarcomas using fluorodeoxyglucose positron emission tomography. Br J Surg 1999;86:550-556.
2. Griffith LK, Dehdashti F, McGuire AH, et al: PET evaluation of soft tissue masses with fluorine-18 fluoro-2-deoxy-D-glucose. Radiology 1992;182:185-194.
3. Schwarzbach MH, Dimitrakopoulou-Strauss A, Willeke F, et al: Clinical value of [18-f] fluorodeoxyglucose positron emission tomography imaging in soft tissue sarcoma. Ann Surg 2000;231:380-386.

4. Messa C, Landoni C, Pozzato C, et al: Is there a role for FDG PET in the diagnosis of musculoskeletal neoplasms? J Nucl Med 2000;41:1702-1703.

5. Adler LP, Blair HF, Makely JT, et al: Noninvasive grading of musculoskeletal tumors using PET. J Nucl Med 1991;32:1508-1512.

6. Nieweg OE, Pruim J, van Ginkel RJ, et al: Fluorine-18-fluorodeoxyglucose PET imaging of soft-tissue sarcoma. J Nucl Med 1996;37:257-261.

7. Schwarzbach MH, Dimitrakopoulou-Strauss A, Mechtersheimer G, et al: Assessment of soft tissue lesions suspicious for liposarcoma by F18-deoxyglucose (FDG) positron emission tomography (PET). Anticancer Res 2001;21:3609-3614.

8. Franzius C, Schulte M, Hillmann A, et al: Clinical value of positron emission tomography (PET) in the diagnosis of bone and soft tissue tumors. 3rd Interdisciplinary Consensus Conference "PET in Oncology": Results of the Bone and Soft Tissue Study Group. Chirurg 2001;72:1071-1077.

9. Schulte M, Brecht-Krauss D, Heymer B, et al: Grading of tumors and tumorlike lesions of bone: evaluation by FDG PET. J Nucl Med 2000;41:1695-1701.

10. Lucas JD, O'Doherty MJ, Wong JCH, et al: Evaluation of fluorodeoxyglucose positron emission tomography in the management of soft-tissue sarcomas. Br J Bone Joint Surg 1998;80-B:441-447.

11. Kole AC, Nieweg OE, van Ginkel RJ, et al: Detection of local recurrence of soft-tissue sarcoma with positron emission tomography using [18F] fluorodeoxyglucose. Ann Surg Oncol 1997;4:57-63.

12. Garcia R, Kim EE, Wong FC, et al: Comparison of fluorine-18-FDG PET and technetium-99m-MIBI SPECT in evaluation of musculoskeletal sarcomas. J Nucl Med 1996;37:1476-1479.

13. Jones DN, McCowage GB, Sostman HD, et al: Monitoring of neoadjuvant therapy response of soft-tissue and musculoskeletal sarcoma using fluorine-18-FDG PET. J Nucl Med 1996;37:1438-1444.

CASE 22 | *Unsuspected recurrent leiomyosarcoma to multiple muscles*

A 37-year-old woman was referred for PET scanning with a history of a low-grade left popliteal fossa leiomyosarcoma, treated with limb-sparing surgery and irradiation 2 years before. Follow-up MRIs showed no evidence of local recurrence. More recent evaluation for entry into a weight loss program identified abnormal liver function tests. CT showed two liver lesions. Biopsy demonstrated fatty change but no evidence of malignancy. PET scan was requested to further evaluate the

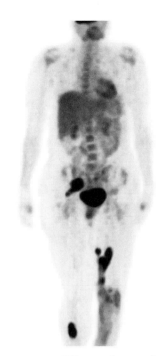

FIGURE 1. Anterior projection PET image shows moderate, diffuse left knee and proximal calf activity, consistent with the prior extensive surgery and radiation therapy. Intense hypermetabolic foci in the right buttock, left medial thigh and right proximal calf were unexpected, and regarded with suspicion for recurrent sarcoma.

liver abnormalities. The patient was otherwise clinically without evidence of disease. PET scanning was extended to the mid-calf level to include the original sarcoma site, which showed diffuse low-level activity (Figure 1). This seemed consistent with the prior surgery and radiation therapy. No focus of more intense activity was seen within the operative bed to suggest a local recurrence. However, multiple other intensely active, completely unexpected and asymptomatic sites were found, including in the right buttock, left thigh, and right calf musculature (Figures 1 to 3, and 11). The PET scan was interpreted as

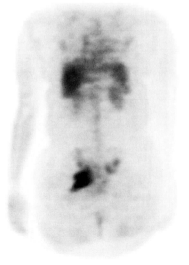
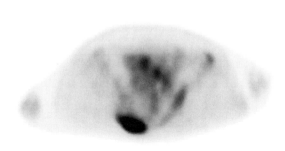

FIGURE 2. Coronal (**A**) and axial (**B**) PET images localize the right buttock activity to the right gluteus.

A   B

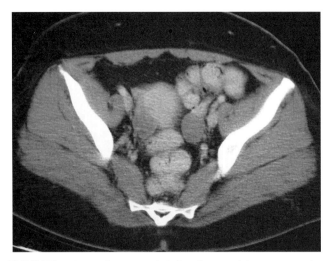

FIGURE 3. Pelvic CT from 3 months before shows no definite corresponding mass.

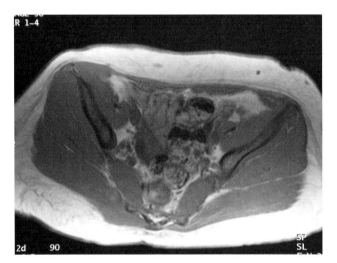

FIGURE 4. Axial T1-weighted MR image shows only subtle loss of muscle striation in the medial right gluteus maximus muscle.

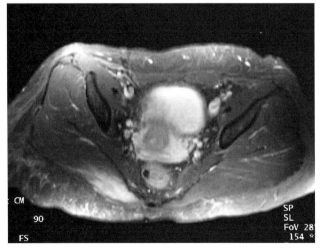

FIGURE 5. Fat-saturated, enhanced T1-weighted axial MR image at the same level shows an enhancing intramuscular mass of the medial right gluteus maximus muscle, corresponding to the PET abnormality. In retrospect, this abnormality is manifested on CT and T1-weighted MR as a subtle contour bulge of the muscle.

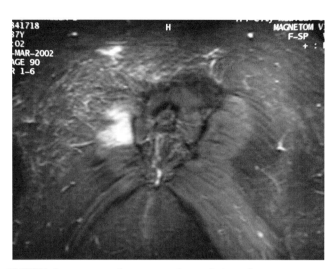

FIGURE 6. STIR coronal MR image of same finding. The sacrum appears unaffected.

extremely suggestive of recurrent sarcoma, and correlation with MRI was recommended. MRIs of the areas in question showed enhancing intramuscular masses, corresponding precisely to the abnormalities on PET (Figures 4 to 10). Surgical excision of these foci confirmed metastatic sarcoma with osteoclast-like giant cells, consistent with the prior histology. Deep margins of resection were all positive, and post-operative radiation therapy was undertaken.

TEACHING POINTS

The PET scan in this patient yielded very unexpected results. This patient was clinically without evidence of active disease, and the study was obtained for reassurance about the liver. No liver abnormalities were found, confirming the benign biopsy results. The intensely hypermetabolic recurrences identified in the right buttock, left thigh, and right calf were completely unexpected. Their identification on PET allowed the subsequent MRI evaluation to be specifically tailored to these levels. PET also enables the site of the original primary lesion to be metabolically evaluated, alleviating the difficulties of MRI follow-up of areas with significant anatomic alterations.

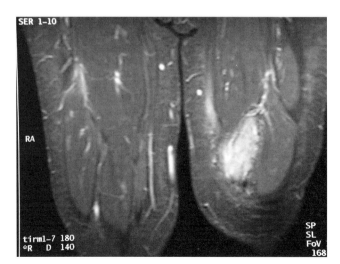

FIGURE 7. STIR coronal MR section through the thighs shows one of two hyperintense ovoid left medial thigh masses, above the level of the prior surgery.

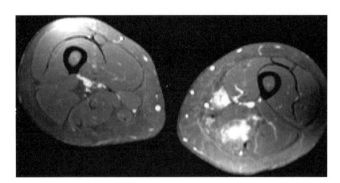

FIGURE 8. Fat-saturated, enhanced T1-weighted axial MR image through the thighs shows the two adjacent, enhancing intramuscular masses.

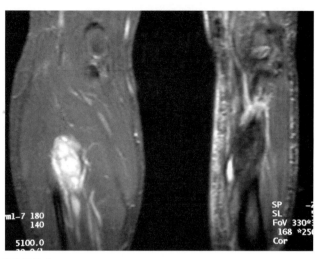

FIGURE 9. Coronal STIR MR image through the proximal calves shows a similar, ovoid, hyperintense intramuscular mass on the right. Note the generalized atrophy on the left, with skin changes of radiation therapy.

FIGURE 10. Fat-saturated, enhanced T1-weighted axial MR image through the proximal calves shows the enhancing right intramuscular calf mass. No abnormal enhancement is seen on the left to suggest local recurrence.

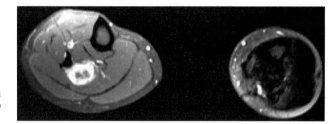

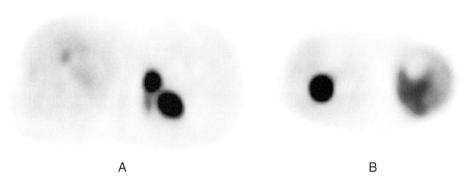

A   B

FIGURE 11. Axial PET sections through the thighs (**A**) and calves (**B**) show very precise correspondence between the PET scan findings and MRI.

CASE 23 | *Synovial sarcoma, metastatic to lung*

A 28-year-old woman with a history of locally advanced left groin synovial sarcoma developed new pulmonary parenchymal nodules on chest CT. The patient's 5-cm left groin mass had been treated with radiation therapy before surgical excision. The margins were clear, with a close (1 mm) medial margin, and two lymph nodes were negative. Postoperatively, the patient was treated with completion radiation therapy and adjuvant chemotherapy, which was discontinued after the third cycle.

Approximately 2 years after diagnosis of the primary tumor, new left lower lobe nodules were found on chest CT, the largest 1.5 cm (Figure 1). Metastatic disease was suspected, and the patient was then evaluated with PET. It showed LLL uptake at the site of the largest nodule, consistent with a metastasis (Figure 2). No pathologic uptake was seen in the left groin surgical bed. The patient underwent left lower lobectomy, which confirmed metastatic synovial sarcoma, with approximately four tumor nodules found, three 5 mm and one 2 cm. Three hilar lymph nodes were negative.

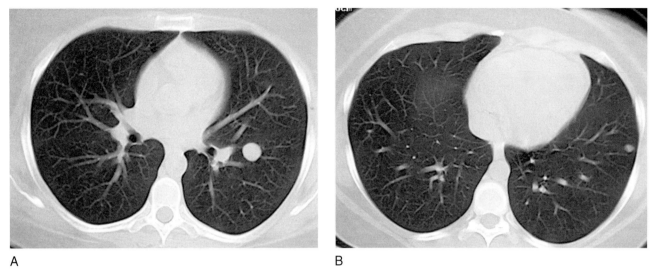

FIGURE 1. CT (lung windows, two levels [**A** and **B**]) shows noncalcified, round new left lower lobe lung nodules, suspicious in this clinical setting for lung metastases.

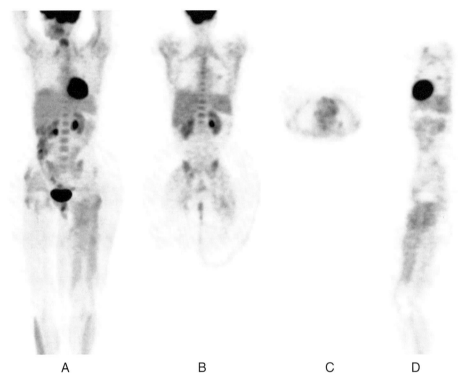

A   B   C   D

FIGURE 2. Metabolic activity is identifiable in the superior segment of the left lower lobe, corresponding to the largest of the LLL nodules seen on CT and consistent with a metastasis. Mild diffuse increased activity is seen in the left thigh musculature, attributable to the prior therapies. The left lower extremity is enlarged compared with the right, secondary to chronic post-treatment lymphedema. Projection (**A**), coronal (**B**), transaxial (**C**), and sagittal (**D**) views are shown.

TEACHING POINTS

Extremity sarcoma follow-ups with MRI are frequently difficult to interpret, owing to the anatomic alterations and distortions from prior resections, as well as edema and thickening associated with radiation therapy. PET scan provides a complementary means for assessing the primary site for local recurrence, as well as an efficient means of whole body surveillance for remote metastatic recurrences. In this case of suspected lung metastasis, the positive PET scan provided noninvasive confirmation, which was pathologically proved.

CASE 24 | *Recurrent intra-abdominal leiomyosarcoma*

A 53-year-old woman with recurrent pelvic leiomyosarcoma was evaluated with PET when CT showed development of a new LUQ mass. She had presented 4 years before with extrauterine extension found at the time of hysterectomy for presumed fibroids. A hysterectomy, oophorectomy, and negative lymphadenectomy were performed, and no additional therapy was given. Just over a year later, a posterior abdominal wall recurrence was identified, surgically excised, and treated with chemotherapy. An additional pelvic recurrence a year later was excised, with very extensive pelvic recurrence from sidewall to sidewall identified 4 months later. This was treated with chemotherapy, with an excellent response, with apparent resolution of disease several months later. On routine CT follow-up a year later, a new, bulky left upper quadrant mass was noted (Figure 1). Another leiomyosarcoma

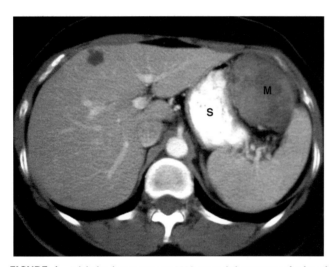

FIGURE 1. A lobular, heterogeneous LUQ mass (M) impresses the lateral aspect of the stomach (S). The mass appears separate from both stomach and spleen. A cyst is noted in the liver, medial segment left lobe.

recurrence was presumed. PET scan showed intense hypermetabolism of the lesion, confirming the impression of recurrence (Figure 2).

TEACHING POINTS

Sarcomas can be variable in metabolic activity level. Relatively aggressive sarcomas, like this recurrent leiomyosarcoma, are metabolically active and very suitable for PET imaging. Other, more indolent sarcomas, such as liposarcomas, are generally less metabolically active and may be less reliably evaluated with PET imaging (see Case 25).

CASE 25 | *Recurrent thoracic liposarcoma*

A 17-year-old high school athlete developed the sudden onset of shortness of breath. His work-up identified a huge mediastinal fatty mass, extending into the right hemithorax. CT-guided biopsy suggested a low-grade liposarcoma. At surgery, the massive tumor occupied the entire anterior mediastinum. It appeared attached to the chest wall and impinged the right lung, which was collapsed. Subtotal resection was performed, which required multiple wedge resections to extricate the tumor from attachments to the right lung. The tumor pathology reported a low-grade myxoid liposarcoma.

The patient initially recovered well, until he developed RUQ and right upper back pain about 6 months after surgery. Chest CT evaluation suggested recurrence of the liposarcoma (Figure 1), at which point he was referred for PET imaging (Figure 2). Subsequent reoperation confirmed the recurrence.

TEACHING POINTS

The utility of PET in the evaluation of sarcomas depends on their inherent metabolic activity. Although many sarcomas are aggressive and highly metabolically active, there are varieties, such as liposarcoma, that generally are relatively low in metabolic rate and may be poor candidates for PET evaluation. In this case, the CT evidence of recurrence, which suggested a more aggressive liposarcoma, prompted PET imaging in this patient. As noted, the modest intrinsic metabolic activity displayed where there is obvious tumor recurrence on CT does not inspire confidence that distant sites of involvement could be recognized if present.

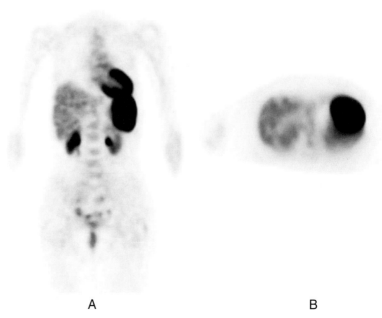

FIGURE 2. Coronal (**A**) and axial (**B**) PET scan images show an intensely hypermetabolic mass corresponding to the new CT finding. A small additional presumed tumor site was identified in the pelvis (not shown), with no clear CT correlate identifiable.

A   B

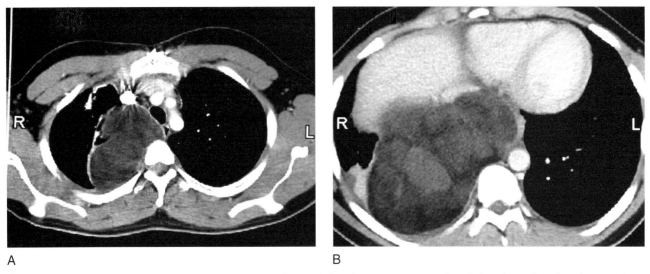

FIGURE 1. Enhanced chest CT sections show heterogeneous, predominantly fatty density tumor mass in the right hemithorax along the right paramediastinal margin and at the posterior costodiaphagmatic level. Findings are consistent with recurrent liposarcoma.

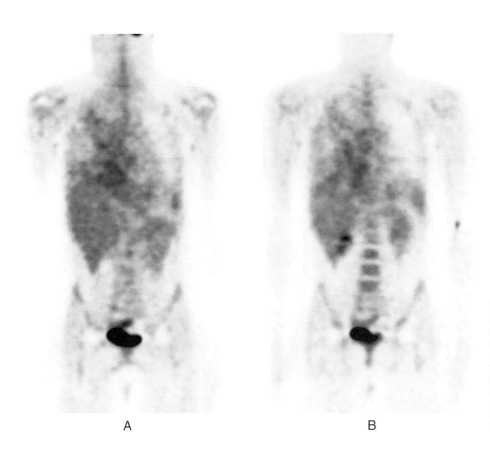

FIGURE 2. Two coronal PET sections (**A** and **B**) show the large right hemithoracic tumor mass to be only modestly metabolically active. Visually, it is easiest to recognize the tumor at the right costophrenic angle level, where there is some contrast to the lower metabolic activity level of the liver. Whereas the right hemithoracic known tumor can be recognized, its relatively low metabolic activity level markedly lowers the confidence level that involvement of distant sites could be recognized.

CASE 26 | Ewing's sarcoma follow-up

A 15-year-old boy with multifocal Ewing's sarcoma was evaluated with PET scanning after chemotherapy for 6 months. He had presented with a swollen right ankle, which worsened with casting. Diagnosis of Ewing's sarcoma was made by biopsy of the ankle. After diagnosis, the patient was staged with bone scan and CT and found to have multiple additional foci of disease, including a lung nodule and multiple osseous sites (Figures 1 to 4). At the time of PET scanning, the patient had shown a good clinical, bone scan, and CT response to chemotherapy, as evidenced by resolution of a presumed pulmonary metastatic nodule. PET scan was requested to see if it could aid in radiation therapy treatment planning (Figures 5 and 6).

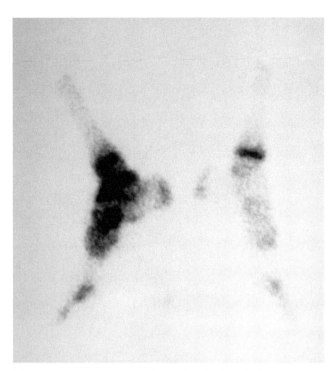

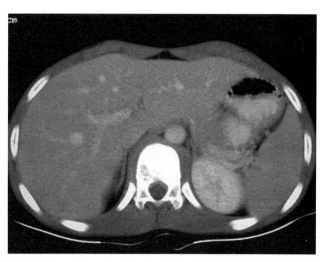

FIGURE 3. Enhanced CT scan through the upper abdomen shows sclerosis and adjacent soft tissue at the T12 level, corresponding to the abnormal bone scan finding.

FIGURE 1. Lateral views of the feet and ankles from the bone scan at the time of diagnosis show intense, diffuse activity in the right ankle, hindfoot, and midfoot. Diagnosis of Ewing's sarcoma was made by biopsy of the ankle. Normal growth plate activity is noted on the left side.

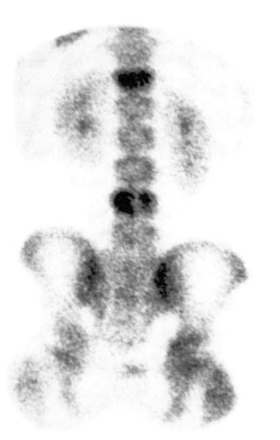

FIGURE 2. Posterior bone scan view of the lumbar spine shows increased activity at the T12 and L4 vertebral bodies, consistent with additional disease sites.

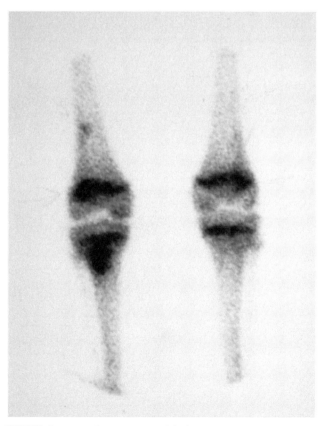

FIGURE 4. Anterior bone scan view of the knees shows additional abnormal foci presumed to be disease sites, including the right distal femoral shaft, the right distal femoral epiphysis, and the right proximal tibial metaphysis.

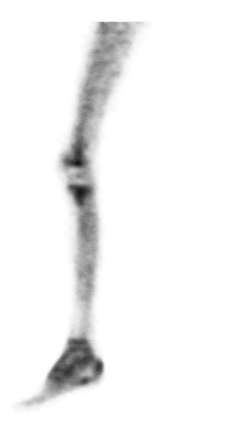

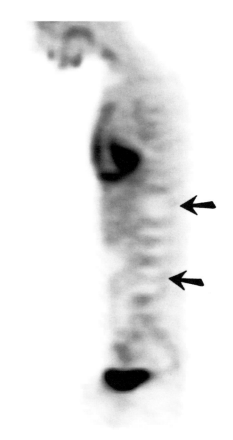

FIGURE 5. Sagittal PET image through the right lower extremity shows asymmetrical diffuse increased activity at the right ankle level, in the same distribution as the abnormal bone scan activity, which had persisted on follow-up bone scans. The increased distal femoral and proximal tibial metaphyseal activity was symmetrical with the opposite side and accompanied by an overall increase in bone marrow activity. This was noted in the proximal humeri, pelvis, and spine and attributable to marrow activation from chemotherapy. The distal femoral diaphyseal site seen on the first bone scan resolved on follow-up scintigraphy and was negative on PET.

FIGURE 6. Sagittal PET scan image through the midline shows the spine with diffuse increased marrow activity, except at the T12 and L4 levels (*arrows*). The diffuse marrow activity is consistent with activated marrow post chemotherapy. The "sparing" is seen at T12 and L4, where bone scan had previously shown evidence of disease activity, which had improved on repeat scintigraphy. The absence of increased activity at these levels was thought to be reassuring regarding tumor activity.

TEACHING POINTS

PET scanning was used to complement other imaging modalities in the treatment monitoring and planning in this patient with metastatic Ewing's sarcoma. At staging, metastases were manifested by multiple active foci on bone scan and a lung nodule. With chemotherapy, the lung nodule resolved and all osseous disease sites, except the presenting ankle, improved or resolved on bone scan. On PET, only the ankle showed increased activity, with other previously identified osseous sites scintigraphically inactive, suggesting that local radiation therapy be directed to the primary site. Whole-body irradiation was also planned.

CASE 27 | *Residual leiomyosarcoma (GIST), postoperative evaluation for residual disease*

A 42-year-old man was referred for PET imaging after undergoing surgical excision of a large leiomyosarcoma that filled the LUQ. He had presented 3 months before with a several-week history of abdominal discomfort and was found to have a palpable epigastric mass. CT examination showed a massive heterogeneous mass, which appeared to arise exophytically from the greater curvature of the stomach (Figure 1). Percutaneous biopsy confirmed a gastrointestinal stromal tumor (GIST), and endoscopy showed no mucosal involvement. At surgery, the tumor was so sizeable that until two necrotic, bloody fluid–containing components were aspirated the abdomen could not be entered or the mass's attachments fully assessed. The mass did arise from the greater curvature of the stomach and compressed the liver, stomach, spleen, and colon. The tumor was eventually freed from the colon, and the involved omentum was excised with the mass, as was a portion of the stomach and the spleen. The final pathology was interpreted as invasive malignant stromal tumor extending from the submucosa of the gastric wall through the full gastric wall thickness. Mucosal margins were free of tumor. A separate omental mass proved to be metastatic gastrointestinal stromal tumor. The patient's postoperative recovery was uneventful. Follow-up CT showed left basilar pleural effusion and reaction, as well as subphrenic nodularity, suggestive of residual tumor (Figure 2). PET imaging was performed 3 months after surgery and showed multiple left subphrenic hypermetabolic tumor foci, consistent with residual or recurrent sarcoma (Figures 3 and 4).

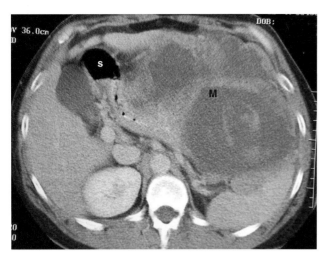

FIGURE 1. Enhanced abdominal CT scan from the patient's initial presentation, showing a heterogeneous massive left upper quadrant mass (M). The mass is contiguous with the greater curvature of the stomach (S), which is severely compressed and displaced to the right. Lower density components of the mass proved at surgery to contain necrotic, bloody fluid, which had to be aspirated in order to evacuate the mass.

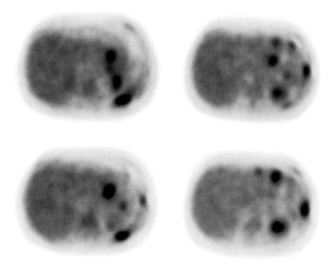

FIGURE 3. Corresponding axial PET images show multiple LUQ foci of hypermetabolism.

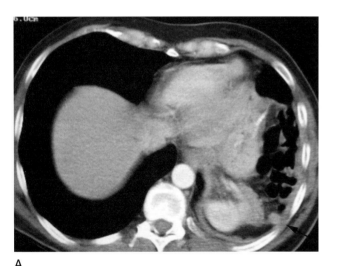

A

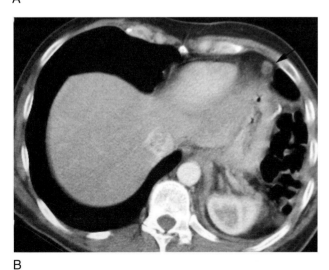

B

FIGURE 2. Postoperative enhanced abdominal CT scan, 3 months later, shows nodular foci, on the order of 1 cm in size, along subphrenic peritoneal surfaces *(arrows)*.

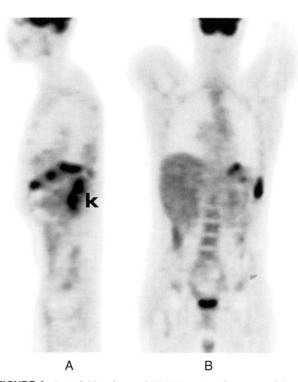

A   B

FIGURE 4. Sagittal (A) and coronal (B) PET sections show many of the subphrenic foci to be aligned along the undersurface of the diaphragm. k, kidney.

TEACHING POINTS

After this patient's massive leiomyosarcoma was surgically evacuated, there remained questions as to what additional therapy should be given and how much residual disease was present. CT follow-up showed the bulk of the mass to be gone, with suspicious subphrenic nodularity and slowly resolving left basilar pleural thickening and reaction. The PET scan results effectively resolved the question of residual disease and provided an ideal modality for the future follow-up and assessment of therapeutic efficacy.

MALIGNANT THYMOMA

CASE 28 | *Malignant thymoma, pleural recurrence*

A 50-year-old woman was referred for PET imaging 6 weeks after finishing six courses of chemotherapy for recurrent thymoma in the pleural space. She had been diagnosed with stage I thymoma 3 years before and treated with surgical excision. Recurrent thymoma was identified in the pleura 2 years later and treated with chemotherapy. Reportedly, a CT performed after concluding chemotherapy showed stable findings. PET scan was requested to assess disease activity. It showed multiple right hemithoracic peripheral foci of activity, consistent with active pleural tumor (Figure 1).

TEACHING POINTS

PET can be very useful is assessing the activity of neoplastic findings that are static on imaging or that fail to resolve completely after therapy. Although this patient's disease initially seemed limited, its recurrence as spread along pleural surfaces is a known pattern of behavior for invasive thymoma.

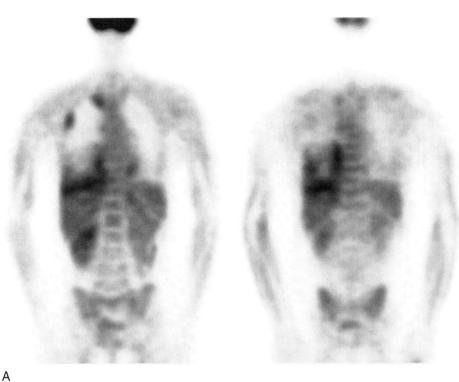

A

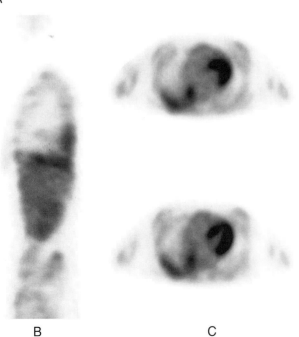

B   C

FIGURE 1. Coronal (**A**), sagittal (**B**), and axial (**C**) PET sections show peripheral, linear right hemithoracic hypermetabolic foci, consistent with active pleural malignant thymoma.

CASE 29 | Pitfall: Inflammatory reaction, suspected anterior mediastinal thymoma

A 64-year-old man was evaluated with PET for suspicion of recurrent thymic carcinoma. One year before he had undergone median sternotomy for excision. He then underwent radiation therapy, which concluded approximately 8 months previously. On a CT follow-up, he was noted to have developed new anterior mediastinal soft tissue, compared with a post-treatment CT 4 months before (Figure 1). Biopsy was considered, but its location adjacent to the aorta was a contraindication. PET scanning was requested to further evaluate this mass (Figure 2). Metabolic activity of moderate intensity (SUV 1.6) was identified at the site on PET. This was regarded with suspicion for recurrent disease given the variability in metabolic activity rates of

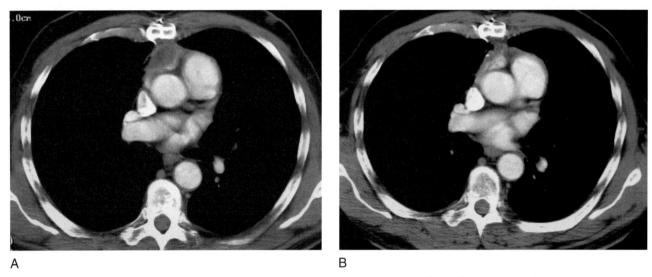

A   B

FIGURE 1. Enhanced chest CT shows low-density prevascular, anterior mediastinal soft tissue or fluid collection (**A**), new from a post-treatment study 4 months before (**B**).

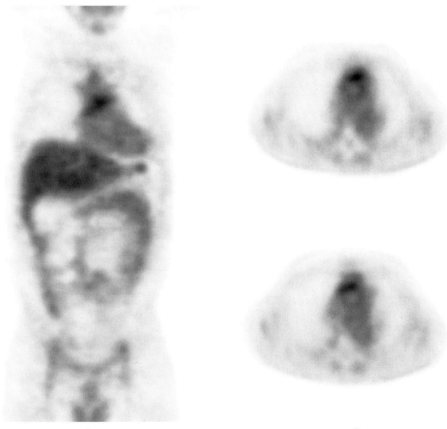

FIGURE 2. Coronal (**A**) and axial (**B**) PET sections show moderate increased metabolic activity at the same level, greater than background mediastinum.

A   B

thymic tumors. The patient underwent surgery for excision of this suspected recurrence via right thoracotomy. The mass was excised as well as a Duraguard pericardial patch and adjacent right and left lung segments. Pathologic findings were intra-alveolar hemorrhage with fibrosis and chronic inflammation but no evidence of residual malignancy.

TEACHING POINT

The mediastinum is used as a visual reference against which to compare suspected abnormalities on FDG PET. This focus was clearly greater in activity level than background mediastinum. The presence of metabolic activity in a new mass in an oncology patient must in general be regarded with suspicion for recurrent tumor until proven otherwise, as it was in this case. The precise explanation for this new finding remains mysterious despite its excision. The modest metabolic activity level it displayed is consistent with the benign, inflammatory pathologic result obtained. Unfortunately, there can and will be overlap with neoplastic masses of relatively low metabolic rate, as this case could easily have proven to be.

MULTIPLE MYELOMA

CASE 30 | *Multiple myeloma, initial staging*

A 60-year-old man who was an avid golfer developed a symptomatic left shoulder and was evaluated with MRI for a suspected rotator cuff tear. MRI showed unsuspected bone lesions, which were new from a prior MRI 2 years before (Figure 1). An expansile soft tissue mass was seen in the acromion, and a second medullary lesion was noted in the proximal humeral shaft. A differential diagnosis of metastases versus myeloma was raised. A whole-body bone scan was obtained next. Increased activity was present in the left acromion and left posterior 10th rib, with faintly increased activity noted in the right proximal humeral shaft and the left skull (Figure 2). Osseous metastatic disease was suspected. A search for an unknown primary lesion was undertaken with chest, abdominal, and pelvic CT scans. These showed abnormal bone findings corresponding to those previously seen but did not identify an occult primary source. PET scan was requested next for suspected carcinoma of unknown primary tumor. This showed multiple hypermetabolic foci, more than had been previously identified by any other study, all localizing to bone (Figure 3). Multiple myeloma was now suggested as the leading diagnosis, because urine protein electrophoresis had by this time identified Bence Jones proteinuria. A subsequent bone marrow biopsy and aspirate demonstrated abnormal plasmacytosis, with morphologic and immunophenotypical findings of multiple myeloma.

TEACHING POINTS

The identification of multiple bone lesions by any imaging modality raises the differential diagnosis of osseous metastases and multiple myeloma. In this case, PET identified more lesions than any other imaging modality obtained in this patient's evaluation. This case also illustrates the known limitations of bone scanning in multiple myeloma, with some lesions demonstrated (the right mid humerus), with other known lesions (left proximal humerus) essentially occult. When multiple myeloma manifests as in this case as discrete focal plasmacytoma type lesions, PET scanning can be an excellent whole-body means of quantifying the disease burden at diagnosis and staging, providing an optimal modality for follow-up during and after therapy. However, PET imaging will have significant limitations in the evaluation of multiple myeloma manifesting as a more diffusely infiltrative process (see Case 32). (Case courtesy of Richard L. Cole, Jr., MD, Naval Medical Center, San Diego.)

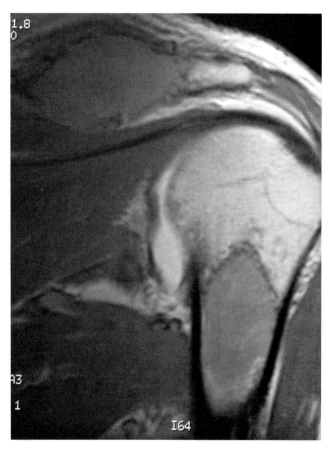

FIGURE 1. Proton density–weighted coronal MR image of the left shoulder shows two focal medullary space bone lesions. The acromial lesion is expansile, whereas the proximal humeral shaft lesion is a central medullary lesion without remodeling. Imaging features of the lesions are nonspecific. Osseous metastases and myeloma are the leading differential diagnostic possibilities.

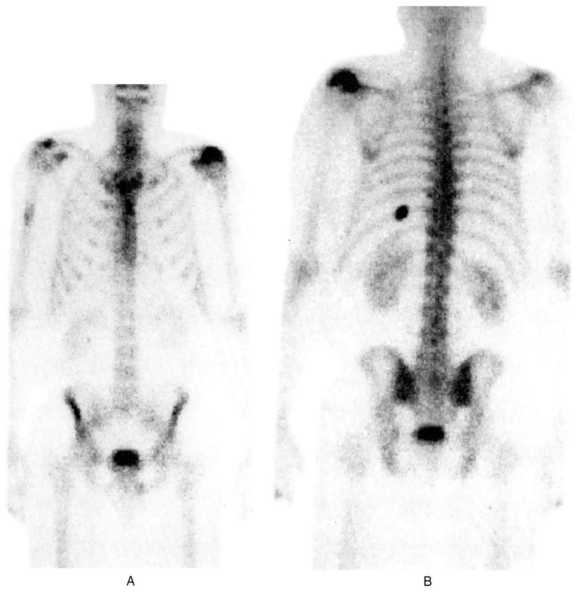

A   B

FIGURE 2. Anterior (**A**) and posterior (**B**) bone scan images show markedly increased activity at the left acromial level, corresponding to the shoulder MRI expansile lesion. The left proximal humeral abnormality is not visualized. There is a focus of increased activity demonstrated at the left posterior 10th rib level, and mildly increased activity is now seen at the right mid-humeral shaft. With these multiple findings, osseous metastases were considered the most likely etiology.

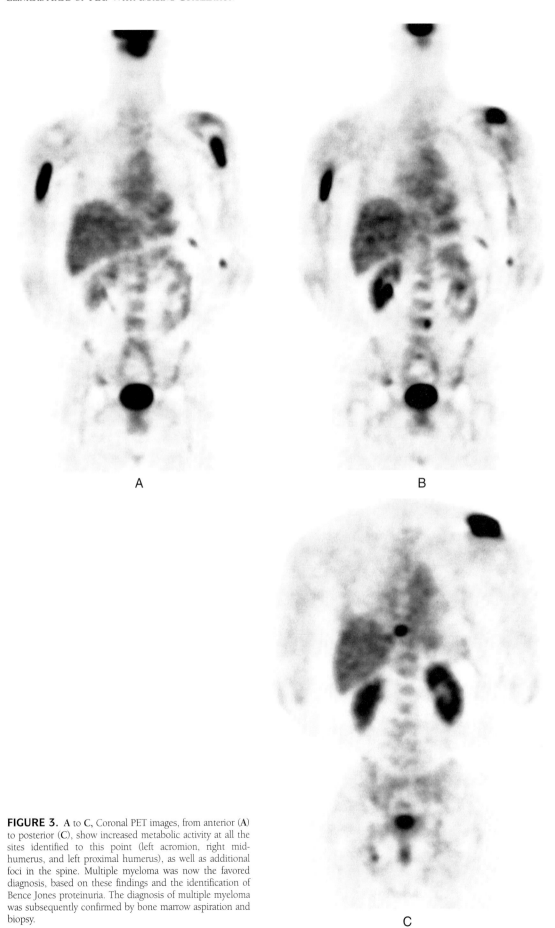

FIGURE 3. **A** to **C,** Coronal PET images, from anterior (**A**) to posterior (**C**), show increased metabolic activity at all the sites identified to this point (left acromion, right mid-humerus, and left proximal humerus), as well as additional foci in the spine. Multiple myeloma was now the favored diagnosis, based on these findings and the identification of Bence Jones proteinuria. The diagnosis of multiple myeloma was subsequently confirmed by bone marrow aspiration and biopsy.

CASE 31 | Multiple discrete myeloma lesions, known disease follow-up

A 59-year-old woman with multiple myeloma initially presented with a left clavicular lump. Her work-up for other lesions was negative, and the patient was irradiated for a plasmacytoma. Approximately 6 months later, lytic lesions were identified in her humeri on skeletal series, and the patient was treated with chemotherapy. She then developed a T11 compression fracture, which was irradiated. These therapies concluded approximately 3 months before PET scan was requested to assess disease activity. PET scanning showed multiple sites of activity, some of which were known disease sites and others that were unsuspected (Figures 1 to 3).

TEACHING POINTS

Multiple myeloma can be difficult to evaluate and follow. Disease activity is gauged by symptoms, biochemistry, and skeletal survey and MRI findings. Unfortunately, nonspecific findings such as osteopenia and compression fractures are frequently the only imaging manifestations of the disease. Bone scan is unreliable. Data are emerging that suggest a role for PET scanning in the assessment of multiple myeloma disease activity. In this case, PET imaging identified a number of sites of increased osseous activity, some of which could be correlated with radiographic findings and some which were not identified on prior radiographic evaluation.

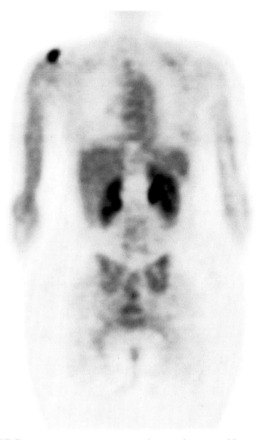

FIGURE 2. A more posterior PET coronal image shows an additional site at the right acromial level.

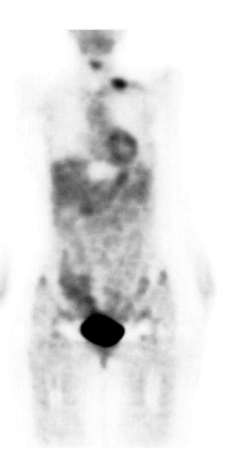

FIGURE 1. Coronal PET image shows a focus of intense activity in the medial left clavicle. This activity correlated with lytic destruction on x-ray evaluation, and the patient developed a subsequent pathologic fracture at this site.

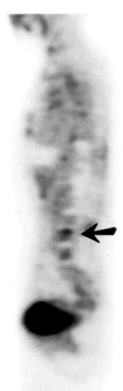

FIGURE 3. Sagittal PET through the lumbar spine shows a more subtle site of presumed disease activity at the L4 level (*arrow*). The sternum is also visualized, suggesting an additional disease site (confirmed radiographically).

CASE 32 | *Multiple myeloma, diffusely infiltrative, poorly demonstrated on PET*

A 66-year-old man with multiple myeloma was diagnosed 4 years previously (Figure 1). He was initially treated with pulse melphalan and prednisone, followed by pulse dexamethasone (Decadron). He subsequently underwent tandem stem cell transplantation, followed by maintenance therapy with interferon-gamma and pamidronate (Aredia). Restaging evaluation showed myeloma in the marrow, and the patient was imaged with lumbar spine MRI and PET (Figures 2 and 3).

TEACHING POINTS

There are reports in the literature that PET scanning may be beneficial in assessing the activity of multiple myeloma and/or follow-up of therapy.

This seems to apply predominantly to those cases in which myeloma manifests as discrete, focal, plasmacytoma-type lesions (see Case 30). In this case, the PET scan findings are not particularly helpful or elucidating. The disease presentation is one of diffuse marrow heterogeneity on MRI with only small discrete lesions on MRI and bone survey. The major manifestations of the disease here are the multiple compression fractures and osteopenia. The heterogeneity of the bone marrow seen on PET may correlate with the marrow heterogeneity on MRI, but with only one data point it is difficult to say whether this appearance is significant. It also is not dramatically different from the mild diffuse marrow heterogeneity seen frequently on normal PET scans. The small size of the discrete, punched-out lytic lesions here is an important limitation, and the prior treatment of this patient may be an additional contributing factor.

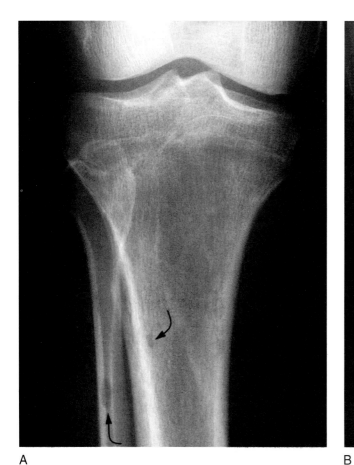

A

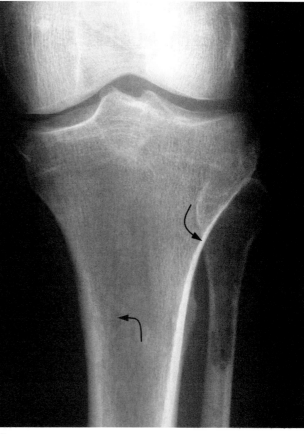

B

FIGURE 1. **A** and **B**, Anteroposterior views of the proximal tibias and fibulas, from a skeletal survey, show typical, sharply demarcated, small, "punched-out" lytic lesions of bone *(arrows)*, best seen in the left proximal fibula.

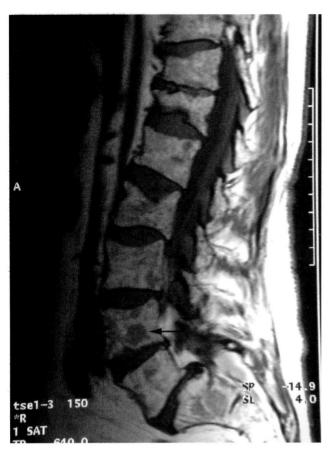

FIGURE 2. T1-weighted sagittal MR image shows heterogeneous bone marrow signal, with a small rounded hypointense focus at L4 (*arrow*). There are multiple compression fracture deformities, with anterior wedging at T11 and T12, and superior end plate invagination at L2.

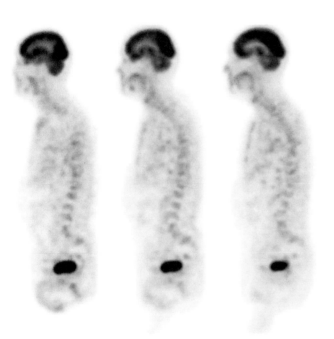

FIGURE 3. Sagittal PET scan images through the spine of this patient show heterogeneity of bone marrow activity.

NONMELANOMA SKIN MALIGNANCIES

CASE 33 | *Kaposi's sarcoma (non-AIDS)*

A 77-year-old man was referred for PET assessment of long-standing and progressive non-AIDS–related Kaposi's sarcoma of the lower extremities. He was first diagnosed 10 years before with involvement of both feet. In recent years, the involvement had progressed proximally and become more confluent, particularly in the right thigh. Initial lesions were surgically excised. As the disease became more extensive, radiation therapy was utilized. Three years before, the right distal lateral calf was treated with radiation, and 3 weeks before the PET scan the patient had completed irradiation to the sole of the right foot and the upper right lateral calf. At the time of PET scanning, systemic therapy with interferon injections had just begun. The patient noted extreme right lower extremity swelling for the 2 preceding months. Doppler evaluation for deep venous thrombosis was negative. On physical inspection, the skin lesions were particularly confluent in the right upper medial calf.

PET scan showed a number of unexpected abnormalities, suggesting nodal involvement of the lower extremities as well as of the mediastinum (Figures 1 to 3). The largest discrete focus in the right popliteal fossa seemed likely nodal. Similarly, nodular to linear foci in

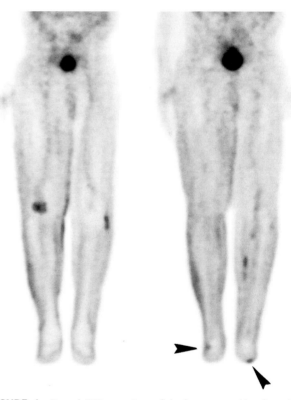

FIGURE 1. Coronal PET scan views of the lower extremities show right popliteal fossa and left proximal calf presumed nodal disease sites. More discrete Kaposi's lesions at the right lateral hindfoot and left plantar hindfoot are identifiable as small punctate foci of activity (*arrowheads*). The entire right lower extremity is swollen compared with the left and shows a diffuse overall increase in skin activity level, as can be seen with lymphedema from any etiology. Skin activity level is most increased at the right medial knee level, where the patient's Kaposi's sarcoma was particularly confluent.

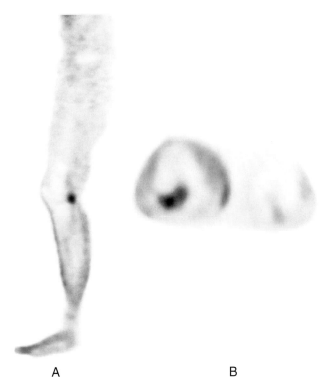

the left proximal calf soft tissues, along vessel courses, also seemed most likely nodal. Small, focal discrete active sites in the right lateral hindfoot and left hindfoot plantar soft tissues corresponded to more discrete and painful Kaposi's lesions. A diffuse increase in the skin activity of the right proximal medial calf correlated with the most confluent skin involvement. There also was increased activity identified in the anterior mediastinum, suggesting nodal activity at this level as well.

TEACHING POINTS

The role PET scanning has to play in imaging of cutaneous malignancies is evolving and has not been entirely defined. Although PET imaging has well established utility in the evaluation of systemic lymphomas, there is less experience with its use in cutaneous lymphomas. Clearly, as in the imaging evaluation of melanoma, the whole-body capability of PET imaging lends itself to the assessment of skin malignancies. However, the process of validating such applications is ongoing. Attenuation-corrected images are preferred over non–attenuation-corrected images to best depict the extremities for assessment of skin abnormalities.

In this case, the most useful information PET imaging provided is evidence of nodal involvement, suggesting the patient may benefit from systemic rather than local therapy.

A   **B**

FIGURE 2. Sagittal (**A**) and axial (**B**) PET sections through the popliteal fossa of the right lower extremity show the focal, nodal-type activity at this level.

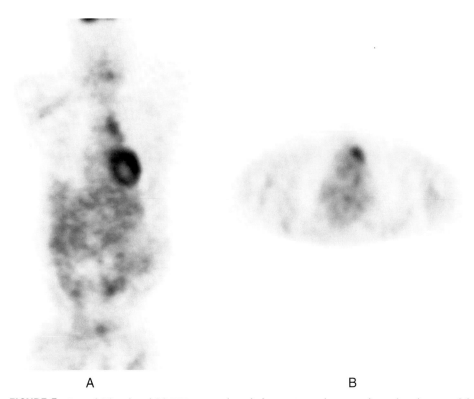

A   **B**

FIGURE 3. Coronal (**A**) and axial (**B**) PET sections through the anterior mediastinum show relatively intense left anterior mediastinal prevascular, presumably nodal, activity, suggesting involvement at this level as well.

CASE 34 | *Bowen's disease (multiple squamous cell carcinoma)*

A 46-year-old Vietnamese woman with a diagnosis of Bowen's disease was referred for PET imaging to assess the activity of known lesions. Bowen's disease is a rare condition of multiple plaques of squamous cell carcinoma, and those affected have an increased propensity for development of systemic malignancy. This patient had previous involvement identified at the left foot instep level 2 years before, with lesions identified 1 year later at the left knee, left thigh, and right shoulder levels.

PET imaging identified two metabolically active disease sites (Figures 1 to 3). One was at the left medial mid-thigh level, corresponding to a lesion. The second was at the left inguinal level, which was not previously known to be involved. Other sites in question were scintigraphically inactive.

TEACHING POINTS

As previously noted, the precise role of PET in assessment of nonmelanoma skin malignancies is evolving. In individual cases, PET's whole-body survey capability may be useful in the evaluation of such patients. Attenuation-corrected images will be preferred when the skin is of particular interest.

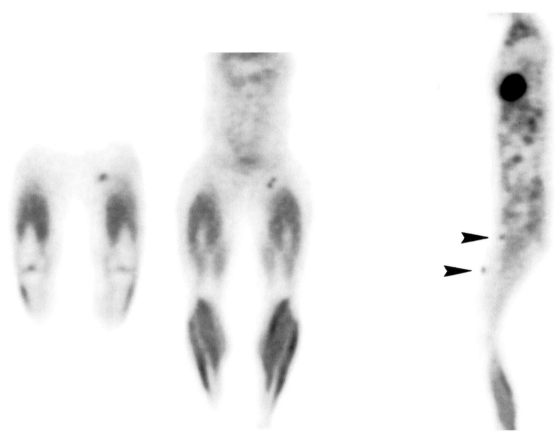

FIGURE 1. Coronal PET sections show small, discrete hypermetabolic foci, one at the medial left thigh level and two at the left inguinal level.

FIGURE 2. Sagittal PET image show the punctate hypermetabolic foci at the inguinal and mid-thigh (*arrowheads*) levels.

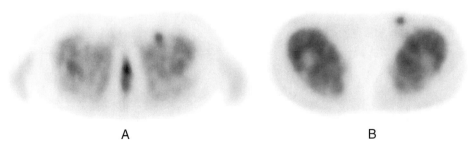

A   B

FIGURE 3. Corresponding axial PET sections through the inguinal (**A**) and mid-thigh (**B**) levels.

Neurologic PET Applications

The use of PET in neurologic disorders can be conveniently divided into four main areas: (1) brain tumors, (2) seizure disorders, (3) dementia, and (4) research applications, such as neuropsychiatric disease, trauma, movement disorders, drug effects, and brain biochemistry/function.

BRAIN TUMORS

PET has shown clinical efficacy in assessing the degree of malignancy, determining prognosis, separating recurrence from therapy-related changes, and monitoring progression.[1] FDG accumulation is typically increased in high-grade gliomas but in only 10% of low-grade gliomas.[2] This can be assessed either visually or semi-quantitatively utilizing standardized uptake values. Although the majority of studies in patients with brain tumors are for the evaluation of gliomas, there is evidence to support the use of FDG-PET to assess aggressiveness and likelihood of recurrence in meningiomas.[3] The initial imaging work-up of suspected brain tumor includes MRI and/or CT; however, PET's unique ability to measure tumor metabolism supports its role as a complementary study in selected cases. Recently, MR spectroscopy has gained increasing acceptance for tumor evaluation. Determination of prognosis can be made with PET. Increased FDG uptake at the site of tumor was found to be predictive of transformation to a higher grade.[4] Conversely, absence of increased uptake at the time of diagnosis was a strong predictor that subsequent transformation was unlikely. There is also some evidence that in high-grade gliomas the level of glucose metabolism is predictive of survival.[4,5] An extension of the use of PET for prognosis is its potential utilization to predict the outcome of radiosurgery by detecting hyperacute changes in tumor glucose metabolism.[6] Much of the work in assessing brain tumors has been done with FDG. Some centers have shown excellent results in low-grade gliomas using ^{11}C-methionine, but close proximity to a cyclotron is necessary, owing to the short 20-minute half-life of carbon-11.[7] The differentiation of therapy-related changes, primarily due to

radiation, from recurrence can be very difficult with anatomic imaging modalities such as MRI or CT. Radiation injury may occur in up to one third or more of patients and, in this group, PET has been shown to be both sensitive and specific in separating recurrence from radiation necrosis. False-negative PET studies in these patients may occur with recent radiation therapy, low histologic grade, or very small tumor volume. False-positive findings result from nonmalignant inflammatory lesions, subclinical seizure activity, or persistent radiation-induced inflammatory response.[8]

SEIZURE DISORDERS

Although most patients with epileptic seizures can be controlled on medication(s), some cannot. These patients are said to have refractory seizures. They may benefit from surgical resection of the epileptogenic focus. PET can be efficacious in locating the epileptogenic zone by showing an area (or areas) of hypometabolism in the interictal phase. This may be particularly helpful in patients with partial complex seizures, a suggestive electroencephalogram, and negative or equivocal MRI. A recent summary of more than 1200 patients showed a benefit for PET in the vast majority of studies.[9] There are also data that show a correlation between PET results and surgical outcome; specifically, an improvement in seizure control after surgical removal of a hypometabolic focus.[10-12]

DEMENTIA

In patients presenting with symptoms of dementia, PET has demonstrated efficacy and cost-effectiveness for diagnosis as well as prognosis.[13-16] The classic metabolic abnormality associated with Alzheimer's disease is bilateral temporoparietal hypometabolism. The reliability of these findings for Alzheimer's disease suggests that other patterns of hypometabolism should prompt alternate diagnoses. One example is the typical finding of hypometabolism in the occipital cortex in diffuse Lewy body disease.[17] Importantly, as with cerebral single photon emission CT (SPECT), a limitation of PET is specificity. To date, few disease-specific patterns have been identified. However, certain findings are highly suggestive (e.g., bifrontal hypometabolism and Pick's disease; multiple, variable-sized regions of hypometabolism and multi-infarct dementia).

RESEARCH APPLICATIONS

Exciting research is ongoing in the use of PET in neuropsychiatric disease, movement disorders (i.e., fluoroDOPA), cerebral trauma, drug effects, and brain biochemistry/function.[18-21]

REFERENCES

1. Coleman RE, Hoffman JM, Hanson MW, et al: Clinical application of PET for the evaluation of brain tumors. J Nucl Med 1991;32:616-622.
2. DiChiro G: Positron emission tomography using [18F] fluorodeoxyglucose in brain tumors: A powerful diagnostic and prognostic tool. Invest Radiol 1986;22:360-371.
3. DiChiro G, Hatazawa J, Katz DA, et al: Glucose utilization by intracranial meningiomas as an index of tumor aggressivity and probability of recurrence: A PET study. Radiology 1987;164:521-526.
4. DeWitte O, Levivier M, Violon P, et al: Prognostic value of positron emission tomography with [18F] fluoro-2-deoxy-D-glucose in the low-grade glioma. Neurosurgery 1996;39:470-477.
5. Patronas NJ, Dichiro G, Kufta C, et al: Prediction of survival in glioma patients by means of positron emission tomography. J Neurosurg 1985;62:816-822.
6. Maruyama I, Sadato N, Waki A, et al: Hyperacute changes in glucose metabolism of brain tumors after stereotactic radiosurgery: A PET study. J Nucl Med 1999;40:1085-1090.
7. Herholz K, Holzer T, Bauer B, et al: ^{11}C-methionine PET for differential diagnosis of low grade gliomas. Neurology 1998;50:1316-1322.
8. Langleben DD, Segall GM: PET in differentiation of recurrent brain tumor from radiation injury. J Nucl Med 2000;41:1861-1867.
9. Gambhir SS, Czernin J, Schwimmer J, et al: A tabulated summary of the FDG-PET literature. J Nucl Med 2001;42:71S-76S.
10. Delbeke D, Lawrence SK, Abou-Khalil BW, et al: Postsurgical outcome of patients with uncontrolled complex partial seizures and temporal lobe hypometabolism on 18FDG-positron emission tomography. Invest Radiol 1996;31:261-266.
11. Heinz R, Ferris N, Lee EK, et al: MR and positron emission tomography in the diagnosis of surgically correctable temporal lobe epilepsy. Am J Neuroradiol 1994;15:1341-1348.
12. Shih YH, Yiu CH, Su MS, et al: Temporal lobectomy in adults with intractable epilepsy. J Formos Med Assoc 1994;93:307-313.
13. Silverman DHS, Small GW, Chang CY, et al: Positron emission tomography in evaluation of dementia. JAMA 2001;286:2120-2127.
14. Silverman DHS, Gambhir SS, Huang H-WC, et al: Evaluating early dementia with and without assessment of regional cerebral metabolism by PET: A comparison of predicted costs and benefits. J Nucl Med 2002;43:253-266.
15. Hoffman JM, Welsh-Bohmer KA, Hanson M, et al: FDG-PET imaging in patients with pathologically verified dementia. J Nucl Med 2000;41:1920-1928.
16. Silverman DHS, Phelps ME: Assessing brain biochemistry in the early evaluation of dementia: Can we afford the improved diagnostic accuracy obtained by incorporating cerebral metabolic data acquired with positron emission tomography into the clinical work-up? Mol Imag Biol 2002; 4:5-9.
17. Albin RL, Minoshima S, D'Amato CJ, et al: Fluoro-deoxyglucose positron emission tomography in diffuse Lewy body disease. Neurology 1996;47:462-466.
18. Newberg A, Alavi A, Reivich M: Determination of regional cerebral function with FDG-PET imaging in neuropsychiatric disorders. Semin Nucl Med 2002;32:13-34.
19. Herscovitch P: Evaluation of the brain by positron emission tomography. Rheum Dis Clin North Am 1993;19:765-793.
20. Phelps ME, Mazziotta JC: Positron emission tomography: Human brain function and biochemistry. Science 1985;228:799-809.
21. Alavi A, Newberg AB: Metabolic consequences of acute brain trauma: Is there a role for PET? J Nucl Med 1996;37:1170-1172.

CASE 1 | *Normal brain PET: guidelines for image interpretation*

An understanding of normal patterns of cerebral metabolism on FDG-PET is critical to accurate image interpretation (Figure 1). This is particularly true with subtle, early abnormalities, such as may be seen in mild cognitive impairment.

The adult brain relies almost exclusively on glucose oxidation for energy metabolism, with synaptic connections being the most expensive of energy functions. Generally, regional cerebral blood flow (rCBF) and local cerebral glucose metabolism are proportional to each other. Metabolic activity in gray matter is on the order of four times greater than that in white matter. The cerebellum is 10% to 30% less metabolically active than the cerebral cortex. Conversely, basal ganglia activity is normally 10% to 30% greater than that of the cortex. Therefore, cerebral cortical activity is typically midway in intensity between normal basal ganglia and the cerebellum.

Highest metabolic activity ↔ lower metabolic activity
Basal ganglia ← gray matter — cerebellum → white matter

The thalamus is usually isometabolic to cerebral cortex. The mesial temporal lobe cortex is generally less metabolically active than the lateral temporal cortex. Commonly seen normal variant regions of locally increased metabolic activity are the frontal eye fields and posterior cingulate cortex. The posterior cingulate activity can normally range up to 30% to 40% greater than the remainder of the cortex. A decline in activity at this level, resulting in isometabolism to the rest of the cortex, can be a subtle clue to identifying early cognitive impairment or Alzheimer's dementia.

There is considerable normal variation of FDG uptake. The normal brain is not completely symmetrical, and the pattern of distribution can be affected by patient activity during the uptake phase. For example, increased visual cortical activity may be observed in studies obtained with a patient's eyes open. Antiepileptic drugs and sedatives are known to reduce cerebral metabolism. It is also important to understand that normal brain metabolism patterns in children differ considerably from those in adults. In the normal newborn, the sensorimotor cortex is metabolically active compared with the rest of the cerebral cortex, producing a pattern that resembles advanced Alzheimer's disease.

TEACHING POINT

Cerebral PET image interpretation can be difficult. A simple technical aid is the inversion of images to white on black or the selection of one

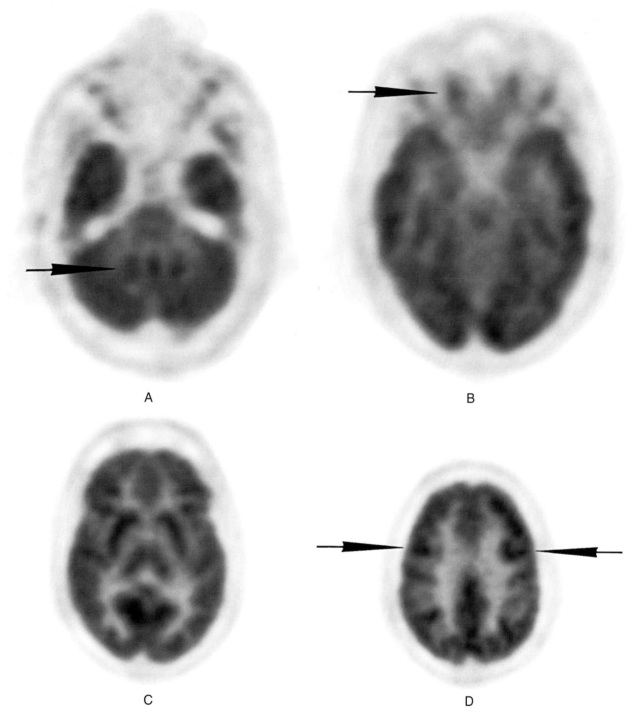

A

B

C

D

FIGURE 1. Axial brain PET sections, from inferior to superior, normal example. **A,** Image through posterior fossa, including inferior temporal lobes, shows dentate nuclei of the cerebellum *(arrow)*. **B,** Higher section, through temporal and occipital lobes, shows the normal higher metabolic activity level of lateral temporal cortex over medial. Note activity in extraocular eye muscles *(arrow)*. **C,** Higher section, through basal ganglia. Caudate head and putamen are of higher metabolic activity normally than cortical gray matter. Thalamus is approximately equivalent in intensity to cortex. Posterior cingulate cortex is commonly relatively hypermetabolic. A decline in activity to isointensity with other cortical regions can be a clue to early Alzheimer's disease. **D,** Superior brain PET slice, through the centrum semiovale, shows another frequently observed normal variant in cortical activity. Frontal eye fields *(arrows)* show relatively increased metabolic activity.

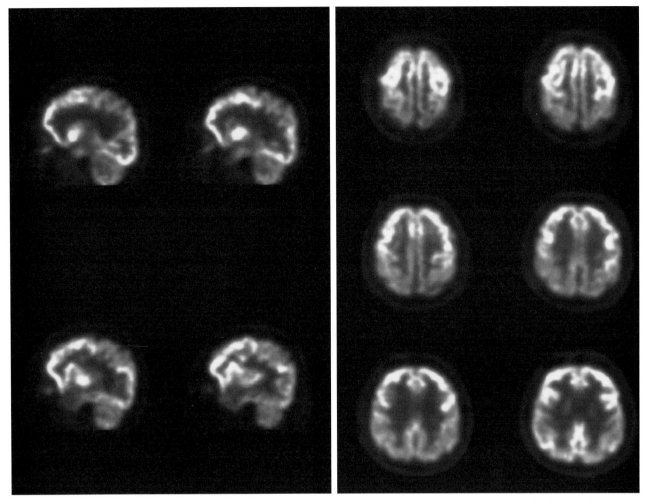

FIGURE 2. Reviewing images with different color scales can be helpful in delineating differential metabolic activity. The parietal and temporal lobes show symmetrically reduced activity, a pattern suggestive of Alzheimer's dementia. Refer to color plate 6 to see this case in a color scheme in which higher metabolic activity is depicted by greater intensity of yellow.

or more color tables to better delineate subtle differences. The following example, with symmetrical biparietal and bitemporal hypometabolism typical of Alzheimer's disease, illustrates the use of color to highlight intensity differences (Figure 2 and color plate 6).

CASE 2 | *Recurrent glioblastoma multiforme (differentiation from radiation necrosis)*

A 46-year-old woman was evaluated with PET imaging when MRI showed findings suggestive of recurrence of glioblastoma multiforme (GBM). The patient had previously undergone a left temporal craniotomy for debulking, followed by radiation therapy. Gamma knife therapy was abandoned when treatment planning scans showed a new adjacent lesion, which was too large. The patient then underwent a repeat left craniotomy for debulking, with the operative specimen reportedly showing only radiation necrosis.

Approximately a year after the last surgery, the patient developed headache, nausea, and vomiting. MRI showed development of a large area of enhancement in the left frontal and temporal lobes, accompanied by vasogenic edema. The mass effect partially effaced the left frontal ventricle and produced 1 cm of midline shift. Recurrent tumor was favored over radiation necrosis in the differential diagnosis. PET scan was requested for differentiation (Figure 1). Intense uptake was present in the temporal lobe, consistent with recurrent GBM.

The patient underwent a partial debulking, confirming recurrent tumor.

TEACHING POINT

The MRI and CT manifestations of recurrent tumor, namely, mass effect, enhancement, and edema, are often indistinguishable from those of radiation necrosis. The development of such suspicious findings in settings altered by prior surgery and radiation therapy effects contributes to the difficulty in morphologic follow-up.

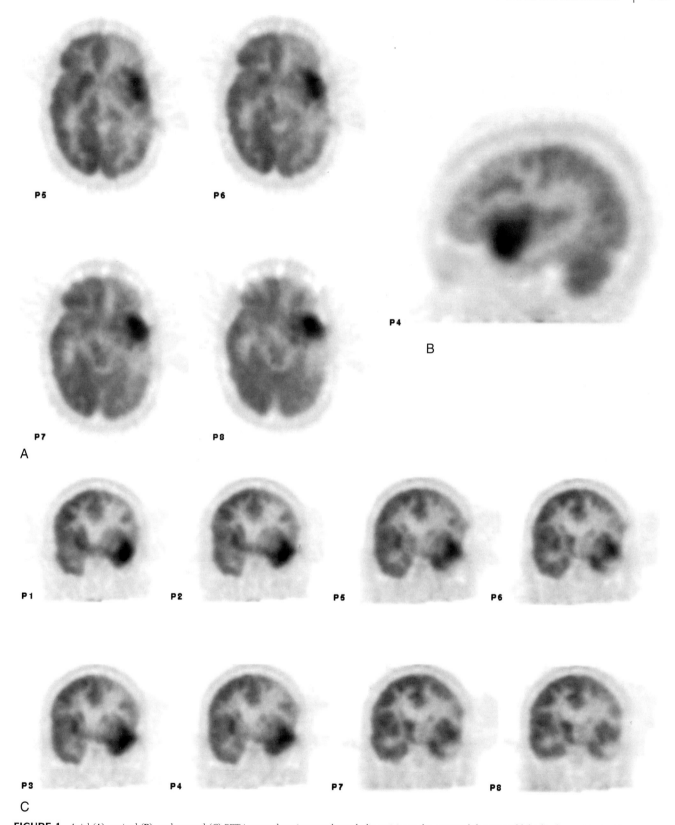

FIGURE 1. Axial (**A**), sagittal (**B**), and coronal (**C**) PET images show increased metabolic activity at the anterior left temporal lobe level, consistent with recurrent glioblastoma multiforme. Diffuse hypometabolism is noted in the left frontal and temporal lobes, attributable to the severe accompanying edema.

PET is an elegant, noninvasive technique that can differentiate between these possibilities with ease. If the enhancing mass on MRI is frankly hypermetabolic, as in this case, the diagnosis of recurrent tumor is readily made. Radiation necrosis will be hypometabolic in the regions of concern. Multiple examples follow in this chapter.

PET can also demonstrate tumor coexisting with post-treatment changes and, in such cases, can be used to identify the most metabolically active tissue for biopsy direction.

CASE 3 | Lung cancer metastasis, gamma knife follow-up

A 57-year-old man, status post right upper lobectomy and radiation therapy for non–small cell lung cancer, developed an enhancing intracranial mass lesion, presumed to be a metastasis (Figures 1 and 2).

Dedicated brain PET study, performed in conjunction with a whole-body scan, demonstrated a corresponding intensely hypermetabolic right frontal mass (Figure 3). He was treated with radiation and gamma knife therapy, and follow-up MRIs showed a progressive decline in the size of the lesion, until only a small enhancing focus could be seen at the site (Figures 4 and 5). The associated edema resolved as well. The follow-up brain PET showed essentially complete reversion to normal (Figure 6). No intracranial disease was evident 1.5 years later.

TEACHING POINTS

PET can be useful in monitoring the course of therapies, such as with gamma knife, especially if the imaging findings are equivocal on follow-up. The initial PET findings in this case are indicative only of the presence of malignancy, but they do not distinguish between hypermetabolic activity from a primary brain tumor versus metastasis.

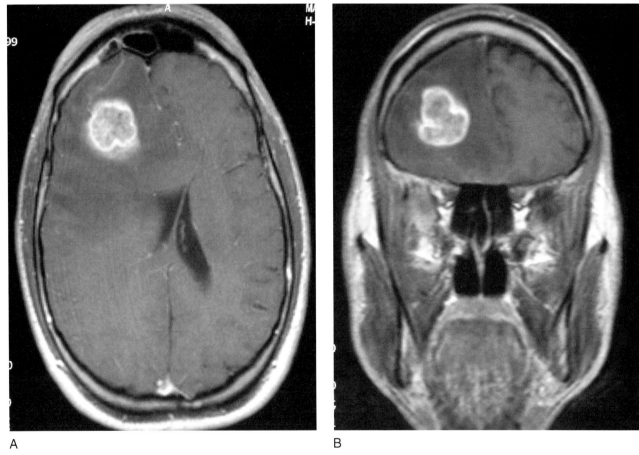

A   B

FIGURE 1. Enhanced T1-weighted axial (**A**) and coronal (**B**) MR images show a lobular, enhancing right frontal mass, associated with a large amount of vasogenic edema and mass effect. There is partial effacement of the right lateral ventricle and midline shift (subfalcine herniation).

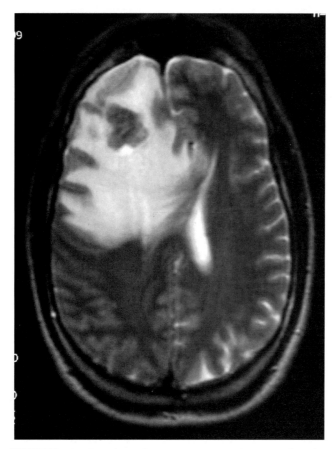

FIGURE 2. On T2 weighting, the mass is isointense to brain parenchyma but is well seen against the extensive right frontal edema. The mass effect on the ventricles and the midline shift are well seen.

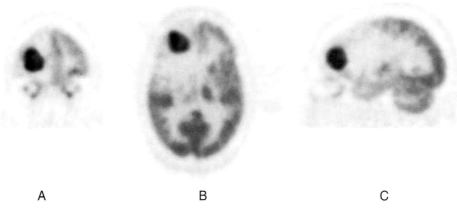

A   B   C

FIGURE 3. PET shows the lesion to be intensely hypermetabolic, confirming its malignant nature. The diffusely decreased metabolic activity of the entire right frontal lobe is attributable to the edema and mass effect. Coronal (**A**), transaxial (**B**), and sagittal (**C**) views are shown.

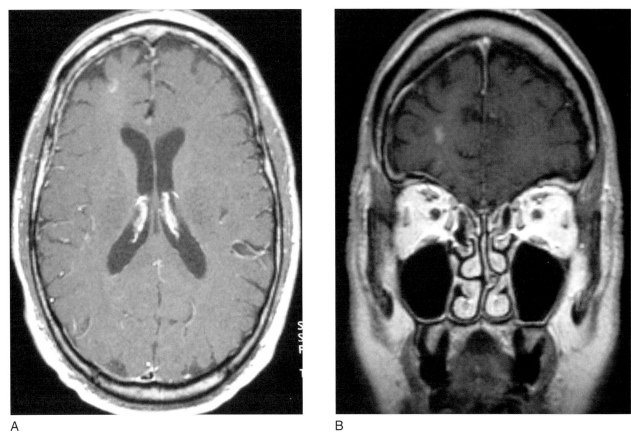

A   B

FIGURE 4. Appearance on MRI 5 months later. Enhanced T1-weighted axial (**A**) and coronal (**B**) MR sections show complete resolution of the edema and mass effect present previously. At the site of the lesion, only a tiny residual enhancing focus remains.

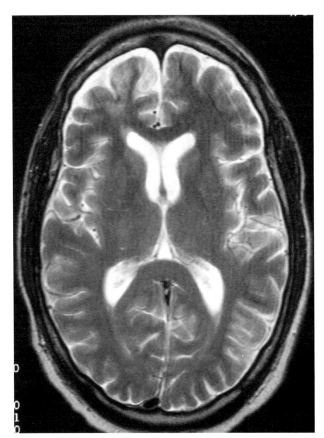

FIGURE 5. T2-weighted fast spin echo axial image also shows near-complete reversion to normal. Minimal cortical hyperintensity remains in the right para-median frontal region.

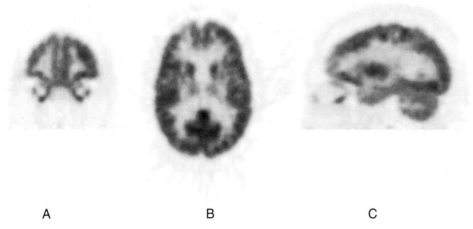

A   B   C

FIGURE 6. Repeat brain PET scan 6 months after the original PET scan also shows essentially complete reversion to normal. No pathologic hypermetabolic activity is now seen, and minimal subtle right frontal cortical hypometabolism is barely perceptible. Coronal (**A**), transaxial (**B**), and sagittal (**C**) views are shown.

CASE 4 | *Low-grade oligodendroglioma, initial diagnosis*

A 35-year-old woman initially sought ENT evaluation for a rushing water sensation in her left ear, noted at night when she rolled to that side in bed. She also complained of frequent headaches. When a trial of sinus disease therapy did not help, she was evaluated with a brain MRI.

The MRI was abnormal, showing a right frontal region of altered parenchymal signal intensity, without much mass effect or enhancement (Figures 1 to 3). A low-grade glioma was favored in the differential diagnosis. PET scan was requested to further evaluate the lesion (Figure 4). No hypermetabolic activity was seen at the lesion site to suggest an alternative diagnosis. The lesion was essentially hypometabolic. Again, a low-grade neoplasm was favored. The patient underwent tumor resection via right frontal craniotomy, with gross total

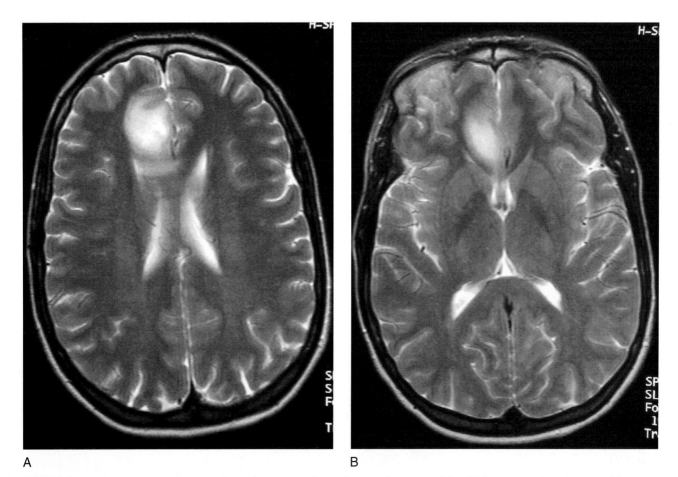

A   B

FIGURE 1. **A** and **B**, T2-weighted fast spin echo axial MR images show a discrete right parasagittal frontal lobe mass, involving the genu of the corpus callosum and the right cingulate gyrus. Mass effect is minimal.

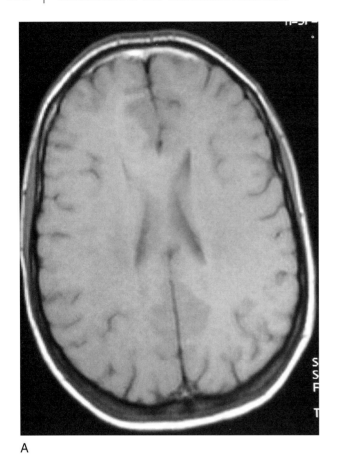

A

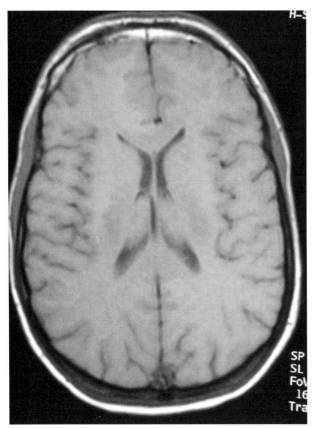

B

FIGURE 2. A and B, The lesion is not well seen on T1-weighted axial MRI.

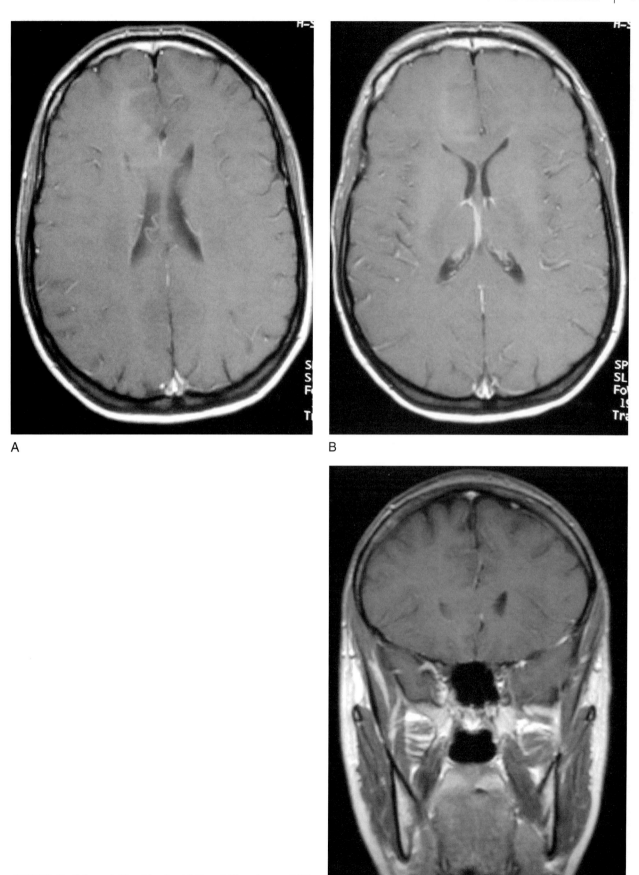

FIGURE 3. Enhanced T1-weighted axial (**A** and **B**) and coronal (**C**) images show minimal enhancement of the lesion.

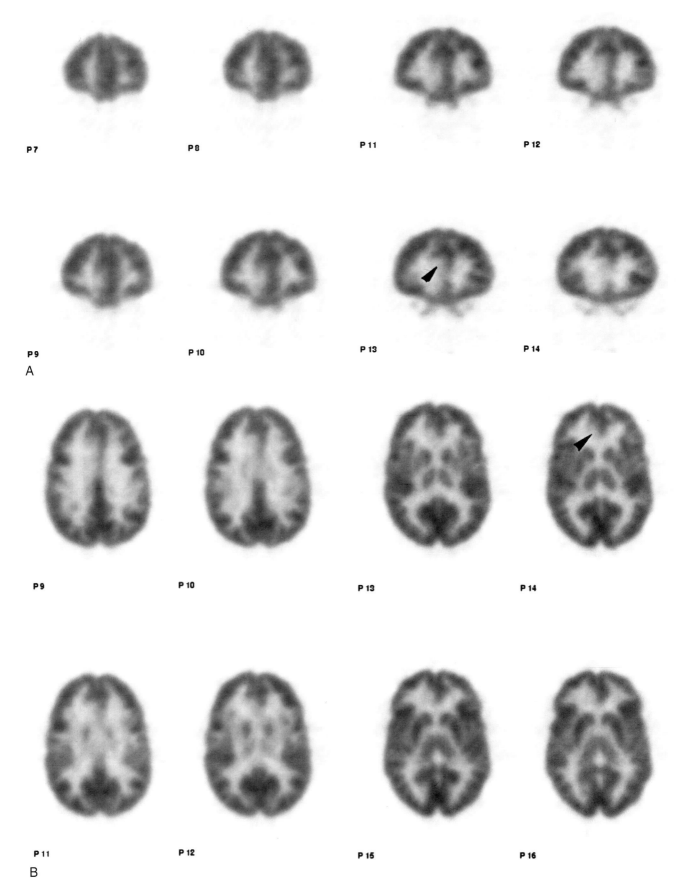

FIGURE 4. **A,** coronal, and **B,** axial. The lesion is hypometabolic on PET (*arrowheads*). There is loss of the normal right parasagittal frontal cortical activity. No hypermetabolism is noted of the lesion.

resection under intraoperative MR guidance. The pathology report indicated a low-grade oligodendroglioma.

TEACHING POINTS

PET can be used as an adjunct to the differential diagnosis of intracranial mass lesions and processes. PET in this case helped to solidify the preoperative impression of a low-grade neoplasm.

Brain PET imaging can also be performed with carbon-11 methionine, if one has immediate access to a cyclotron. Target-to-background levels in the brain offer an advantage over FDG-PET, but low metabolic rate tumors may still be difficult to visualize.

CASE 5 | *Oligodendroglioma, tumor differential diagnosis*

A 75-year-old man presented with nausea, vomiting, confusion, headache, and visual impairment. On examination, he was noted to have a left hemianopsia and left-sided neglect. His past medical history was remarkable for a similar episode of acute symptoms over a year before, with abnormal right parieto-occipital findings on MRI, which were thought to be ischemic.

When his relatively acute neurologic symptoms recurred, the patient was evaluated with brain CT and MRI. MRI showed abnormal signal intensity and edema in the right parieto-occipital region, with only localized mass effect and little enhancement (Figures 1 and 2). Comparison of the MRI to the study performed 14 months before showed the findings were progressive (Figure 3). An infiltrative, relatively low-grade neoplastic process was suspected. The lesion was growing and no longer conformed to a vascular territory. Spectroscopy showed alterations trending toward, but not diagnostic of, tumor.

PET was requested to aid in the differential diagnosis. It showed the mass to be hypometabolic (Figure 4). No hypermetabolic components were identified. A low-grade neoplasm was again favored.

Biopsy was recommended. However, the patient refused, as he rapidly improved and soon became relatively asymptomatic again. He was followed with serial MRIs for an additional 4 months. The lesion demonstrated slight increasing enhancement, and repeat spectroscopy now displayed a tumor signature.

The patient then underwent biopsy, confirming a well-differentiated, low-grade glioma, with features consistent with an oligodendroglioma.

TEACHING POINTS

This patient initially presented with an episode of acute neurologic symptoms, which was attributed to a stroke. Abnormal signal on MRI approximated a vascular territory. When he presented again 14 months later with a similar episode, his initial nonenhanced head CT was interpreted similarly. However, work-up with MRI and comparison with the prior MR study demonstrated that the questioned "stroke" was

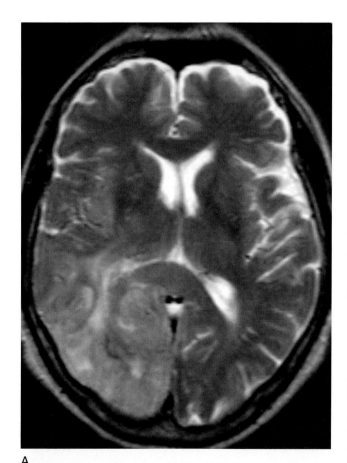
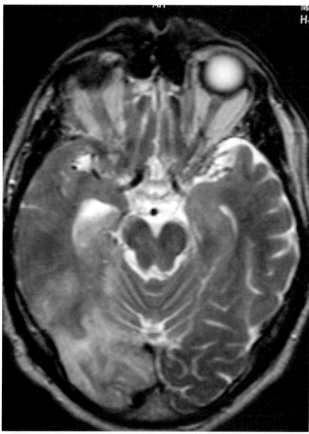

A

B

FIGURE 1. **A** and **B**, T2-weighted axial MR images show abnormal parenchymal signal intensity in the right parieto-occipital region, extending to the posterior temporal level. Note the involvement of the right periatrial white matter and encroachment on the splenium of the corpus callosum.

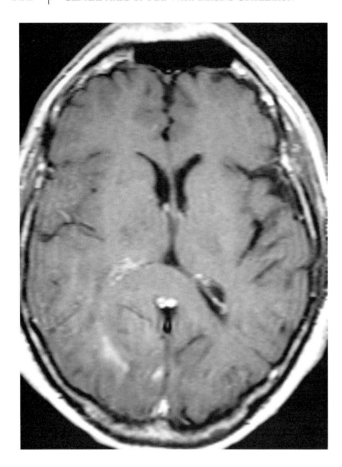

FIGURE 2. Enhanced T1-weighted axial image shows little lesional enhancement. Mass effect is noted, with effacement of the atrium of the right lateral ventricle.

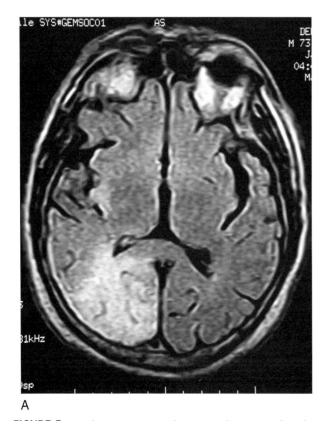

A

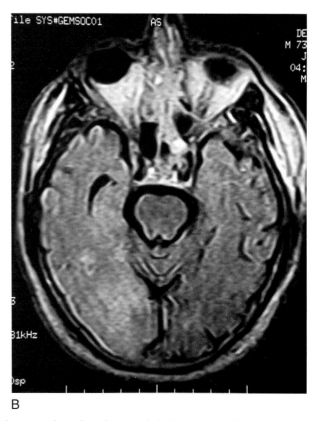

B

FIGURE 3. **A** and **B,** Comparison with FLAIR axial MR images from the outside prior study, performed 14 months before, shows the lesion is progressive and infiltrating more anteriorly. The lesion was previously thought to conform to posterior cerebral artery territory and was therefore most likely ischemic. Diffusion was not performed at the time.

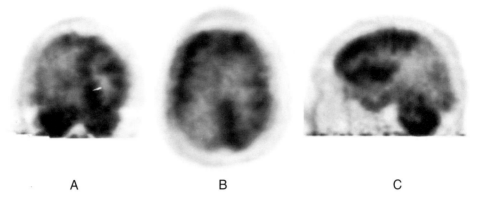

FIGURE 4. PET image quality is degraded by motion artifact but shows the lesion to be hypometabolic. Coronal (**A**), transaxial (**B**), and sagittal (**C**) views are shown.

progressive and had been present and smaller over a year before. Based on the serial MRIs, an infiltrative, low-grade neoplasm was suspected. Unfortunately, initial spectroscopy was only suggestive, but not diagnostic, of tumor. PET was requested to aid in the differential diagnosis. The lesion was hypometabolic, which is typical of low-grade gliomas. No hypermetabolic elements were found on PET to guide biopsy of any particular portion of the lesion.

CASE 6 | *Low-grade glioma, transformation*

A 42-year-old woman presented with new onset of grand mal seizure. A head CT and MRI identified a right frontal lobe mass lesion without enhancement. The diagnosis of low-grade glioma was made by stereotactic biopsy. The size of the lesion precluded gamma knife therapy. She was maintained on anticonvulsants and followed without further

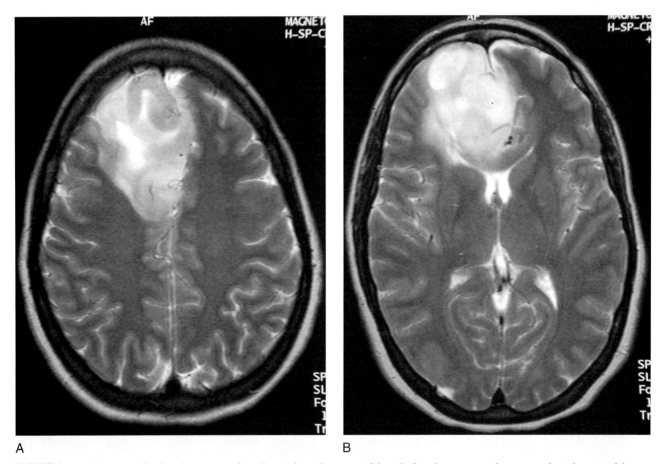

FIGURE 1. **A** and **B**, T2-weighted axial MR images show abnormal signal intensity of the right frontal region, extending posteriorly to the genu of the corpus callosum and across the midline to the left frontal paramedian level.

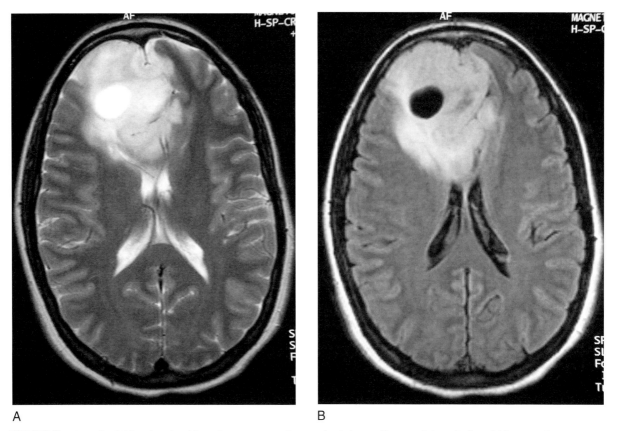

FIGURE 2. T2-weighted (**A**) and FLAIR (**B**) axial MR images at the same level show infiltration of the right frontal lobe, extending across the midline to the left and posteriorly infiltrating the corpus callosum. The intratumoral cyst is best demonstrated on FLAIR (**B**).

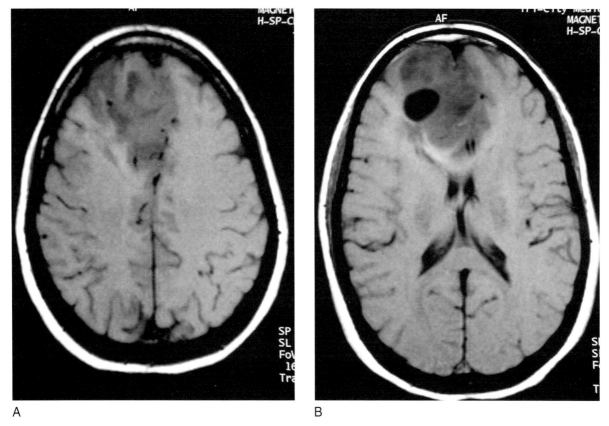

FIGURE 3. **A** and **B**, Unenhanced T1-weighted axial MR images show the lesion to be hypointense and nonhemorrhagic, with an intratumoral cyst.

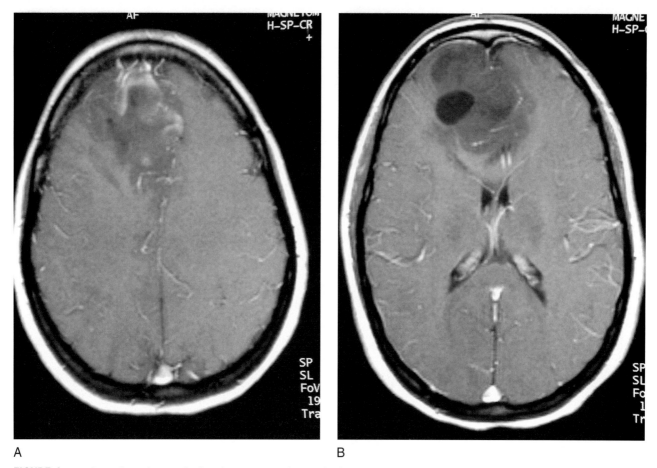

FIGURE 4. **A** and **B,** Enhanced T1-weighted axial MR images at the same levels as Figure 3 show little enhancement of most of the lesion. The cephalad section (**A**) shows enhancement at the superior margin of the lesion.

treatment for 3 years. The patient was functional and minimally symptomatic, with clumsiness and falls. Serial MRIs showed eventual development of intratumoral cysts, growth of the lesion, and, finally, development of enhancement (Figures 1 to 6). PET scan was requested when the lesion began to display increased mass effect and enhancement on MRI, to aid in treatment decision making (Figures 7 and 8).

TEACHING POINTS

Lower-grade neoplasms (low to intermediate grade, grade I to II gliomas) generally are hypometabolic on PET imaging. Higher-grade,

more aggressive gliomas, especially glioblastoma multiforme, are associated with increased mass effect and enhancement. These lesions frequently display areas of hypermetabolism, often corresponding to enhancement demonstrable on CT and/or MRI. Transformation of a relatively indolent, low-grade neoplasm was suspected in this patient based on morphologic changes of the tumor. The PET appearance of this lesion correlated well with the changing morphologic picture and served to confirm the impression of increasing aggressiveness of the lesion.

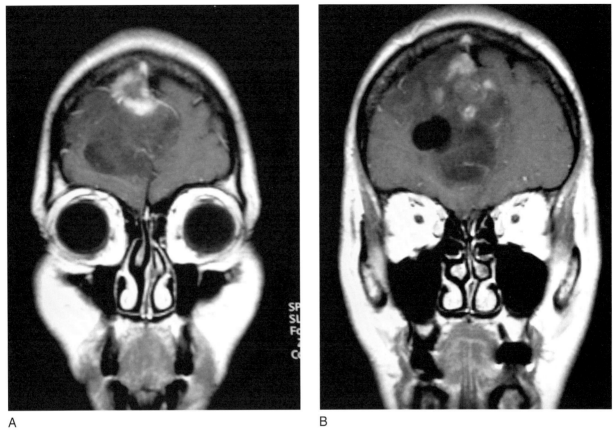

A   B

FIGURE 5. **A** and **B**, Coronal enhanced T1-weighted MR images show the right frontal infiltrative lesion crossing the midline and the associated cyst. Enhancement associated with the lesion is concentrated in the superior aspect of the lesion, at the right paramedian and midline levels.

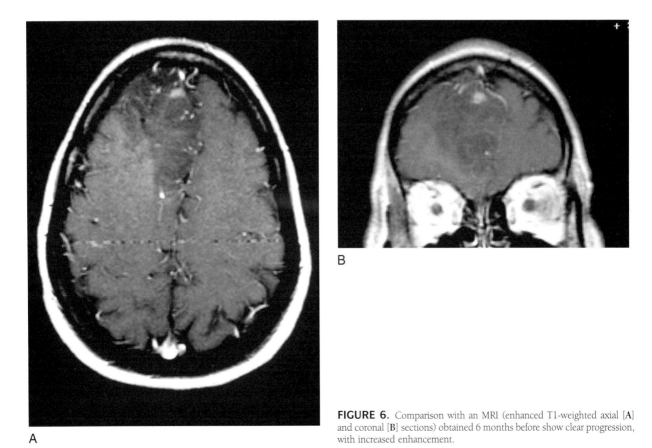

B

A

FIGURE 6. Comparison with an MRI (enhanced T1-weighted axial [**A**] and coronal [**B**] sections) obtained 6 months before show clear progression, with increased enhancement.

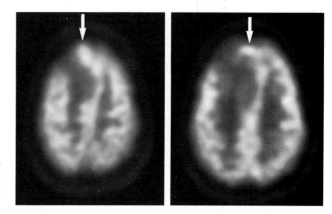

FIGURE 7. Axial PET sections show the right frontal mass lesion is largely hypometabolic. However, foci of hypermetabolism are noted at the superior right paramedian margin of the tumor, corresponding to the progressive enhancement on MRI (*arrows*).

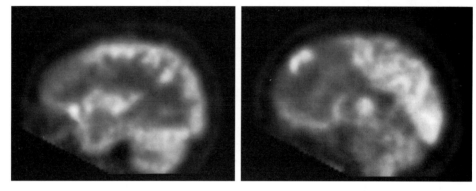

FIGURE 8. Sagittal PET sections through the right side again show the dominant hypometabolism of the frontal mass. The focal marginal hypermetabolism is well seen in this plane and corresponds to the increasing enhancement on MRI.

CASE 7 | *Middle cerebral artery infarct*

A 40-year-old woman was referred for PET imaging on suspicion of recurrent meningioma. She had undergone gross total resection of a left frontal meningioma 4 years before without additional treatment. Three months before presentation, the patient developed a transient episode of right hand numbness. One week before, the hand numbness recurred and the patient was unable to speak. MRI evaluation showed stable post-surgical encephalomalacia and gliosis at the site of the resected meningioma (Figure 1). However, immediately adjacent to this, in the frontotemporal region, new parenchymal edema was identified with enhancement (Figure 2). The enhancement consisted of increased dural thickening and a small, dural-based, mass-like focus, suggesting a small, plaque-like meningioma (Figures 3 and 4). There was also enhancement within the edematous parenchyma. The region of new abnormal signal was also hyperintense on diffusion, suggesting an ischemic etiology. However, the enhancement was regarded as suggestive of a recurrent en plaque meningioma, and for this reason a PET scan was requested. On PET imaging, the region of new abnormal signal and increased diffusion signal was hypometabolic (Figure 5).

The patient was followed with repeat MRI in 6 months (Figures 6 to 8). This showed resolution of the increased diffusion signal, as well as the parenchymal edema and the enhancement, indicating that the findings noted previously had been ischemic and secondary to an infarct in the middle cerebral artery territory. The dura-based, mass-like focus of enhancement showed interval growth, adding to the evidence of a slowly growing small recurrent meningioma.

TEACHING POINTS

This case illustrates an additional etiology for brain parenchymal hypometabolism, namely, ischemia. Although retrospective review of this case with the benefit of the follow-up MRI makes the diagnosis of evolving left middle cerebral artery infarct seem obvious, the initial evaluation was complicated by the coexistent second process of the previously operated meningioma with suspicion of recurrence. The nearly confluent locations of these two processes served to complicate the assessment.

In terms of PET's utility with regard to questions of recurrence of meningioma, there are several limitations. Meningiomas vary in metabolic activity and generally would be expected to be hypometabolic to isometabolic compared with brain tissue. The relatively rare aggressive meningioma that incites edema might be expected to be metabolically active, but it would be quite unusual to be hypermetabolic compared with metabolically active normal brain. This particular recurrence was detected early, and its small size effectively precludes visualization, quite apart from its intrinsic metabolic activity.

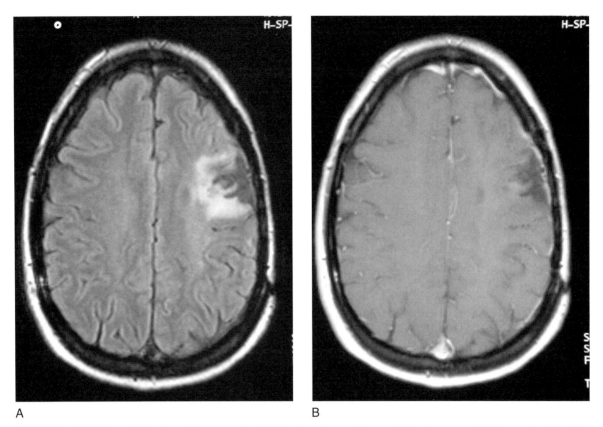

FIGURE 1. FLAIR (**A**) and T1-weighted (**B**) enhanced axial MR sections show a left posterior frontal post-surgical defect, with gliosis of the bordering parenchyma, subjacent to a craniotomy flap. These findings were stable compared with prior postoperative studies. No pathologic enhancement is seen at this level, with stable, relatively thick, and presumably postoperative dural enhancement noted.

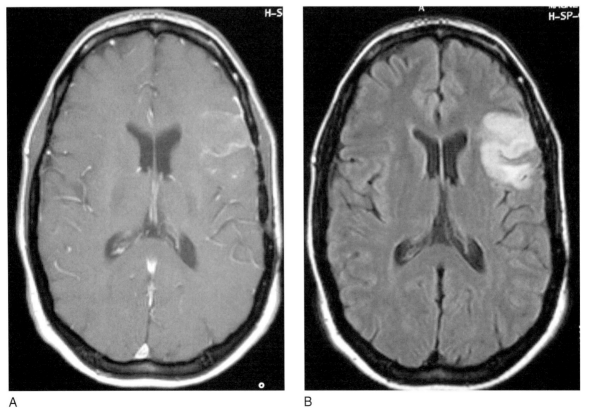

FIGURE 2. Enhanced T1-weighted (**A**) and FLAIR (**B**) axial MR sections at the same level through the lateral ventricles show new left posterior frontal findings. There is swelling and edema of a wedge-shaped region of tissue, with a localized increase in vascular enhancement.

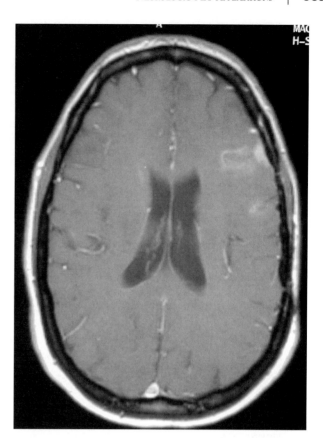

FIGURE 3. Another enhanced T1-weighted axial MR image from the same study shows more of the luxury perfusion. In addition, there is a small, dural-based, plaque-like focus of enhancement. This raised the suspicion of meningioma recurrence.

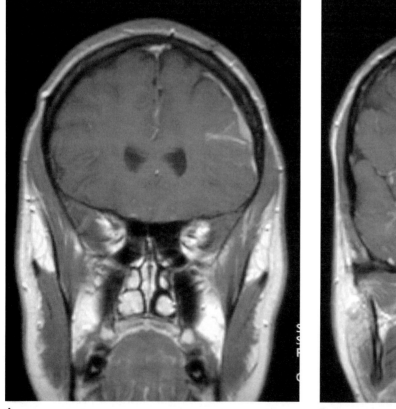

A

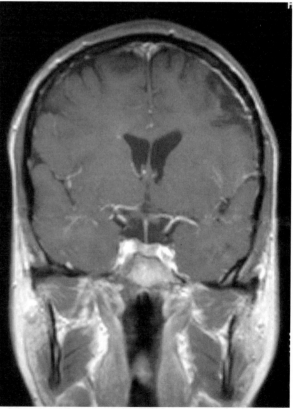

B

FIGURE 4. Enhanced T1-weighted coronal MR images show the enhancement in the left frontotemporal region. The more anterior section (**A**) shows the plaque-like region of focal, dural-based enhancement, suggestive of early recurrent meningioma. The more posterior section (**B**) shows the post-surgical defect.

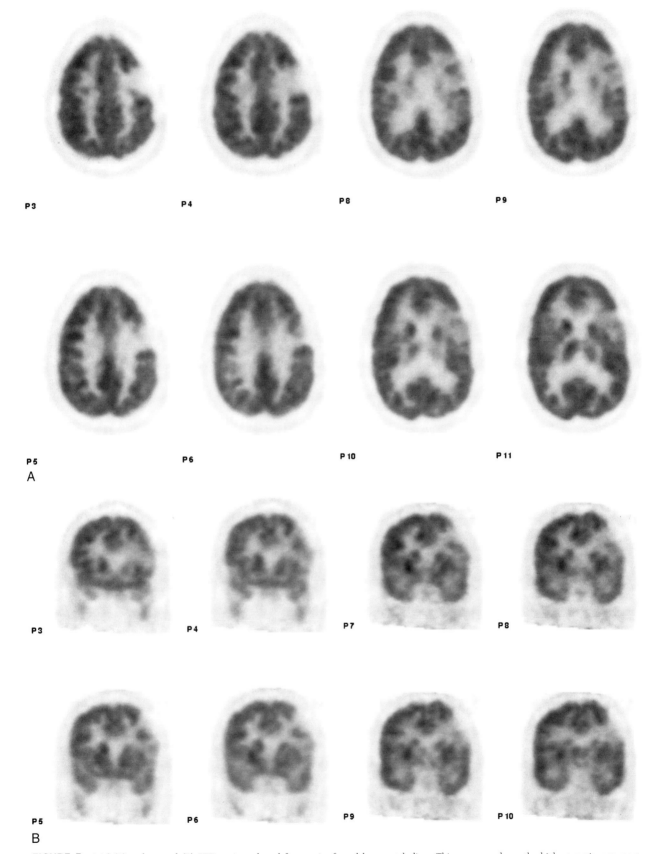

FIGURE 5. Axial (**A**) and coronal (**B**) PET sections show left posterior frontal hypometabolism. This corresponds on the highest sections to post-surgical encephalomalacia and gliosis but is continuous with the more inferior left middle cerebral artery infarct findings.

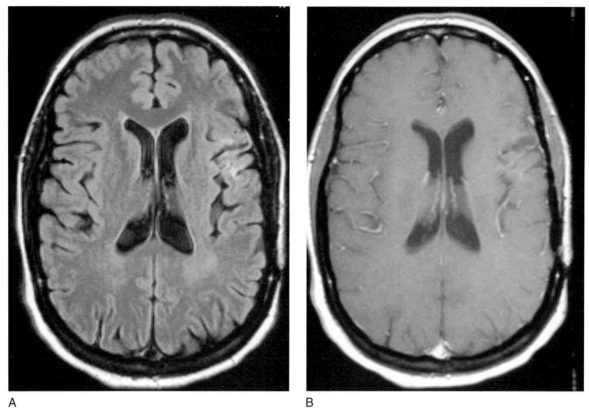

FIGURE 6. Repeat MRI scan, 6 months later: FLAIR (**A**) and enhanced T1-weighted (**B**) axial MRI images through the opercular region show resolution of both the abnormal signal and the enhancement, consistent with evolution of an infarct.

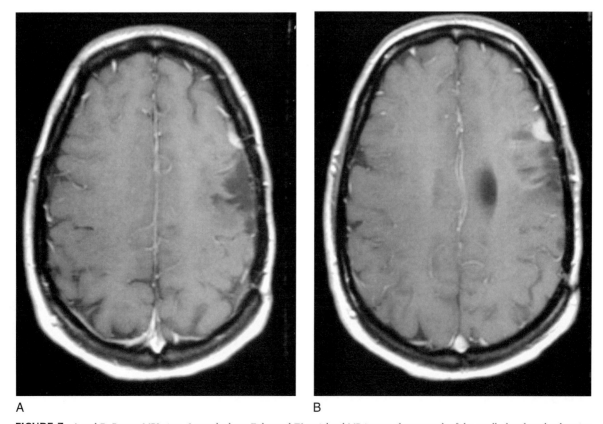

FIGURE 7. A and **B,** Repeat MRI scan, 6 months later. Enhanced T1-weighted MR images show growth of the small, dura-based enhancing mass, consistent with a slow-growing meningioma.

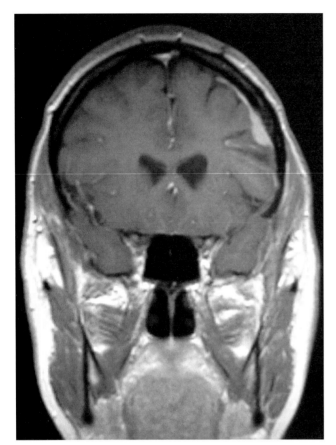

FIGURE 8. Repeat MRI scan, 6 months later. Enhanced T1-weighted coronal MRI section depicts the smoothly marginated, dura-based, recurrent extra-axial growing meningioma, with increased localized dural thickening.

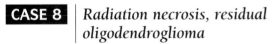

CASE 8 | *Radiation necrosis, residual oligodendroglioma*

A 38-year-old man with a prior history of treated low-grade oligoden-droglioma developed increased enhancement in the left frontal opera-tive bed on CT. He was diagnosed 3 years before when he presented with a seizure, with histology established by CT-guided biopsy. He was treated with fractionated radiation. On follow-up 2 years later, a grow-ing ring of enhancement and edema was identified on imaging. This was treated with gamma knife radiotherapy. A few days later, he pre-sented with lethargy and weakness and inability to walk. A left frontal craniotomy was performed for debulking, with a small amount of resid-ual glioma identified within extensive radiation necrosis at pathology. About 9 months later, increased enhancement was again noted in the surgical bed on CT (Figures 1 and 2). He was referred for PET scan-ning to differentiate between radiation necrosis and tumor. PET scan showed diffuse left frontal hypometabolism, with mild metabolic activ-ity posteriorly at the site of the enhancement on CT. The PET result suggested the enhancement was secondary to residual oligoden-droglioma, with the more extensive left frontal findings attributable to radiation necrosis (Figure 3). This impression seems confirmed by sub-sequent CT follow-ups showing later regression of the mass effect (Figure 4).

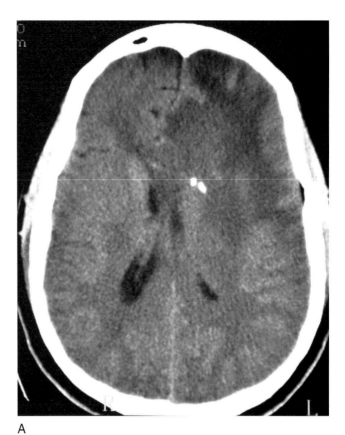

A

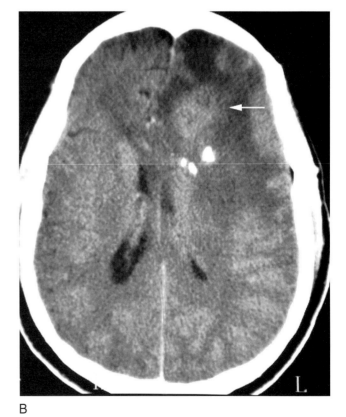

B

FIGURE 1. Unenhanced (**A**) and enhanced (**B**) head CT scans at the same lateral ventricular level show extensive left frontal edema and mass effect, with subfalcine herniation. Foci of calcification are noted, and ill-defined enhance-ment is seen anterior to the calcifications (*arrow*).

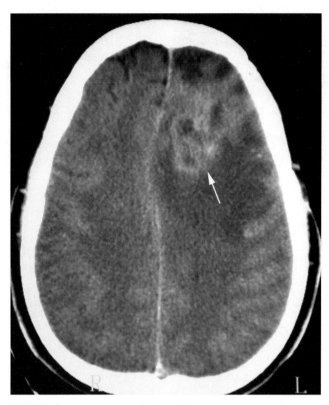

FIGURE 2. A more superior enhanced head CT section shows more of the ill-defined enhancement in the left frontal lobe (*arrow*), with edema and midline shift.

TEACHING POINTS

The PET scan in this patient demonstrated predominant hypometabolism, with very mild metabolic activity identifiable where CT showed enhancement. This patient had biopsy-proven oligodendroglioma, treated by irradiation, with proven residual tumor and radiation necrosis.

The PET result in this case was thought consistent with coexisting residual metabolically active low-grade tumor and radiation necrosis and was probably most useful in reassuring his physicians that the progressive enhancement noted on CT did not signify transformation to a more aggressive histology.

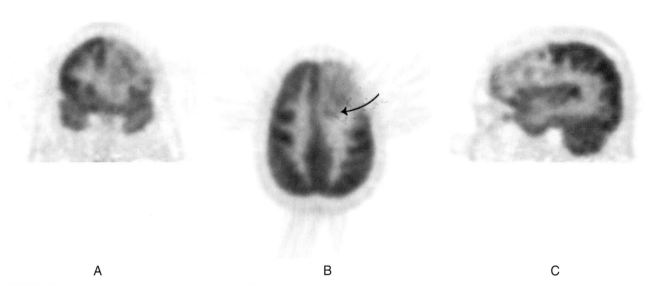

A   B   C

FIGURE 3. Dedicated brain PET shows diffuse left frontal hypometabolism. At the posterior margin, there is a ring of mild metabolic activity (*arrow*), corresponding to enhancement on CT. Coronal (**A**), transaxial (**B**), and sagittal (**C**) views are shown.

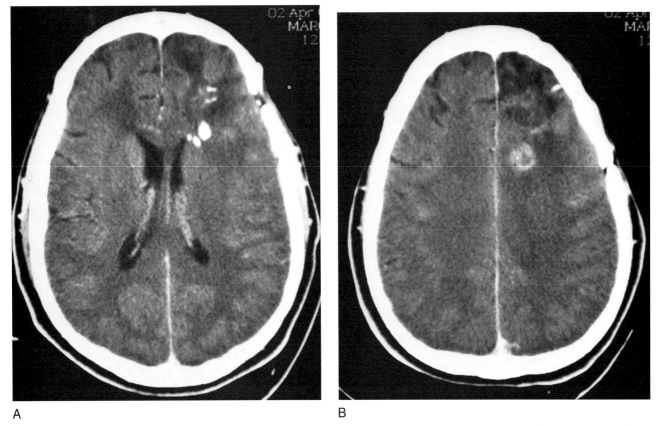

A   B

FIGURE 4. **A** and **B**, Head CT examination from over a year later, without additional therapy other than dexamethasone (Decadron), shows improved mass effect and smaller region of enhancement.

CASE 9 | Radiation necrosis, status post scalp melanoma therapy

A 63-year-old woman with Clark's level IV melanoma of the scalp was treated with surgery and radiation therapy. Approximately 8 months after completion of radiation therapy, she developed confusion and experienced episodes of right hand and arm spasms. She was evaluated with MRI, which showed an unusual pattern of asymmetrical biparietal convexity hyperintensity and enhancement, subjacent to scalp changes related to prior surgery (excision and skin grafting, with tissue expanders) (Figures 1 to 4). A dedicated brain PET, performed in conjunction with a whole-body study, was normal (Figure 5). Repeat brain MRI, 1 month later, showed progression of nodular and gyriform biparietal enhancement and edema, and the possibility of leptomeningeal involvement was raised. Meanwhile, the patient's symptoms had progressed to right hemiparesis. A repeat dedicated brain PET, 2 months after the first study, showed new hypometabolism in the same distribution (Figure 6). The patient's subsequent repeat MRI showed progressive heterogeneous enhancement, now associated with greater edema and mass effect, including midline shift, with increasingly characteristic findings of radiation necrosis (Figures 7 to 10).

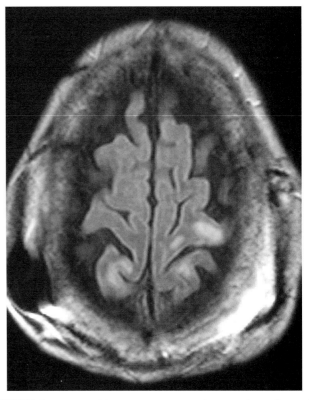

FIGURE 1. FLAIR axial brain MRI image near the vertex shows abnormal, asymmetrical, biparietal parenchymal hyperintensity (left greater than right).

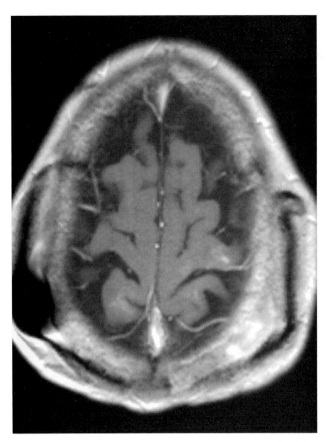

FIGURE 2. Enhanced T1-weighted axial MR image at the same level shows faint vaguely gyriform enhancement.

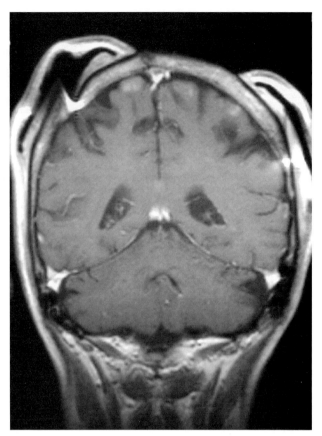

FIGURE 3. Enhanced T1-weighted coronal image shows the faint enhancement of cortex subjacent to a large scalp defect. Scalp tissue expanders are seen on either side of the defect.

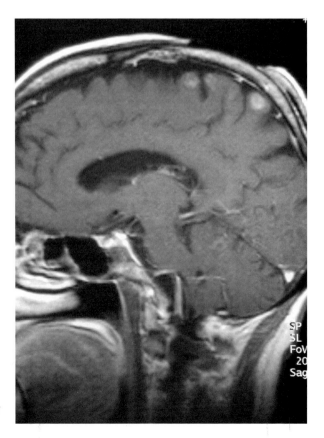

FIGURE 4. Enhanced T1-weighted sagittal MR image shows the vaguely nodular cortical enhancement, subjacent to the scalp defect.

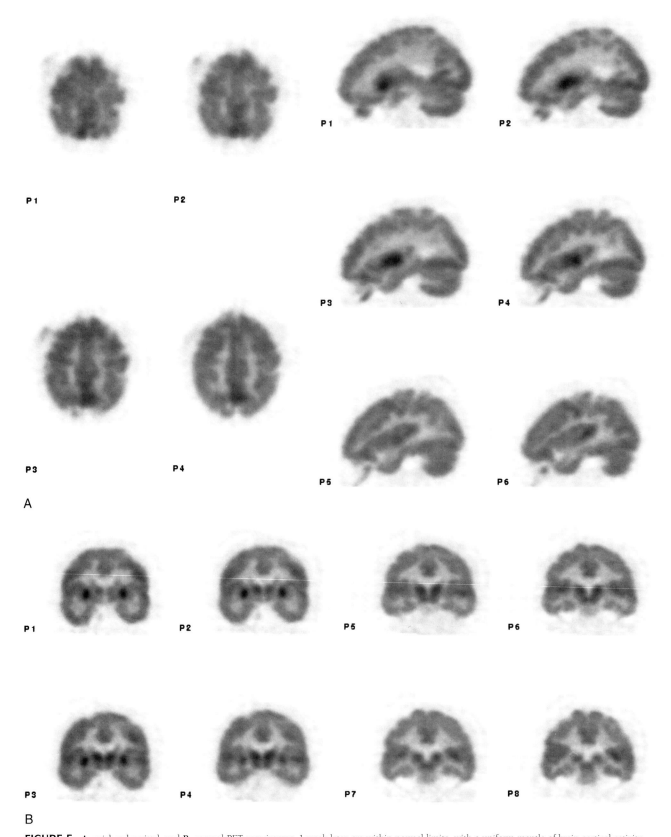

FIGURE 5. **A**, axial and sagittal, and **B**, coronal PET scan images, 1 week later, are within normal limits, with a uniform mantle of brain cortical activity.

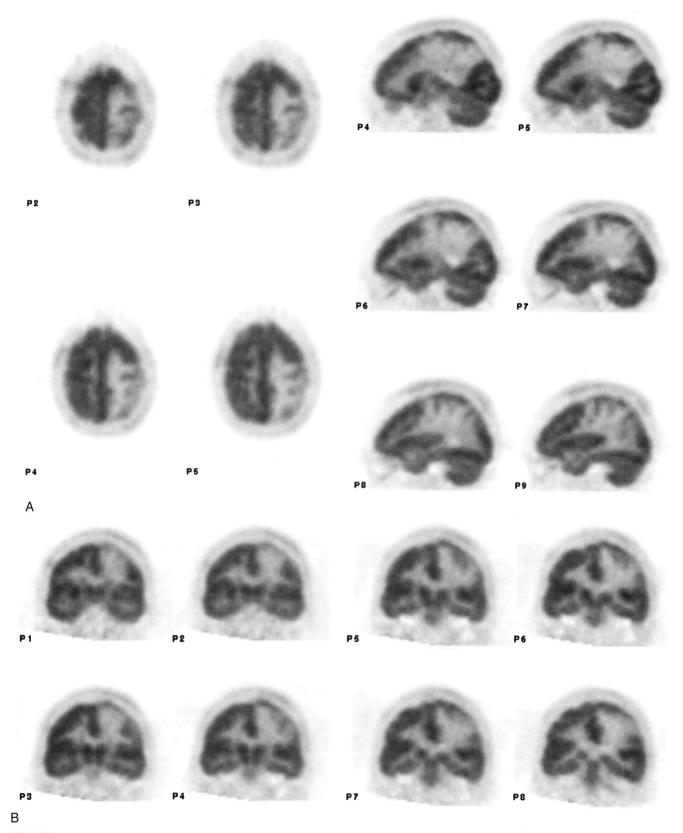

FIGURE 6. **A,** axial and sagittal, and **B,** coronal. Repeat brain PET study, 2 months later, shows new hypometabolism extensively in the left parietal lobe. The axial sections at the vertex show a ribbon of hypometabolism crossing the midline to involve the right paramedian parietal lobe as well.

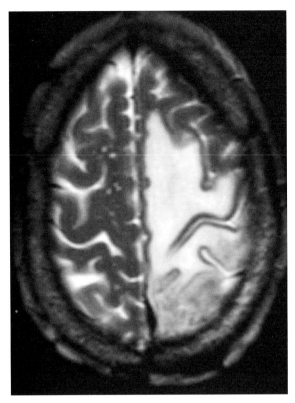

FIGURE 7. Follow-up MR image shows progressive findings of radiation necrosis. T2-weighted fast spin echo axial section shows biparietal parenchymal hyperintensity (left greater than right) now accompanied by a large amount of edema on the left.

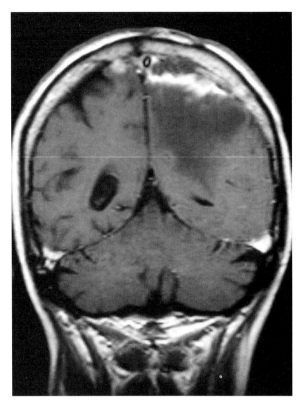

FIGURE 9. Enhanced T1-weighted coronal image shows the enhancement to be irregularly geographic, crossing the midline to involve the paramedian right parietal lobe. The extensive accompanying left parietal edema is also well seen, with mass effect effacing the left lateral ventricle and sulci.

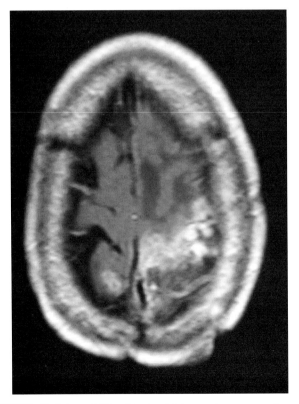

FIGURE 8. Enhanced T1-weighted axial image shows progression and change in the enhancement pattern with a nodular, more confluent sheet of enhancement.

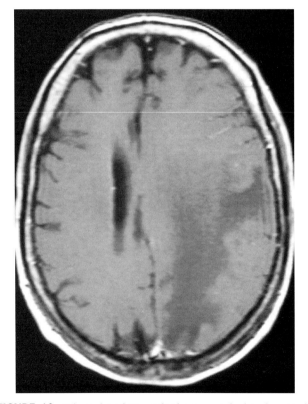

FIGURE 10. Enhanced axial T1-weighted image, at the lateral ventricular body level, shows extensive left parietal edema, with effacement of the left lateral ventricle and sulci and midline shift.

TEACHING POINTS

In this case, radiation therapy changes, which subsequently progressed to frank radiation necrosis, were visible on MRI before they became apparent on PET. PET did help to reassure the clinicians involved in this patient's care that the bizarre enhancement pattern seen on MRI was not an unusual manifestation of the patient's malignancy. The PET scan changes, concurrent with the MRI progression to fairly characteristic findings of radiation necrosis, served to confirm the presumptive diagnosis. Further confirmation came on an MRI follow-up examination, 7 months later, which showed marked regression of these findings.

CASE 10 | *Bitemporal radiation necrosis, status post nasopharyngeal carcinoma therapy*

A 53-year-old man presented with headaches, confusion, memory impairment, left-sided weakness, abnormal gait, and a left hand tremor. MRI evaluation showed bitemporal enhancement and mass effect (Figures 1 to 3). Radiation necrosis was favored as the etiology, given a history of radiation therapy in Asia for nasopharyngeal carcinoma 4 years before. PET scan was requested for further evaluation. Hypometabolism was found in the temporal lobe regions of the abnormal enhancement (right more pronounced than left), noninvasively confirming the diagnosis of presumed radiation necrosis (Figure 4).

TEACHING POINTS

Brain parenchymal enhancement and mass effect always raise the specter of neoplasia when encountered on MRI examinations, particularly when there is a prior history of malignancy. If the available clinical data are incomplete, additional possibilities such as radiation necrosis may not be initially considered in the differential diagnosis. In this case, the past history of radiation therapy for nasopharyngeal carcinoma was not known initially to the MRI interpreter. A multifocal neoplastic process was suspected until the relevant history became known, which better explained the unusual distribution. Confirmation of the diagnosis of radiation necrosis in the past would have required a biopsy or prolonged follow-up. Today, PET scanning offers a noninvasive means to assess metabolic activity of a variety of processes and, in the proper setting, may help confirm a suspected diagnosis of radiation necrosis.

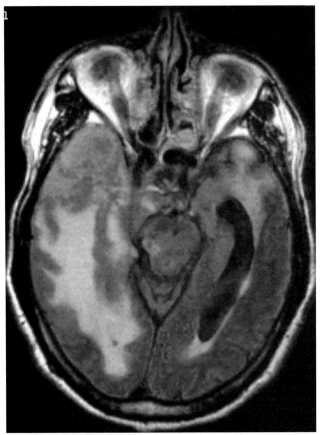

A

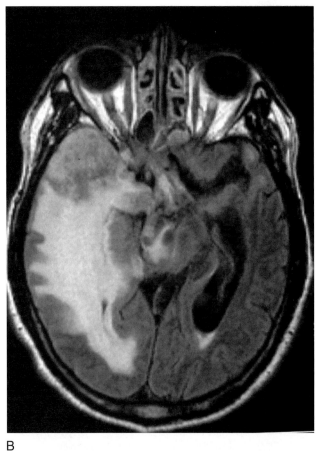

B

FIGURE 1. **A** and **B,** FLAIR axial MR sections show abnormal parenchymal increased signal intensity of the anterior temporal lobes (right greater than left). Marked accompanying edema is noted on the right, extending posteriorly to the occipital lobe and medially to the brainstem. Swelling and mass effect of the right temporal lobe deviate the brainstem to the left. Ethmoidal sinus mucosal thickening is noted.

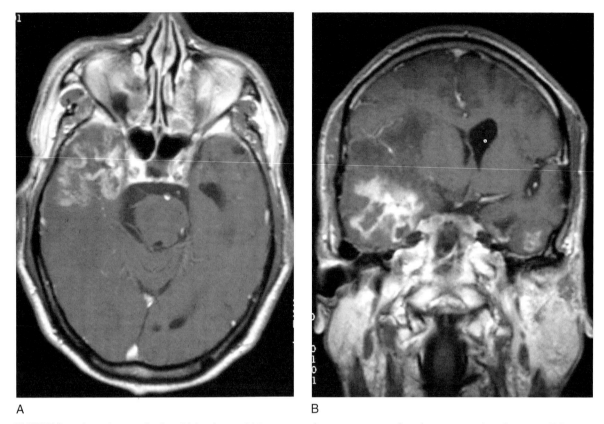

A   B

FIGURE 2. Enhanced T1-weighted axial (**A**) and coronal (**B**) MR images show extensive, irregular enhancement in the right temporal lobe anteriorly. Accompanying edema and mass effect efface the right lateral ventricular temporal and frontal horns. The midline shift and subfalcine herniation are well seen on the coronal image. A small focus of enhancement in the left temporal lobe is also seen on the coronal view.

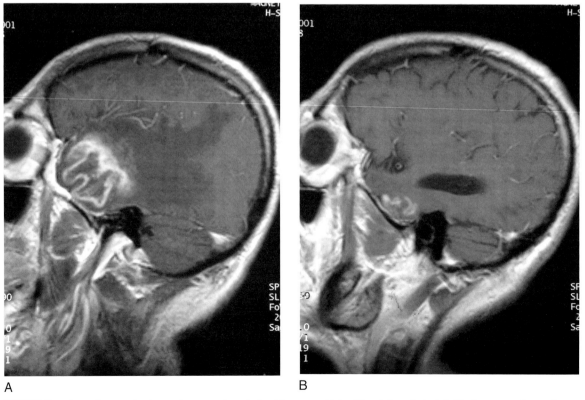

A   B

FIGURE 3. Enhanced T1-weighted sagittal sections through the right temporal lobe (**A**) and through the left (**B**), showing gyriform enhancement, right greater than left. Extensive edema accompanies the changes on the right.

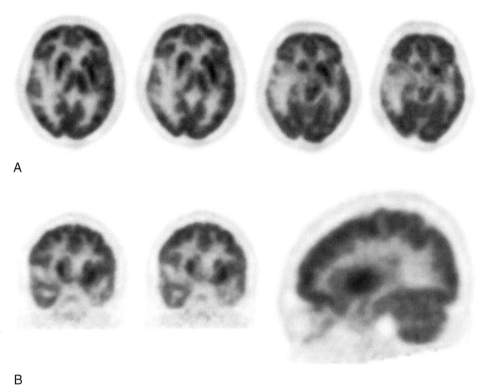

A

B

FIGURE 4. PET images show hypometabolism of the areas in question. Right temporal hypometabolism is best seen on the axial sections (**A**). Coronal and sagittal images (**B**) demonstrate hypometabolism of the anterior left temporal lobe as well, in the region of the abnormal MRI enhancement. No hypermetabolic activity is seen in these regions to suggest an alternative diagnosis.

CASE 11 | *Temporal radiation necrosis, status post preauricular basal cell carcinoma therapy, abnormal brain SPECT*

An 80-year-old man developed difficulty with speech, grasping objects, and writing 8 years after extensive surgery and radiation therapy for a left preauricular basal cell carcinoma. The neurologic evaluation noted right-sided weakness and numbness, as well as progressive dysarthria. MRI showed an enhancing, irregular left posterior temporal lesion, with edema. High-grade neoplasm versus radiation necrosis was entertained in the differential diagnosis. A thallium brain SPECT was abnormal, with focally increased left frontoparietal activity, favoring tumor (Figure 1). PET imaging showed diffuse left frontoparietal hypometabolism in the regions of the MRI abnormality and SPECT activity, consistent with radiation necrosis (Figure 2). The patient died 1.5 years later.

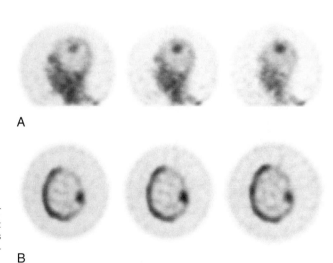

A

B

FIGURE 1. Sagittal (**A**) and axial (**B**) images from a thallium brain SPECT show a round focus of increased activity, within an extensive region of left frontal and parietal hypoperfusion. Tumor activity was suspected based on this study, but because radiation necrosis was favored based on MRI, PET was suggested to help differentiate.

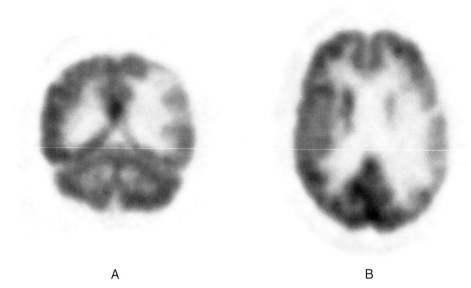

A   B

FIGURE 2. Coronal (**A**) and axial (**B**) PET images through the region in question on MRI show diffuse left frontal and parietal hypometabolism. No hypermetabolism is seen to suggest a high-grade neoplastic process or to correlate with the activity seen on brain thallium SPECT. PET findings are consistent with radiation necrosis.

TEACHING POINTS

Brain SPECT and PET frequently parallel each other in expected findings of many, but not all, neurologic processes. Brain SPECT reflects perfusion and PET metabolic activity, and in processes such as Alzheimer's disease, in which perfusion and metabolic activity decline, the studies generally display comparable findings. However, radiation necrosis consists of tissue that is metabolically dead although still enhances and is perfused. In such processes, the two study's findings may well diverge, as in this case.

CASE 12 | *Alzheimer's disease*

A 54-year-old woman underwent neurologic evaluation for a 5-year history of short-term memory impairment, with progression per the patient's husband, for the preceding 6 to 8 months. The patient was no longer able to hold a job and could not recall conversations from a few hours before or why she went into a room. On the Folstein Mini-Mental Status examination, the patient scored 19.5 of 30.

Imaging evaluations included brain MRI and brain SPECT scans. The brain MRI was within normal limits for age (Figure 1). The SPECT perfusion scan was abnormal, with regions of reduced perfusion on the left, greater in the parietal region than in the frontal area (Figure 2). PET scan was obtained to confirm the suspected diagnosis of Alzheimer's type dementia (Figure 3). The PET brain scan was also abnormal and correlated well with the brain SPECT scan, with hypometabolism notable in the parietal lobes, with lesser changes in the frontal lobes.

TEACHING POINTS

This case illustrates the constellation of clinical and imaging findings of an asymmetrical and early onset, but otherwise typical, Alzheimer's type dementia. The clinical history of progressive cognitive impairment and abnormal Mini-Mental Status examination, with normal laboratory evaluations and brain MRI, are typical. The findings of neurodegenerative processes such as Alzheimer's dementia on brain SPECT and PET scans generally parallel each other, with SPECT showing hypoperfusion where PET depicts hypometabolism. PET scans of the brain are easier to interpret than brain SPECT scans, owing to the inherent higher resolution of PET imaging. Given the devastating nature of such a diagnosis, particularly in a younger patient, the argument can be made that the higher confidence level of interpretation possible with PET favors its use in these circumstances, despite the higher study cost.

A more advanced case of Alzheimer's disease usually shows more symmetrical findings, with a predilection for involvement of the parietal lobes, followed by the posterior temporal and frontal lobes. Advanced cases often show sparing at the sensorimotor cortical level, which aids in recognition.

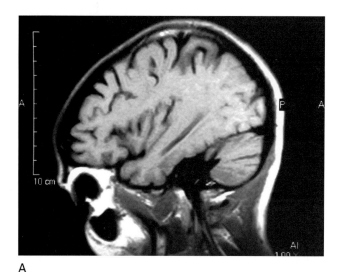

A

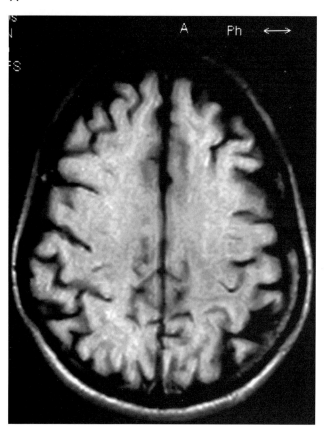

B

FIGURE 1. T1-weighted sagittal (**A**) and axial (**B**), and FLAIR (**C**) axial images from a brain MRI study show no structural abnormalities. The ventricles are normal in size.

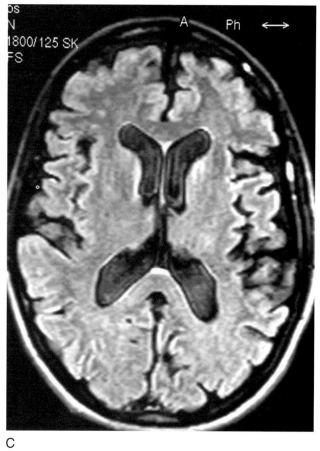

C

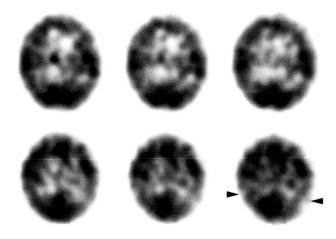

FIGURE 2. Brain SPECT with ^{99m}Tc Neurolite shows parietal regions of hypoperfusion, most readily apparent on the left (*arrowheads*).

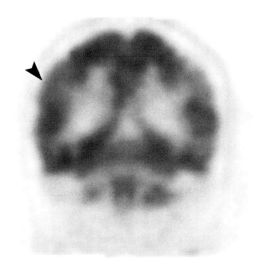

P2

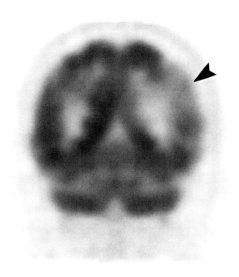

P3

A

FIGURE 3. Coronal (**A**), axial (**B**), and sagittal (**C**) PET sections (sagittal through left hemisphere) confirm the abnormal brain SPECT findings, with hypometabolism in the parietal and frontal lobes (*arrowheads*), flanking a spared sensorimotor cortical strip (left greater than right).

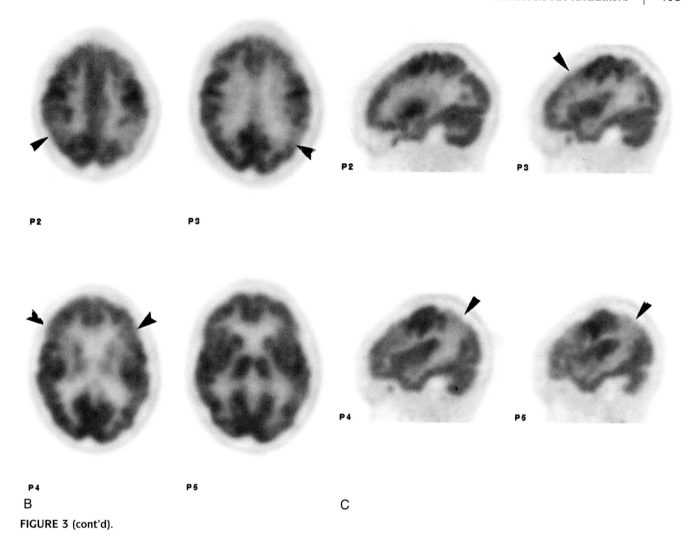

P2

P3

P4

P5

B

P2

P3

P4

P5

C

FIGURE 3 (cont'd).

CASE 13 | *Alzheimer's disease*

A 78-year-old man was evaluated with PET for memory difficulty and dizziness. Dedicated brain PET imaging confirmed fairly symmetrical reduced metabolism of the parietal and temporal lobes (Figure 1). The symmetry and distribution are consistent with the suspected diagnosis of Alzheimer's type dementia.

TEACHING POINTS

Alzheimer's dementia has historically been a diagnosis of exclusion. Patients with cognitive dysfunction are evaluated with a history and physical examination, laboratory studies, memory and language testing, and head CT or MRI to exclude structural abnormalities, such as stroke.

Until the era of clinical PET, there was little available to assess a patient's brain functionally. Brain SPECT is utilized to assess cortical perfusion, and hypoperfusion in a characteristic distribution may help to confirm the suspected diagnosis of Alzheimer's or other neurodegenerative processes. However, the resolution of brain SPECT is limited, and clinical experience and utilization vary widely by region. PET offers a high-resolution alternative that has been shown to be a highly sensitive predictor of progressive dementia in patients with suspicious cognitive symptoms. A study published by Silverman and colleagues[13] of 210 patients with brain PET findings of a progressive dementing process documented subsequent progression in 91%, either by longitudinal clinical follow-up or histopathologically at autopsy. Symptomatic patients with focal cortical hypometabolism not accounted for by cerebrovascular ischemia had progressive dementia at a 4.5-fold greater frequency than those with nonsuspicious metabolic patterns.

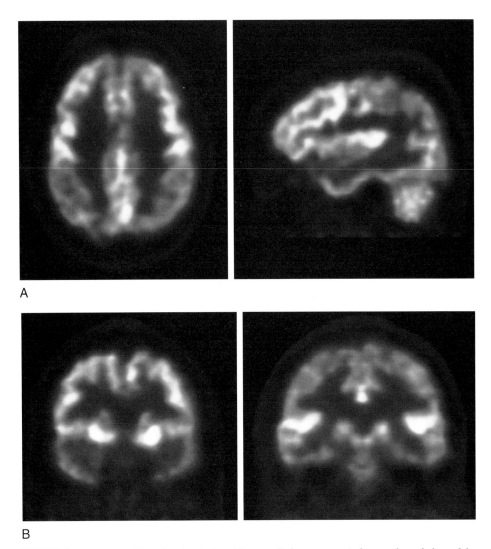

FIGURE 1. PET sections (**A**, axial and sagittal, and **B**, coronal) show comparatively normal metabolism of the frontal lobes, with reduced metabolism of both parietal and temporal lobes. Patients with advanced cases of Alzheimer's disease frequently show frontal involvement as well. See color plate 7.

CASE 14 | Pick's disease (frontotemporal dementia)

A 73-year-old female college administrator was referred for brain PET imaging for impaired job performance and suspicion of Alzheimer's disease. PET imaging demonstrated profound bifrontal and temporal hypometabolism, consistent with Pick's disease, or frontotemporal dementia (Figure 1).

TEACHING POINTS

Brain cortical hypometabolism in characteristic distributions correlates with a variety of neurodegenerative processes, most commonly Alzheimer's disease. Of course this presumes that there is no identifiable structural abnormality on CT or MRI to provide an alternative explanation. Brain parenchymal hypometabolism can be observed with lower-grade neoplasms (see examples of grade I to II astrocytomas and oligodendrogliomas in this chapter), with swelling and edema associated with other processes and with radiation necrosis. In the absence of such processes, brain hypometabolism that is symmetrical and characteristic in location correlates with progressive dementias, including Alzheimer's and Pick's diseases. Alzheimer's disease displays a predilection for parietal and temporal involvement, usually but not invariably symmetrical, with variable frontal lobe involvement. Frontal lobe involvement is more likely to be present in more advanced cases. This case illustrates a less common type of progressive dementia, with the decided frontal and temporal distribution lending it its name of frontotemporal dementia, also known as Pick's disease.

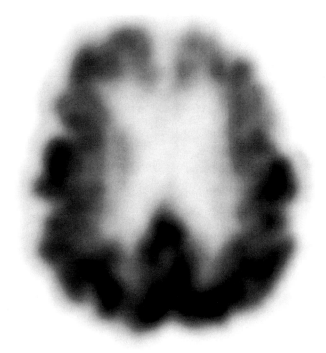

A

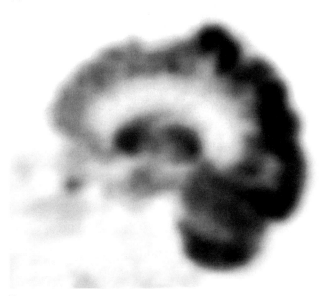

B

FIGURE 1. Axial (**A**) and sagittal (**B**) PET sections show symmetrical, profound bifrontal hypometabolism. The sagittal image also shows diminished temporal lobe metabolism. This distribution is a dementia pattern typical of Pick's disease (frontotemporal dementia).

CASE 15 | *Primary cerebellar degeneration*

A 54-year-old man sought neurologic consultation regarding dizziness and ataxia. His work-up included MRI, which showed profound and isolated cerebellar atrophy, disproportionate with the patient's age (Figures 1 and 2). PET scanning was also obtained and showed corresponding findings of isolated, striking cerebellar hypometabolism (Figure 3).

TEACHING POINTS

PET scanning can provide a functional, alternative means of assessing a neurodegenerative process, such as in this case of primary cerebellar degeneration. It is important to recognize that cerebellar activity is typically equal to or less than the cerebrum on PET, the opposite of SPECT.

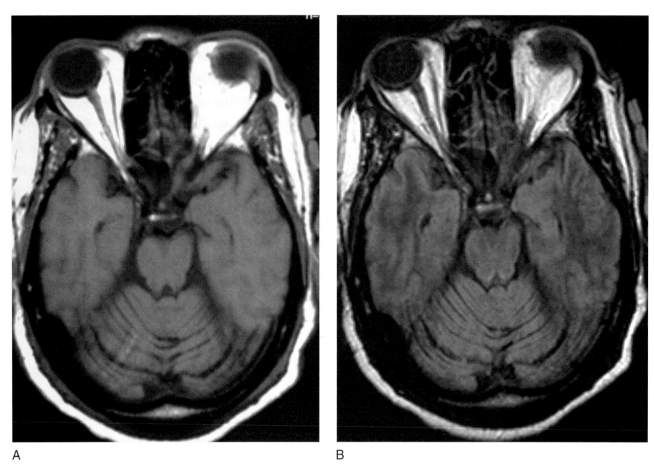

A   B

FIGURE 1. T1-weighted (**A**) and FLAIR (**B**) axial MR images of the cerebellum show pronounced atrophy. Supratentorial findings were normal for age.

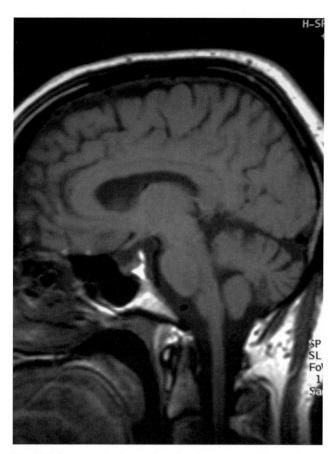

FIGURE 2. T1-weighted sagittal midline image shows disproportionate cerebellar sulcal size, compared with normal supratentorial findings.

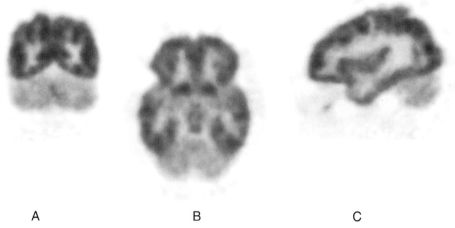

A   B   C

FIGURE 3. A to C, PET scan images (*A*, coronal; *B*, axial; *C*, sagittal) show marked disparity in metabolic activity levels between the cerebellum and the cerebrum, with the cerebellum strikingly hypometabolic here.

CASE 16 | *Temporal lobe hypometabolism*

A 51-year-old woman was referred for PET brain imaging for increasing difficulty of medical control of long-standing epilepsy. Electroencephalograms reportedly were abnormal in the right temporal region. Brain MRI also reportedly showed an abnormality at this level. Dedicated brain PET imaging identified right temporal hypometabolism (Figures 1 and 2).

TEACHING POINTS

Dedicated brain PET imaging can be an important noninvasive component of the evaluation of epilepsy patients, particularly those being assessed for surgical extirpation of seizure foci. Patients with partial (complex or simple) seizures may be considered for surgical therapy in a variety of scenarios, such as when seizures are refractory on appropriate antiepileptic drug therapy, when side effects of adequate medical therapy are intolerable, or in pediatric patients when there is developmental delay. The incorporation of PET into the work-up of candidates for epilepsy surgery aids in the localization and lateralization of seizure foci and may replace invasive monitoring in certain cases. The findings on brain PET in epilepsy depend on whether imaging is performed in the ictal or interictal state. In interictal state imaging, the seizure focus is hypometabolic. Ictal state imaging shows the activated focus as hypermetabolic. The most common indication for surgery is temporal lobe epilepsy, secondary to mesial temporal sclerosis. Hypometabolism will be seen in mesial and lateral temporal lobe structures on PET. Whereas PET is accurate in identifying the location of abnormalities, the degree of hypometabolism does not reliably predict which patients will benefit from surgery, with some subtle cases responding better than those with more profound hypometabolic abnormalities.

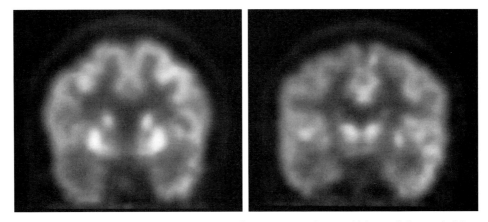

FIGURE 1. Coronal PET views of the temporal lobes show asymmetry of temporal lobe metabolism, with diffuse hypometabolism on the right.

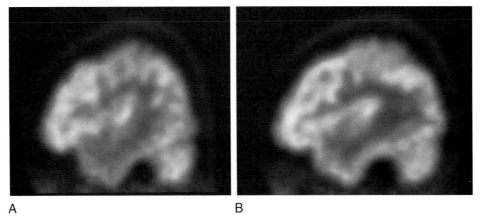

A   B

FIGURE 2. Sagittal PET sections through the temporal lobes (**A**, right temporal lobe; **B**, left temporal lobe) show the diffuse hypometabolism of the right temporal lobe compared with the normal appearance of the left.

CHAPTER

12

Cardiac PET Applications

In research settings, cardiac PET can be used to assess function. For institutions with close proximity to a cyclotron or rubidium generator, elegant perfusion studies are possible. However, the overwhelming majority of centers performing heart studies with PET are limited to utilization of FDG for evaluation of viability.

Perfusion studies can be performed with ^{13}N ammonia, ^{15}O water, or rubidium-82. These studies have a high sensitivity and specificity and provide extremely high quality images.[1-3] They also have an approximately 10% higher diagnostic accuracy than single photon emission computed tomography (SPECT).[3] Studies can be performed at rest or after pharmacologic stress to identify patients with coronary artery disease (CAD).

Myocardial viability can be assessed with SPECT, MRI, and PET. PET has shown significantly better accuracy than thallium rest-redistribution SPECT,[4] and although MRI is promising, it is thus far limited in availability. PET also identifies viable myocardium in patients with and without impaired left ventricular function.[5] Unfortunately, flow measurements alone cannot discriminate between potentially salvageable and irreversibly damaged myocardium.

The myocardium can utilize many substrates for metabolism, primarily free fatty acids and glucose. Ischemia results in preferential utilization of glucose and therefore enhanced myocardial FDG uptake. However, acute and chronic phase uptake of FDG may differ. In the first few days after infarction there may be increased FDG concentration in nonviable tissue secondary to white blood cell accumulation.[5] The predicted pattern of reduced/absent FDG uptake then develops and allows differentiation of viable from nonviable myocardium.

FDG may be utilized alone or in conjunction with a perfusion agent to predict viability, as well as prognosis.[6-10] The use of a perfusion agent (i.e., ^{13}N ammonia, rubidium-82, technetium-based SPECT radiopharmaceuticals) and FDG allows patients to be categorized as having a matched or mismatched pattern. Matched reduction in perfusion and FDG accumulation connotes nonviability. Mismatch (decreased perfusion with relatively normal FDG uptake) suggests viability and predicts functional recovery. Therefore, normal perfusion and mismatch patterns are believed by many to be the best predictors

of revascularization success. Using this approach, Auerbach and associates[6] found that revascularization might improve patient prognosis in 55% and result in improved left ventricular function in 27% of all patients with ischemic cardiomyopathy. PET has also been shown to be of great value in separating dilated, nonischemic cardiomyopathy from ischemic cardiomyopathy.[1] In the former, ^{13}N ammonia and FDG appear relatively equal/normal, whereas in the latter ^{13}N ammonia uptake is reduced and FDG is either normal, reduced, or heterogeneous. A summary of more than 400 patients showed PET sensitivity for viability of 89%, specificity of 73%, and overall accuracy of 79%.[12]

Multiple protocols exist for performing FDG viability studies. Most centers use glucose loading, either oral or intravenous. Typically, nondiabetic patients fast overnight, have their blood sugar measured on arrival to the department, and then receive a glucose load based on the results. Non–insulin-dependent diabetics are generally advised to fast and take their oral agent(s). Insulin-dependent diabetics can usually adhere to their normal insulin and dietary regimen, although some centers recommend fasting with reduction of the normal insulin dose (measurement of serum glucose and careful monitoring are mandatory). Our protocol for patient preparation follows.

The major sources of energy for cardiac metabolism in the resting state are free fatty acids (FFA) and glucose. The goal of viability imaging with FDG is to encourage the heart's preferential use of glucose. Cardiac FDG uptake is related to plasma levels of FFA, glucose, and insulin. Elevated insulin levels promote FDG uptake and suppress FFA. Many protocols exist for patient preparation for myocardial viability studies. These include oral glucose loading, hyperinsulinemic euglycemic clamping, and the use of nicotinic acid derivatives to reduce competing FFA. In designing our protocol, we considered the recommendations of many centers experienced in cardiac imaging (UCLA, Brigham and Women's Hospital, University of Iowa, University of Tennessee, Northern California P.E.T. Imaging Center). The following protocol uses oral glucose loading, accepting the fact that a percentage (may be up to 25%) of studies may be suboptimal and that latent diabetes may be uncovered.

NONDIABETICS

I. NPO after midnight
II. One hour before arrival, consume a low-carbohydrate breakfast
III. Blood sugar measured on arrival to department
    A. If glucose level is less than 120 mg/dL, give 50 g oral glucose and re-measure glucose level after 45 to 60 minutes.
    B. If glucose level is 120 to 150 mg/dL, inject FDG.
    C. If glucose level is greater than 150 mg/dL, give 3 U insulin, wait 15 minutes, and recheck glucose. Once the level is less than 150 mg/dL, inject FDG and image after 30 minutes.*

DIABETICS†

I. Non-insulin dependent
    A. Stay NPO after midnight.
    B. Take oral antidiabetic medication as usual.
    C. Measure blood glucose on arrival to department.
        1. If blood glucose level is less than 120 mg/dL, give 50 g oral glucose, wait 45 to 60 minutes, and recheck glucose level.
        2. If blood glucose level is 120 to 150 mg/dL, inject FDG, wait 30 minutes, and image.
        3. If blood glucose level is greater than 150 mg/dL, give 3 U insulin, wait 15 to 20 minutes and recheck glucose level. If it is less than 150 mg/dL, inject FDG, wait 30 minutes, and image.*
II. Insulin-dependent
    A. Adhere to normal dietary and insulin schedule.
    B. Measure blood glucose on arrival to department
        1. If blood glucose level is less than 120 mg/dL, give 50 g oral glucose, wait 45 to 60 minutes, and recheck glucose level.
        2. If blood glucose level is 120 to 150 mg/dL, inject FDG, wait 30 minutes, and image.

        3. If blood glucose level is greater than 150 mg/dL, give 3 U insulin, wait 15 to 20 minutes, and recheck glucose level. If it is less than 150 mg/dL, inject FDG, wait 30 minutes, and image.*

If images are suboptimal, one may consider re-imaging 2 to 3 hours later, administering 3 to 5 U of insulin (monitor glucose levels), and re-imaging or repeating the study on another day.

Clinically, the most common requests for FDG cardiac studies are for assessment of viability in patients whose SPECT studies are inconclusive or at odds with the expected results (e.g., no good history or evidence of infarction), the separation of ischemic from nonischemic cardiomyopathy, and evaluation of patients before revascularization or cardiac transplantation.

REFERENCES

1. Bergmann SR: Cardiac positron emission tomography. Semin Nucl Med 1998;28:320-340.
2. Gould KL: PET perfusion imaging and nuclear cardiology. J Nucl Med 1991;32:579-606.
3. Schwiger M: Myocardial perfusion imaging with PET. J Nucl Med 1994;35:693-698.
4. Mesotten L, Maes A, Vande Werf F, et al: PET radiopharmaceuticals used in viability studies in acute myocardial infarction: A literature survey. Eur J Nucl Med 2002;29:3-6.
5. Maddahi J: Role of thallium-201 and PET imaging in evaluation of myocardial viability and management of patients with coronary artery disease and left ventricular dysfunction. J Nucl Med 1994;35:707-715.
6. Auerbach MA, Shoder H, Hoh C, et al: Prevalence of myocardial viability as detected by positron emission tomography in patients with ischemic cardiomyopathy. Circulation 1999;99:2921-2926.
7. Akinboboye OO, Idris O, Cannon PJ, et al: Usefulness of positron emission tomography in defining myocardial viability in patients referred for cardiac transplantation. Am J Cardiol 1999;83:1271-1274.
8. Schaiger M, Hicks R: The clinical role of metabolic imaging of the heart by positron emission tomography. J Nucl Med 1991;32:565-578.
9. Schelbert HR: Positron-emission tomography: Assessment of myocardial blood flow and metabolism. Circulation 1985;72:122-133.
10. Bax JJ, Visser FC, El Hendy A, et al: Prediction of improvement of regional left ventricular function after revascularization using different perfusion-metabolism criteria. J Nucl Med 1999;40:1866-1873.
11. Schelbert HR: Myocardial ischemia and clinical applications of positron emission tomography. Am J Cardiol 1989;64:46E-53E.
12. Gambhir SS, Czernin J, Schwimmer J, et al: A tabulated summary of the FDG PET literature. J Nucl Med 2001;42:70S-71S.

---

*If glucose level remains greater than 150 mg/dL, may repeat this step with 2 to 3 U insulin until glucose level is less than 150 mg/dL.
†Preferably studied in the morning.

CASE 1 | *Myocardial viability study: normal example*

Exquisite detail can be obtained from myocardial FDG-PET studies (Figure 1).

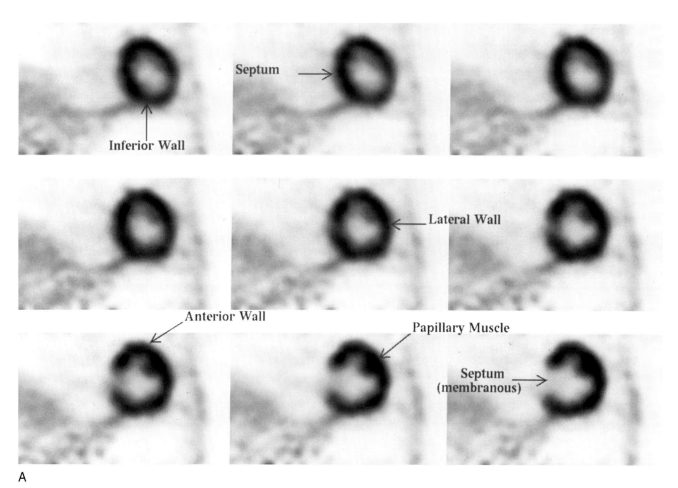

A

FIGURE 1. Views from a normal myocardial FDG-PET study (short axis [A], vertical long axis [B], and horizontal long axis [C]) show the exquisite detail that can be obtained. Note ease of visualization of papillary muscle. Even with careful attention to patient preparation and glucose loading, such intense and uniform FDG utilization by the myocardium may not be achievable in up to 25% of patients. *(Continued)*

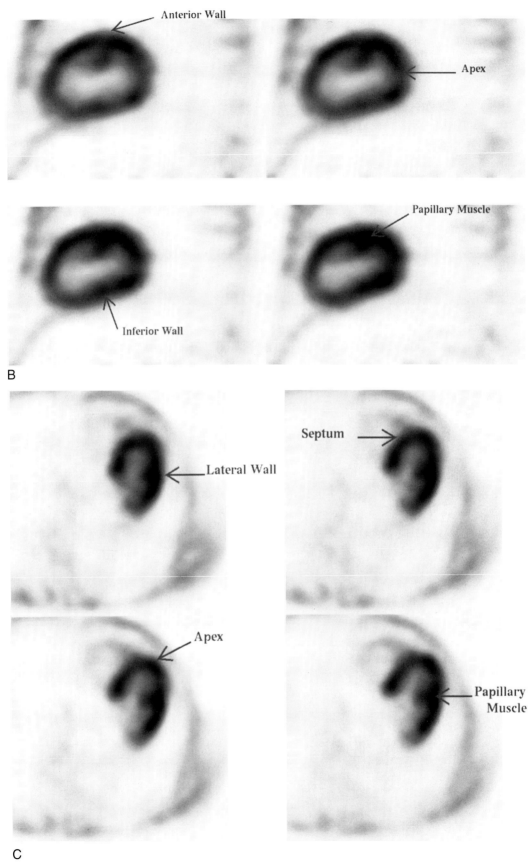

FIGURE 1 (cont'd).

CASE 2 | *Myocardial viability study: patient with non–Q wave myocardial infarction and congestive heart failure, with abnormal thallium viability study*

A 78-year-old woman was hospitalized with a non–Q wave myocardial infarction and congestive heart failure. Coronary angiography identified a high-grade left anterior descending stenosis. The patient had a normal myocardial perfusion imaging (MPI) study 2 years before. A thallium resting myocardial perfusion study, with 24-hour delay, showed a large left ventricle and a large fixed apical perfusion defect, which extended to include the periapical distal anterior and inferior walls and distal septum (Figures 1 and 2). PET imaging was requested to assess the apex for viability and showed myocardial activity, where the thallium study showed a fixed defect, indicating hibernating myocardium (Figures 3 and 4). Based on this result, she underwent revascularization with coronary artery bypass grafting.

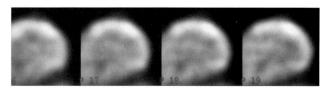

FIGURE 3. FDG-PET VLA images clearly show myocardial activity in the apex, indicating viability. Diminished myocardial activity is seen of the inferior wall, which was normally perfused on thallium viability study. This may reflect localized myocardial fatty acid, rather than glucose, utilization.

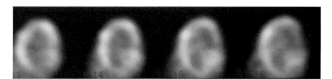

FIGURE 4. HLA views from the same FDG-PET study also show clear myocardial activity in the apex.

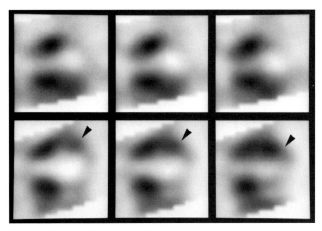

FIGURE 1. Vertical long axis (VLA) views from a thallium resting MPI study show a large fixed apical perfusion defect, suggesting scar. Redistribution is seen of the distal anterior wall (*arrowheads*).

TEACHING POINTS

This case illustrates well a myocardial perfusion/metabolism mismatch, with FDG-PET demonstrating metabolic activity (and thereby viability), of the large fixed apical defect noted on thallium rest/redistribution imaging. A matched defect (absent perfusion and hypometabolism on FDG-PET) would indicate scar, and nonviability, with no expectation of improved contractile function with revascularization. Myocardial perfusion/metabolism mismatches identify ischemic myocardium with impaired contractile function, which stands to improve if revascularized.

FDG-PET assessment of myocardial viability is predicated on the preferential utilization of glucose over fatty acids by ischemic myocardium. Study quality is optimized by glucose loading to encourage myocardium to utilize glucose. This can be achieved by a variety of protocols. Even with such preparations, myocardial uptake may not be entirely uniform, which can complicate the interpretation. This is demonstrated here in the inferior wall, which showed normal perfusion and is presumably viable.

CASE 3 | *Myocardial viability study: patient with known coronary artery disease, post myocardial infarction and percutaneous transluminal coronary angioplasty, with recurrent angina and abnormal SPECT*

A 72-year-old man with coronary artery disease, 6 years post myocardial infarction and percutaneous transluminal coronary angioplasty, developed increasing angina. Myocardial SPECT imaging (not shown) identified a large fixed apical perfusion defect and partially reversible anteroseptal and inferior wall perfusion defects. Left ventricular ejection fraction, by gated SPECT analysis, was estimated to be 36%. FDG-PET imaging showed only a small area of anteroapical hypometabolism (Figure 1). At coronary angiography, the left anterior descending artery was occluded and there was a 70% left circumflex stenosis. The left ventricle was dilated, and left ventricular ejection fraction was estimated to be 35% to 40%.

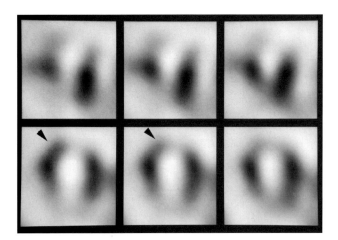

FIGURE 2. Horizontal long axis (HLA) views from the same study show the large fixed apical perfusion defect. Subtle redistribution is seen of the distal septum, bordering the large presumed apical scar (*arrowheads*).

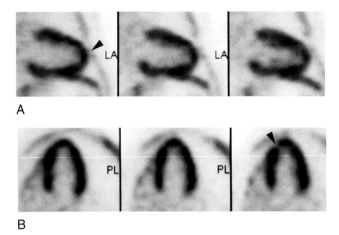

A

B

FIGURE 1. Vertical (**A**) and horizontal (**B**) long-axis views from FDG-PET viability study show only a small anteroapical region of hypometabolism (*arrowheads*).

The patient was treated with coronary artery bypass grafting. Five months after surgery, echocardiography showed improved function, with an ejection fraction of 55%.

TEACHING POINTS

Myocardial viability scan interpretation can be subtle. Normal uptake indicates tissue viability. Absent activity is consistent with nonviable scar. Relatively decreased activity (compared with surrounding myocardium) may occur with subendocardial infarction. Timing of PET imaging is another important factor to consider in myocardial assessment. FDG uptake differs between acute and chronic phases of myocardial injury. Early on (<48 hours), there can be increased FDG concentration in nonviable myocardium owing to leukocyte accumulation. There may also be a temporary decrease in FDG accumulation in acute infarction with successful thrombolysis, thought by some to indicate metabolic "stunning."

CASE 4 | *Myocardial viability study: patient with chronic congestive heart failure post myocardial infarction, being considered for percutaneous revascularization for fatigue and chest pain*

A 64-year-old woman was referred for PET myocardial viability assessment with complaints of fatigue and atypical chest pain. She was 2 years post myocardial infarction, which resulted in chronic congestive heart failure and a left ventricular ejection fraction estimated to be 40%. Angiographic evaluation at the time of myocardial infarction showed inferior infarction and significant left anterior descending artery disease. Myocardial viability study was requested specifically to assess the anterior wall and apex.

FDG-PET showed the anterior wall to be viable and confirmed inferior wall scar (Figures 1 and 2). Based on these results, the patient was treated with stenting of the left anterior descending artery, with dramatic improvement in her energy level and relief of her chest pain.

TEACHING POINTS

Based on the information provided by PET of anterior wall viability, this patient proceeded to angioplasty revascularization, with improvement in symptoms of angina and congestive heart failure. Objective evidence of the efficacy of revascularization, and hence the prognostic value of FDG-PET–demonstrated viability, is most often provided by a measured increase in ejection fraction, reflecting improved contractile function.

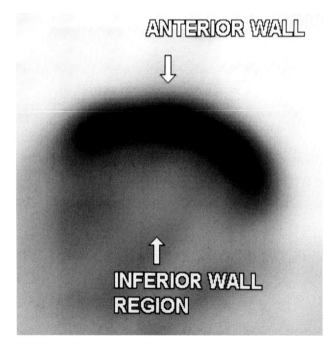

FIGURE 1. VLA view from FDG-PET viability study shows anterior wall myocardial activity, indicating viability. Inferior wall scar is confirmed.

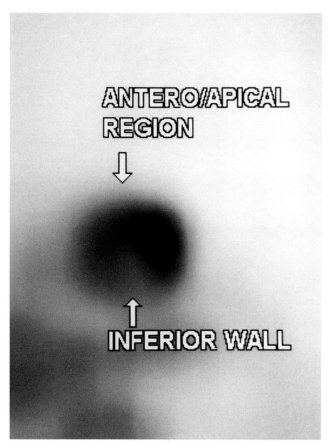

A

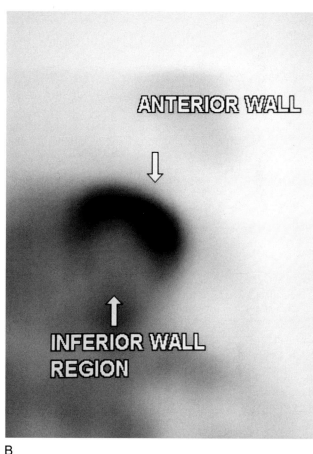

B

FIGURE 2. Distal (A) and proximal (B) short-axis views from myocardial viability study show corresponding findings of inferior scar and anterior wall viability.

CASE 5 | Myocardial viability study: nonsurgical candidate patient with recurrent symptoms, with abnormal SPECT, being considered for repeat percutaneous intervention

A 76-year-old woman with a long history of coronary artery disease was referred for PET myocardial viability assessment because of progressive debility and intermittent chest pain on maximal medical therapy. Her past medical history included prior coronary artery bypass grafting, congestive heart failure, myocardial infarction, and multiple stent placements. Eight months before referral for myocardial PET, she had been evaluated with adenosine perfusion imaging, which showed fixed apical and a partially reversible anterolateral wall perfusion defects (Figure 1). FDG-PET imaging showed a small anterolateral scar, with the rest of the myocardium viable (Figure 2). The patient was recatheterized. Percutaneous transluminal coronary angioplasty and atherectomy were accomplished of the left circumflex artery, and the left anterior descending artery was re-stented. One month later, the patient's symptoms had significantly improved, with no clinical evidence of congestive heart failure and relief of chest pain.

TEACHING POINT

Repeat coronary artery bypass grafting was not an option for this patient. FDG-PET was utilized to identify sufficient myocardial viability to justify catheterization and intervention.

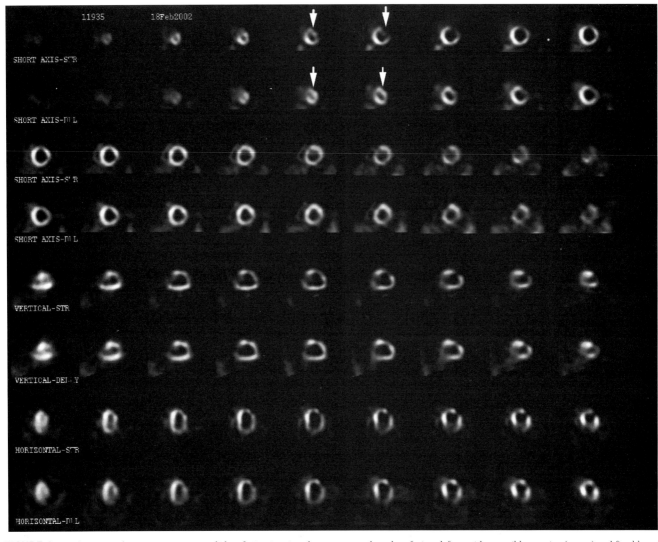

FIGURE 1. Dual isotope adenosine stress myocardial perfusion imaging shows an anterolateral perfusion defect, with reversible anterior (*arrows*) and fixed lateral components. Fixed reduced apical perfusion is also noted.

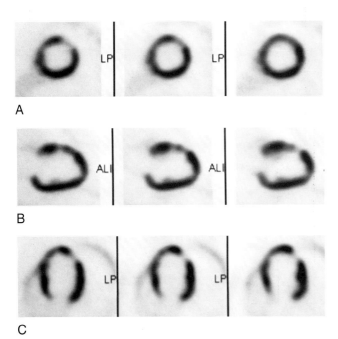

FIGURE 2. **A** to **C**, PET myocardial viability study shows the small anterolateral nonviable scar but is otherwise normal, including in the apex. **A**, Short axis; **B**, vertical long axis; **C**, horizontal long axis.

CASE 6 | *Myocardial viability study: diabetic patient with multivessel coronary artery disease and ischemic cardiomyopathy, being considere for revascularization by coronary artery bypass grafting*

A 68-year-old diabetic man was admitted with ventricular tachycardia. Catheterization confirmed multivessel coronary artery disease, with occlusion of the left anterior descending and right coronary arteries, as well as left circumflex arterial disease. Left ventricular ejection fraction was depressed at 30%, consistent with an ischemic cardiomyopathy. PET myocardial viability study was performed and showed the majority of the myocardium to be viable, with only small regions of reduced metabolism (Figure 1). Based on this result, the patient underwent revascularization with coronary artery bypass grafting.

TEACHING POINTS

Heart failure is a growing public health issue of paramount importance. Approximately two thirds of patients with heart failure have coronary artery disease as the underlying etiology. The prognosis for these patients with ischemic cardiomyopathy is poor. A carefully selected subset of these patients (about one third of the total) with viable myocardium may derive significant functional and survival benefit from revascularization. Preoperative myocardial viability assessment helps in selecting those patients most likely to benefit from revascularization. It is also recognized that patients with ischemic cardiomyopathy with viable myocardium who are managed medically have a high cardiac event rate.

CASE 7 | *Myocardial viability study: patient with prior myocardial infarction, coronary artery bypass grafting, percutaneous transluminal coronary angioplasty, and ischemic cardiomyopathy, with matched perfusion/metabolism defects*

A 52-year-old man with ischemic cardiomyopathy was evaluated with FDG-PET for myocardial viability. He was 11 years post myocardial infarction and coronary artery bypass grafting. He subsequently underwent percutaneous transluminal coronary angioplasty of a LIMA (left internal mammary artery) graft and right coronary artery but had persistent exertional angina. Two years before FDG-PET, myocardial perfusion imaging (MPI) showed anteroapical scar, involving adjacent septum and inferoapical myocardium (Figure 1). An FDG-PET study showed the inferior wall and approximately half the lateral wall to be viable, but with extensive apical, septal, and anterior wall scar (Figure 2).

TEACHING POINTS

Patients with ischemic cardiomyopathy are at high risk for perioperative mortality, and the risk increases with worsening degrees of left ventricular dysfunction. Because of this risk, preoperative identification of those who are most likely to benefit from revascularization is desirable. Because those without viable myocardium are not likely to benefit from revascularization, they may be spared unnecessary operative procedures and their attendant risk.

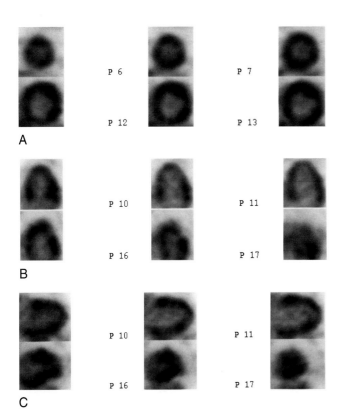

FIGURE 1. Short-axis (**A**), horizontal long-axis (**B**), and vertical long-axis (**C**) views from the FDG-PET viability study show all wall segments and apex to be metabolically active, with only small foci of diminished activity, attributed to his cardiomyopathy.

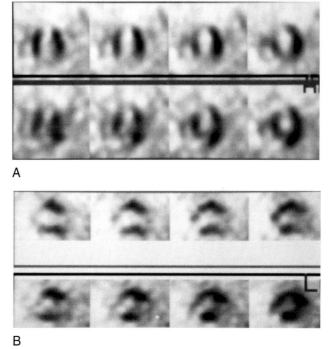

FIGURE 1. Dual isotope (thallium/^{99m}Tc Myoview) MPI (horizontal [**A**] and vertical long-axis [**B**] projections) shows a large fixed apical perfusion defect, involving inferoapical and adjacent septal myocardium.

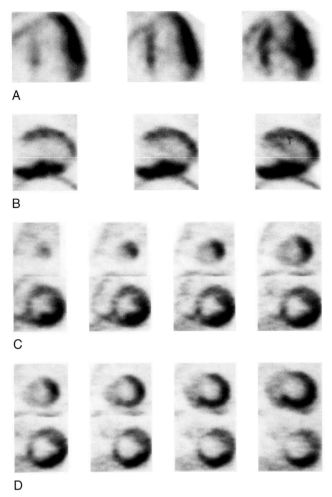

FIGURE 2. **A** to **D,** FDG-PET imaging shows the inferior wall to be viable, as well as an adjacent portion of the lateral wall. However, large swaths of myocardium, including the apex, anterior wall, and septum, are hypometabolic and nonviable. **A,** Horizontal long axis; **B,** vertical long axis; **C,** short axis (distal); **D,** short axis (proximal).

| **CASE 8** | *Myocardial viability study: patient with long-standing coronary artery disease, post multiple revascularization procedures, with persistent angina and dyspnea and recurrent disease by angiography* |

A 53-year-old man with long-standing coronary artery disease was referred for PET imaging for persistent angina with dyspnea, despite multiple interventions. His history included myocardial infarction 17 years before, with coronary artery bypass grafting subsequently and re-do 4 years later. Four years before, he had been evaluated with thallium MPI, which showed a large fixed apical perfusion defect and a reversible area of inferior ischemia, for which he was stented (Figures 1 and 2). His most recent catheterization showed the right coronary artery to be open, with occlusion of the circumflex graft and 90% LIMA stenosis. PET myocardial imaging showed a smaller apical region (predominantly inferoapical and distal septal) of hypometabolism than

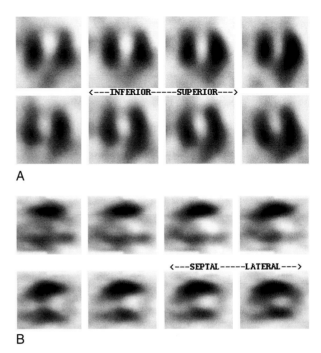

FIGURE 1. Persantine thallium perfusion imaging, with reinjection, shows on HLA (**A**) and VLA (**B**) projections a large fixed apical perfusion defect, involving anteroapical and inferoapical myocardium and suggestive of scar. Perfusion at stress is also reduced to the inferior wall, with improvement at rest, indicating inferior wall ischemia.

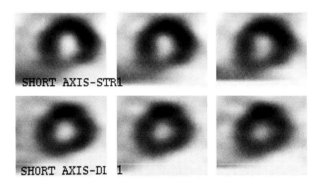

FIGURE 2. Short-axis views from the same study show the reversible inferior wall perfusion defect.

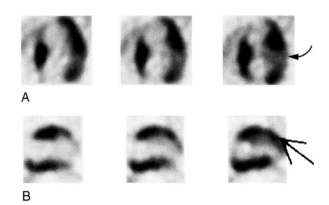

FIGURE 3. HLA (**A**) and VLA (**B**) views from FDG-PET viability study show a much smaller apical perfusion defect than seen on MPI. Apex and adjacent inferoapical and distal septal myocardium are nonviable, but anteroapical viability is demonstrated where MPI suggested scar (*arrow*). A small additional midlateral wall region of nonviability is seen on HLA views (*curved arrow*).

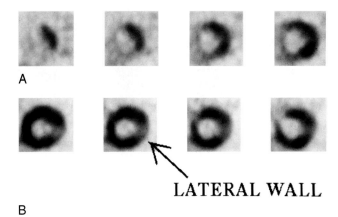

A

B

LATERAL WALL

FIGURE 4. **A,** Distal, and **B,** proximal short-axis views from the same FDG-PET study show the nonviable inferoapical and distal septal regions, as well as the midlateral wall scar (arrow).

had been suggested to be scar on MPI, as well as a small nonviable scar of the midlateral wall. Viability was demonstrated by PET of anteroapical myocardium that had appeared fixed on MPI (Figures 3 and 4).

TEACHING POINTS

Discrepancies between myocardial perfusion imaging and FDG-PET viability studies result in perfusion/metabolism mismatches and offer the opportunity to identify patients with potentially reversible ischemic left ventricular dysfunction. Results from this study suggest this patient is a suitable candidate for further attempts at revascularization.

CASE 9 | *Myocardial viability study: diabetic, vasculopathic, high surgical risk patient, with abnormal SPECT and poor left ventricular function, being considered for coronary artery bypass grafting*

A 59-year-old diabetic man with vasculopathy was admitted with syncope and a non–Q wave myocardial infarction. He initially was clinically unstable but responded to nitrates and beta blockers. He had been catheterized 2 months before, identifying 100% right coronary and left circumflex occlusions, with left to right and left to left collateral filling of the posterior descending artery and obtuse marginal branches via septal collaterals. Seventy percent and 50% left anterior descending arterial stenoses were noted, as well as 4+ mitral regurgitation and anterolateral and inferior hypokinesis. Left ventricular ejection fraction was estimated to be 30%. The patient's past medical history of vascular disease included prior right carotid endarterectomy, left carotid occlusion, and prior aortobifemoral bypass.

He was initially evaluated with a resting thallium myocardial perfusion study, followed by 24-hour delayed imaging (Figure 1). A large inferior and inferolateral perfusion defect appeared predominantly fixed. PET imaging was requested to assess viability before possible revascularization. It showed the inferior and inferolateral regions in question to be metabolically active and, therefore, viable (Figure 2 and color plate 8). The patient underwent coronary bypass grafting and mitral valve replacement the following day.

TEACHING POINTS

This case illustrates well a situation in which utilization of PET helped in medical decision making and optimized management of a high-risk patient. This vasculopathic patient was known to have two occluded coronary arteries, with severely impaired cardiac function. He was admitted in extremis but successfully resuscitated. He had been previously evaluated and turned down for coronary bypass grafting. Another cardiothoracic surgeon agreed to consider him for surgery if enough viable myocardium could be identified to warrant the risk. The demonstration on PET that a large volume of ischemic myocardium was viable, and thereby potentially salvageable by revascularization, convinced his physicians that the patient's best chance lay in surgery.

The timing of this study, 5 days after non–Q wave myocardial infarction, allowed the results to be confidently interpreted. Recall that false-positive studies for myocardial viability have been reported in the first 48 hours after infarction. This is thought to be secondary to white blood cell accumulation at the site of acute injury.

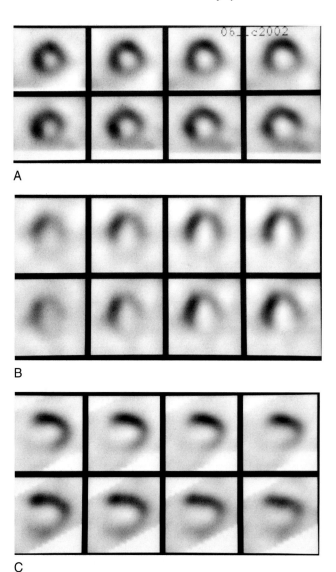

A

B

C

FIGURE 1. **A** to **C,** Resting thallium myocardial viability study, with 24-hour delay, shows a large fixed inferior and inferolateral perfusion defect, with normal perfusion of the septum and anterior wall. **A,** Short axis; **B,** horizontal long axis; **C,** vertical long axis. Top rows = rest; bottom rows = 24-hour.

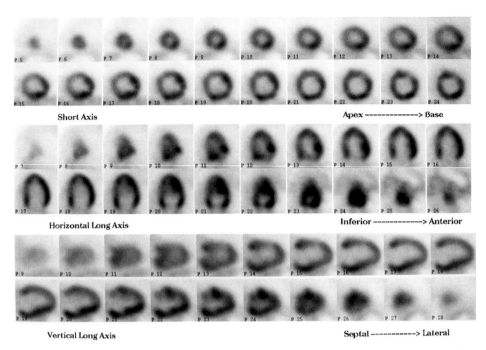

Short Axis   **Apex ------------> Base**

Horizontal Long Axis   **Inferior ------------> Anterior**

Vertical Long Axis   **Septal -----------> Lateral**

FIGURE 2. PET myocardial viability study, obtained 5 days after admission with a non–Q wave myocardial infarction, shows the inferior and inferolateral walls to be viable. Myocardial metabolic activity at these levels is actually greater than in the anterior wall and septum, presumably reflecting the predilection of ischemic myocardium for glucose as a substrate. See color plate 8.

Index

Note: Page numbers followed by f refer to figures.